CURRENT PROGRESS IN BIOLOGICAL RESEARCH

Edited by **Marina Silva-Opps**

Current Progress in Biological Research
http://dx.doi.org/10.5772/45632
Edited by Marina Silva-Opps

Contributors

Hikmet Y. Çoğun, Mehmet Şahin, Serhat Ursavaş, Mustafa Yildiz, Dilek Tekdal, Selim Çetiner, Yelda Emek, Bengi Erdağ, Göksel Doğan, Nazime Mercan Dogan, Gülümser Acar Doganlı, Yasemin Gürsoy, Ayt, Meral Ünal, Canan Usta, Feyza Candan, Özlem Barış, Mehmet Karadayı, Derya Yanmiş, Medine Güllüce, Hugo H. Mejia-Madrid, Valerio Ketmaier, Adalgisa Caccone, Mercedes Sara Lizarralde De Grosso, Dolores Casagranda, Alexander Monastyrskii, Alexander Sizykh, Xianguang Guo, Yong Huang, Yuezhao Wang

Published by InTech

Janeza Trdine 9, 51000 Rijeka, Croatia

Publishing Process Manager Iva Lipovic
Technical Editor InTech DTP team
Cover InTech Design team

Additional hard copies can be obtained from orders@intechopen.com

Current Progress in Biological Research, Edited by Marina Silva-Opps
p. cm.
ISBN 978-953-51-1097-2

For EU product safety concerns:
IN TECH d.o.o., Prolaz Marije Krucifikse Kozulić 3, 51000 Rijeka, Croatia,
info@intechopen.com or visit our website at intechopen.com.

Meet the editor

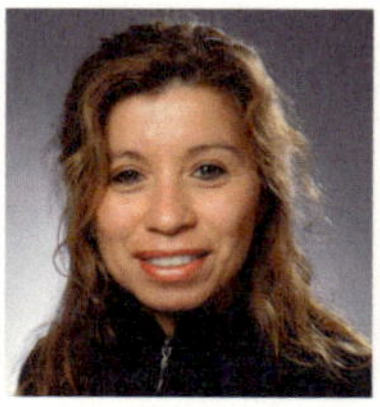

Marina Silva-Opps received her Ph.D. in Biological Sciences from the Université de Montréal, Canada in 1996. She is currently an Associate Professor at the University of Prince Edward Island in Canada. Over the course of her research career, Dr. Silva-Opps has acquired a rare combination of ecological expertise that she uses to study the patterns of abundance, species richness, movement, and body size of mammals and birds across spatial scales. Dr. Silva-Opps is proficient in statistics, GIS spatial analysis, and manipulation and analysis of large databases for macroecological studies. Since her arrival at the University of Prince Edward Island, Dr. Silva-Opps has published several technical reports, as well as papers in high impact national and international journals.

Contents

Preface

Biological sciences focus on the general question of the nature life at different temporal and spatial scales. Such diverse areas as bioscience, ecology, plant biology, genetics, biogeography and conservation biology are all part of what are called biological sciences. During the last decades, there has been unprecedented scientific progress in many of these biological disciplines, explaining the need for more publications that report the work and progress made by researches throughout the world.

Current Progress in Biological Research is a book that focuses on presenting recent scientific advances made in a variety of biological disciplines, including biogeography, plant biology, evolutionary biology, pest control, as well as health and biosciences. Each chapter presented in this book has been carefully selected in an attempt to present original studies conducted by excellent researchers from different parts of the world. The quality of the research that characterizes each one of the chapters composing this book is of high-class. In terms of its content, the book is subdivided into two sections and 16 chapters. The first section of the book, *"Biogeography, Ecology and Evolutionary Biology"*, includes 9 chapters dealing with topics such as historical biogeography, spatial distribution of organisms, genomic rearrangement and evolution as well as in vitro propagation of critically endangered species. The second section of the book, *""Biosciences, Genetic and Health"*, is divided into 7 chapters that covered a variety of topics including plant karyology, microorganisms and pest control, antibiotic susceptibilities and plant sexual reproduction.

Current Progress in Biological Research is a well-documented book that is suitable for academics, graduate students and other scientists who wish to enhance their knowledge in biological sciences. It is our hope that this book will stimulate discussion that will result in more scientific progress in biological sciences.

Dr. Marina Silva-Opps
Associate Professor
Department of Biology
University of Prince Edward Island

Section 1

Biogeography, Ecology and Evolutionary Biology

Chapter 1

Areas of Endemism: Methodological and Applied Biogeographic Contributions from South America

Dra Dolores Casagranda and
Dra Mercedes Lizarralde de Grosso

Additional information is available at the end of the chapter

http://dx.doi.org/10.5772/55482

1. Introduction

The geographic distribution of organisms is the subject of Biogeography, a field of biology that naturalists have carried out for over two centuries [1-6]. From the observation of animal and plant distribution, diverse questions emerge; the description of diversity gradients; delimitation of areas of endemism; identification of ancestral areas and search of relationships among areas, among others, have become major issues to be analyzed, worked out and solved. In this way, biogeography has turned into a multi-layered discipline with both theoretical and analytical frameworks and far-reaching objectives.

However, at the beginning it was closely related to systematics. Taxonomists were the ones who took a keen interest in the geographical distribution of taxa. In other words, because the connection is so close, several analytical tools applied to the treatment of biogeographical problems are adaptations or modifications from methods oriented to solve systematics questions. This apparent panacea may also represent one important analytical obstacle for biogeography. Although some biogeographical questions require systematic information to be solved, the object of study of biogeography, that is, spatial distribution of taxa, as well as its concepts and problems, are different from those of systematics. Hence, methods taken from systematics are not appropriate for the treatment of biogeographical problems. The need for its own methods and its own analytical framework have promoted prolific theoretical discussions and methodological developments throughout the last 20 years. In this context, the concept of areas of endemism is being widely debated and several methods have been proposed to attempt to identify these patterns. Areas of endemism have a central role in biogeography as they are the analytical units in historical biogeography, and are also considered quite relevant for biodiversity conservation [7]. It is the aim of this chapter to introduce the major discussions around the concept of areas of endemism and focus on analytical problems associated with its identification. A brief revision of contributions on endemism in South America is presented and some limitations associated to empirical analysis are highlighted in order to give an overall picture on the current state of affairs on this controversial subject.

2. Areas of endemism, its importance

In biogeography, the term "area of endemism" is used to refer to a particular pattern of distribution delimited by the distribution congruence of, at least, two taxa [8). Given that the range of distribution of a taxon is determined by historical, as well as current factors, it can be assumed that those taxa which show similar ranges have been affected by the same factors in a similar way [9]. The identification of areas of endemism is an essential first step to elaborate hypotheses that help to disclose the general history of biota and the places where they inhabit. Because of this, recognition of these patterns has been central to biogeography. Oddly enough, and despite its indisputable importance, endemism involves several problems which reach even its definition (semantic field), not to mention those resulting from the absence of a clear framework (conceptual problem) or those associated to the identification of areas of endemism (analytical issues) [9, 11-19]; While the first two problems are briefly dealt with in the present chapter, identifying and assessing the main areas of endemism will be the main focus.

2.1. Defining the term

The idea of endemism dates back to more than 200 years, and has been employed, as it is actually understood, by de Candolle [1]). Since then, the concepts of endemicity and areas of endemism have been widely discussed. Some problems around these concepts emerge from the diverse uses and interpretations given to them in literature (e.g. [16, 20-21], Harold and Moii [21], Although differences between diverse uses as regards connotations could seem minor, the lack of precision in the definition of these concepts hinders an unambiguous interpretation and causes confusion. Additionally, numerous expressions, such as "generalized track", "track", "biotic element", "centers of endemicity", "units of co-ocurrence", among others, are commonly used as synonyms of area of endemism, [16, 21-23]. Although basically related with the term "areas of endemism", these concepts refer to different patterns of distribution and are defined on different theoretical grounds.

3. A clear conceptual framework

As it usually happens in other fields such as morphology and embryology, in the field of biogeography, the identification and description of patterns precede the inference of the causes of its occurrence. However, some biogeographers assume that vicariance must be involved [12, 17]). According to this idea, a pattern of sympatry among species could be defined as area of endemism only if it emerged from a vicariant event. This assumption entails new difficulties for the identification of areas of endemism: the causes which originate the patterns must be known a priori, or else, the identification of patterns and processes should be performed simultaneously. Fortunately, most biogeographers follow the generalized concept, which supposes that multiple factors affect and define current patterns.

4. Identifying areas of endemism

The identification of such areas has been a major challenge in biogeography and deals with several difficulties, some of them related with the two questions mentioned above. However, in the last decades, several methods for identification of these patterns have been proposed [9, 15-16, 18, 24-25] In general, current methods for recognizing areas of endemism can be classified on the basis of whether they aim to determine (i) species patterns, i.e. groups of species with overlapping distributions, or (ii) geographical patterns, i.e. groups of area units with similar species composition. These approaches assess closely related but slightly different aspects of biogeographical data. Methods dealing with species patterns group species with similar distributions and result in clusters -which may or may not define obvious spatial patterns-. Instead, methods oriented to define geographical patterns, are more related to the classical notion of area of endemism, resulting in geographical areas defined by species distributions.

The methods currently in use are many and heterogeneous. While reflecting the multiple conceptions of areas of endemism, these proposals differ in their theoretical bases as well in its mathematical formulations. Following are three of them: Parsimony Analysis of Endemicity (PAE [15]), Biotic Elements (BE; Hausdorf and Hennig, 2003[24]), and Endemicity Analysis (EA; Szumik et al., 2002[9]; Szumik and Goloboff, 2004[18]). Although several modifications of PAE, as well as other hierarchical methods have been proposed (see [16, 26]), this method has been selected as a representative of hierarchical methods because it remains the most widely used in empirical analyses ([27-33].

PAE. The Parsimony Analysis of Endemicity (PAE) was the first method proposed to formally identify areas of endemism[15]. The input data for PAE consist of a binary matrix in which the presence of a given species (rows) in an area unit (columns) is coded as 1 and its absence as 0. Analogous to a cladistic analysis, PAE hierarchically groups area units (analogous to taxa) based on their shared species (analogous to characters) according to the maximum-parsimony criterion. Therefore, PAE attempts to minimize both "dispersion events" (parallelisms) and "extinctions" (secondary reversions) of species within a given area. Areas of endemism are defined from the most-parsimonious tree (or strict consensus) as groups of area units supported by two or more "synapomorphic species" (i.e. endemic species [15]). In its most classical formulation, species that present reversions (i.e. are absent in any of the area units) and / or parallelisms (i.e. are present elsewhere) in their distributions are not considered endemic. Therefore, PAE is especially strict when penalizing the absence of a species within an area, which makes it more likely to fail to detect a relatively large number of areas of endemism.

Despite the well-known limitations of hierarchical classification models in the delimitation of areas of endemism [9, 33-34]), PAE remains the most widely used method for describing biogeographical patterns [31- 32, 35]).

BE. Hausdorf [17] considers areas of endemism in the context of the vicariance model, and argues for the use of "biotic elements" defined as "groups of taxa whose ranges are significantly more similar to each other than to those of taxa of other such groups" (p. 651[17]), rather than the more traditional areas of endemism [24]). This method is implemented in the R package Prabclus by Hennig [36], which calculates a Kulczynski dissimilarity matrix [37]) between pairs of species which is then reduced using a nonmetric multidimensional scaling (NMDS; [38]). A Model-Based Gaussian clustering (MBGC) is applied to this matrix to identify clusters of species with similar distributions, or biotic elements. In spatial terms, a biotic element is equivalent to the spatial extent of the distributions of all species included in the cluster.

EA. In 2002, Szumik and colleagues proposed an optimality criterion to identify areas of endemism by explicitly assessing the congruence among species distributions. This proposal, improved by Szumik & Goloboff [17]), is implemented in NDM/VNDM by Goloboff [39] and Szumik and Goloboff [9]). The congruence between a species distribution and a given area is measured by an Endemicity Index (EI) ranging from 0 to1. The EI is 1 for species that are uniformly distributed in the area under study, and only within that area ("perfect endemism"), and decreases for species that are present elsewhere, and / or poorly distributed within the area. In turn, the endemicity value of an area (EIA) is calculated as the sum of the EIs of the endemic species included in the area. Therefore, two factors contribute to the EIA: the number of species included in the area and the degree of congruence (measured by the EI) between the species distributions and the area itself (for details see [9]).

The emergency of quantitative methods that allow describing these patterns objectively has represented an important advance in the discussion of endemism. However, the contrast between different methodological proposals introduced new questions: are the hypothesis resulting from different analysis homologous? Is there a better method to identify areas of endemism? A few recent contributions attempt to elucidate these queries by testing and exploring the behaviour of some methods, e.g. [34, 40]. Several comparisons between methods have been performed by using real data [41-43]). However, real data provide only a limited assessment of the differences between the procedures. Some characteristics of the distribution of species, e.g. geographical shape or number of records, affect pattern recognition in uncertain ways. Furthermore, sampling bias, which often affects available distributional data, causes problems in the identification of biogeographical patterns [44]). As it is often difficult to distinguish whether the identified patterns result from singularities of the data or properties of the methods, an evaluation based on real datasets, or data simulated under realistic conditions, is not enough to establish general conclusions on the performance of the methods.

Recently, Casagranda et al.[19]) states a comparison by using controlled -hypothetical distributions, pointing differences, advantages and limitations of Endemicity Analysis (EA), Parsimony Analysis of Endemicity (PAE), and Biotic Elements Analysis (BE) In their study, these authors measured the efficiency of the methods according their ability to identify hypothetical predefined patterns. These patterns represent nested, overlapping, and disjoint areas of endemism supported by species with different degrees of sympatry.

This comparison shows how the application of different analytical methods can lead to identification of different areas of endemism, and reveals some undesirable effects produced by methodological idiosyncrasies in the description of these patterns. Following are the main results reported in this contribution:

PAE shows a poor performance at identifying overlapping and disjoint patterns. In all cases, PAE is able to recover areas defined by perfectly sympatric species, but its performance decreases as the incongruence among the species distributions increases (Figure 1)

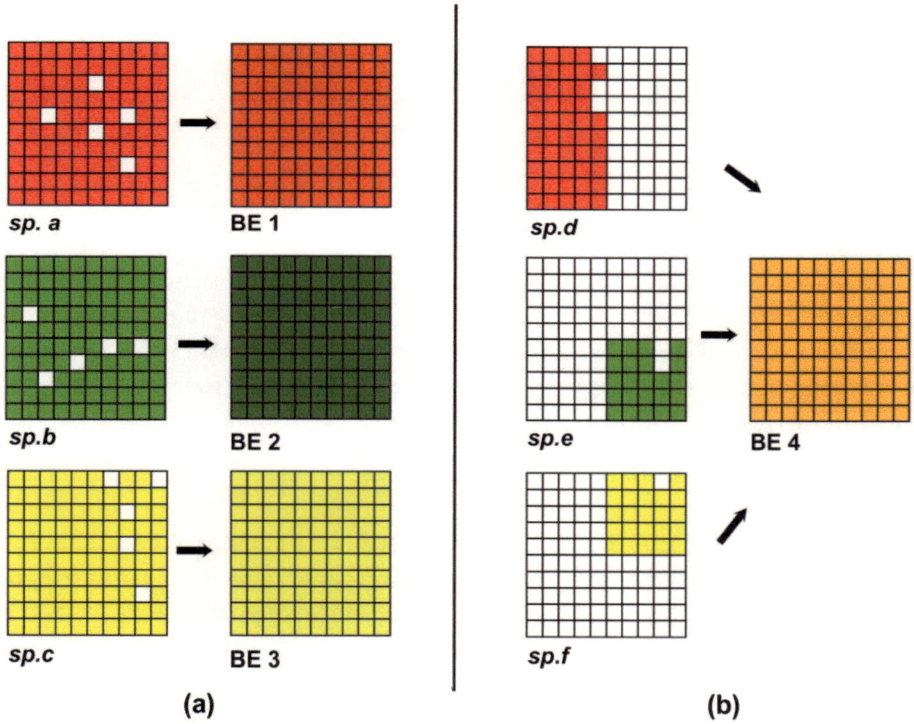

Figure 1. Noise effect on identification of areas of endemism, results using PAE (Modified from Casagranda *et al.*, 2012.)

As regards BE, it is very sensitive to the degree of congruence among the distributions of the species that define an area, showing a counterintuitive behaviour: while the method cannot recognize patterns defined by perfectly sympatric species, its performance improves with increasing levels of incongruence between the species distributions. BE often report multiple distinct biotic elements for species which actually have very similar distributions (Figure 2 a) as well as reporting a single biotic element including species with completely allopatric distributions (Figure 2 b). These examples show discordance between the theoretical basis of the approach [16]) and its practical implementation. Together, these limitations suggest the users should exercise caution when interpreting the results generated by this method.

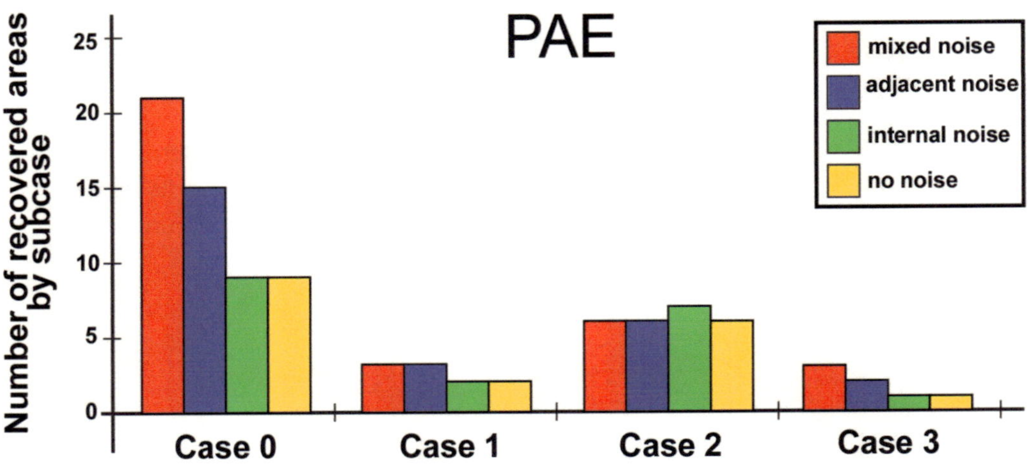

Figure 2. Special results found by biotic elements. (a) Three species with similar distributions (sp.a, sp.b. and sp.c) are separated in different biotic elements (BE 1, BE 2 and BE 3); (b) three species with completely allopatric distributions (sp.d, sp.e. and sp.f) are grouped in the same biotic element (BE 4) (Modified from Casagranda *et al.*, 2012.).

Regarding EA, it shows a high percentage of success in the recovery of predefined areas with no discrimination of case, whether nested, overlapping or disjoint, of degree of congruence between distributions of species. EA reports frequently redundant "twin" areas that have only slight differences in spatial structure and/or in their species composition.

Taking into account that overlapping and disjoint patterns are relatively common in nature, and that, in general, sympatry between species varies widely, PAE is probably not the most suitable method to describe areas of endemism based on real distributional data. Although ideal cases are not frequently observed on the spatial scale used for most biogeographical analyses, the inability of BE to identify a perfect case of the pattern which the method intends to describe is questionable. The flexibility to recognize areas displayed by EA is associated with the fact that, in contrast to the other methods considered here, EA uses both the number of species and the overlap between their distributions as optimality criteria to search for areas of endemism.

One serious problem is that the method relies on an algorithm that is ineffective for its intended purpose. PAE, for example, is a hierarchical method implying that each cell is included in at least one area of endemism; consequently, PAE cannot describe overlapping patterns, such as nested areas. Additionally, the maximum parsimony criterion aims to minimize the number of homoplasies, resulting in PAE hardly identifying any disjoint areas.

Similarly, BE model-based inference requires a series of distributional assumptions which, if not satisfied, may lead to unreliable or erroneous conclusions. Thus, even if, in theory, a biotic element is defined as a "group of taxa whose ranges are significantly more similar to each other than to those of taxa of other such groups", the method may both group totally allopatric species and fail to recognize biotic elements defined by totally sympatric species (see Fig. 2).

An inescapable consequence of the application of an optimality criterion is that multiple hypotheses may be obtained in an analysis; in the case of EA, the "twin" areas represent small variations of single cells. The ambiguity in the input data often results in multiple "best" solutions according to an optimality criterion. The reported alternative and equally optimal patterns often force the researcher to more conservative interpretations.

Conclusions of Casagranda et al. show that EA, in conjunction with consensus areas, is the best available option for endemicity analyses, despite other studies indicating that EA is rather sensitive to certain aspects of the data, such as spatial gaps of information [34]. The advantages of EA over other methods are related to considering spatial information during the identification of areas, as well as using the classical definition of area of endemism as the basis for the analysis: [an area of endemism]... is identified by the congruent distributional boundaries of two or more species, where congruent does not demand complete agreement on those limits at all possible scales of mapping, but relatively extensive sympatry is a prerequisite [8].

5. Areas of endemism in South America

The knowledge about the distribution of species, as well as the geographical patterns, constitute crucial information for biodiversity conservation [7]. Because of this, the study of both species distributions and the mechanisms that give them rise have increased since the awareness of biodiversity crisis.

In the last few years, endemicity has acquired importance in conservation biology since it is considered an outstanding factor for delimitation of conservation areas [45-47]).

Due to its particular history and its huge biodiversity, South America is interesting from a biogeographical point of view. Numerous contributions have been made to address diverse aspects of the distribution of South America's biota ([47], [48-49] [50-55] ; however, quantitative studies are relatively recent.

The development of computational methods [8, 14, 17 23, 35] together with the availability of biodiversity data-bases, such as CONABIO[57] GBIF, [58] y SNDB [59], and Jetz contribution [60] has promoted the advance of empirical analyses dealing with the description of areas of endemism. It is reflected in numerous publications focused on different methodological perspectives and including diverse taxa, in various places of South America [33, 40, 61-64]. A remarkable example of these studies is the recent contribution of Szumik et al (2012) [63], framed between parallels 21 and 32 S and meridians 70 and 53 W, (Figure 3) in the North region of Argentina.

Although the idea of an area of endemism implies that different groups of plants and animals should have largely coincident distributions, most studies of this type are focused on analyzing a restricted number of taxa. In this sense, the analysis of Szumik et al. (2012) represents an atypical example because the number and diversity of taxa included, more than 800 species of mammals, amphibians, reptiles, birds, insects and plants, representing one of the first approximations to the analysis of total evidence in a biogeographical context.

The quality and structure of data influence the identification of biogeographical patterns [19, 43]. Since the knowledge about distribution of organisms is scarce and taxonomical misidentification and georreferencing errors are commonly observed in available distributional data, an appropriate revision and correction of input information is essential to perform reliable biogeographical descriptions. In this sense, the above mentioned analysis differs from similar studies because the traits of the analyzed data set : "unique among biogeographical studies not only for the number and diversity of plant and animal taxa, but also because it was compiled, edited, and corroborated by 25 practising taxonomists, whose work specializes in the study region Thus, it differs substantially from data sets constructed by downloading data from biodiversity websites" (Szumik et al 2012, p.2[63]; see Figure 3).).

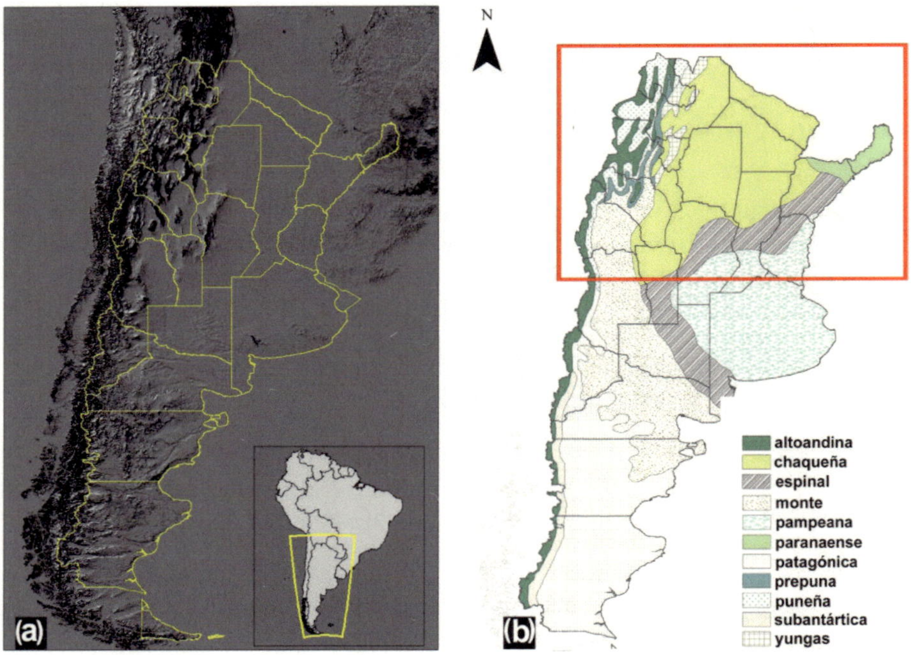

Figure 3. Maps of Argentina: a) relief map; b) biogeographical divisions of Argentina according to Cabrera and Willink (1973); the study region is framed in the red square.

The results reported by these authors indicate that when all the evidence is analysed for a given region, it is possible to obtain areas supported by diverse taxonomic groups (Navarro et al., 2009[63]): half of 126 found areas are supported by three or more major groups. Examples of areas of endemism defined by multiple taxa are the Atlantic Forest (Selva Paranaense—Neotropical, Figure 4) and the north Yungas forest sector (tropical Bermejo- Toldo-Calilegua, two of the most diverse ecorregions of the region.

The patterns of distribution recognized here depict almost all the main biogeographical units proposed in previous studies [26, 47, 49, 51, 53, 54, 55, 60] the Atlantic Forest the Campos (Grasslands) District, the Chaco shrubland (Fig. 5a), the deciduous tropical Yungas forest the Puna highland, and the tropical tails entering Argentina in two disjoint patches[63]. Each of these tropical tails represents part of a broader area that extends towards the north of the South American subcontinent.

Additionaly, the species that support the various areas are consistent in general with previous biogeographical studies based on individual groups (plants [32]; snakes [66]; mammals:[66]; insects: [63]; birds: [65,67]), and should be noted that several of these species are currently on red lists of threatened species [68-73]).

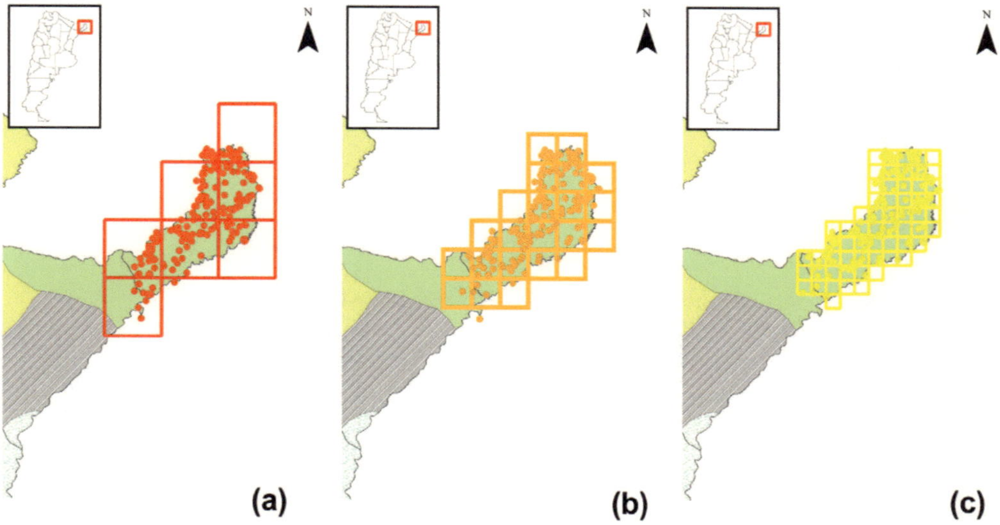

Figure 4. An example of an area of endemism identified under differents grids sides (results of Szumik *et al.*, 2012)

6. Final comments

The necessity of quantitative methods that allow a formal description of nature on the basis of available evidence has been an important subject in modern biology. In the last 30 years, both the advances in the field of informatics and the development of computational methods to explore diverse biological questions have been remarkable [74-76].

Biogeography is not foreign to these important advances. When having to compare and evaluate alternative biogeographical hypotheses, biogeographers hold no doubts over the importance of quantitative methods. However, unlike other research areas such as systematics, the richness of biogeography is quite noticeable as far as the number and variety of methodological proposals are concerned in the attempt to solve a given biogeographical problem. In contrast, those studies where the capacity to explain differences between methods or the quality of the results are put to the test are scarce, as well as anecdotal. The case referred to in the present chapter on the identification of areas of endemism clearly demonstrates the urge of serious and critical studies on biogeography. The formal recognition of areas of endemism is a complex issue; quite a lot has been done in the last few years in order to understand it, but there is still a lot to be done.In addition, the current impending threat on biological diversity urges for methodological improvements conducive to more realistic descriptions of biogeographical patterns.

Acknowledgements

We thank authors of references, specially our colleagues of INSUE. Helpful comments, constructive criticism and generosity from Claudia Szumik are greatly appreciated. Luisa Montivero helped with the English text and Andres Grosso with illistrations. This work was supported by grant PIP-Conicet Nº 1112- 200801-00696

Author details

Dra Dolores Casagranda[1,2] and Dra Mercedes Lizarralde de Grosso[2,3]

1 Instituto de Herpetología, Fundación Miguel Lillo, Tucumán, Argentina

2 Consejo Nacional de Investigaciones Científicas y Técnicas, Tucumán, Argentina

3 Instituto Superior de Entomología (INSUE)-Universidad nacional de Tucumán, Tucumán, Argentina

References

[1] Candolle A P De. Géographie botanique. In:Dictionnaire des Sciences Naturelles, 1820; 18 359–422.

[2] Sclater P L. On the general geographical distribution of the members of the class Aves. Journal of the Proceedings of the Linnean Society. Zool. 1858; 2 130–145. DOI: 10.1111/j.1096-3642.1858.tb02549.x

[3] Sclater P L. On the distribution of marine mammals. Proceedings of Zoological Society of London 1897; 349–359. DOI: 10.1111/j.1469-7998.1897.tb00021.x.

[4] Croizat L. Manual of Phitogeography. Junk, The Hague; 1952

[5] Darlington P J. Jr. Zoogeography: the geographical distribution of animals. John Willey & Sons, New York;1957

[6] Darlington P J Jr. Biogeography of the southern end of the world. Distribution and history of the far southern life and land with assessment of continental drift. Harvard Univ. Press, Cambridge Mass.; 1965 236 pp.

[7] Grehan J R. Conservation biogeography and the biodiversity crisis: a global problem in space/time. Biodiversity Letters 1993; 1 134–40. Stable URL: http://www.jstor.org/stable/2999686

[8] Platnick N I. On areas of endemism. Australian Systematic Botany 1991; 4 xi-xii Preface

[9] Szumik C, Cuezzo F, Goloboff P, Chalup A. An optimality criterion to determine areas of endemism. Systematic Biology 2002; 51 806-816. DOI: 10.1080/10635150290102483

[10] Henderson I M. Biogeography without area? Australian Systematic Botany 1991; 4 59-71. DOI: 10.1071/SB9910059

[11] Anderson S. Area and Endemism. The Quarterly Review of Biology 1994; 69 451-471. http://www.jstor.org/stable/3036434.

[12] Andersson L. An Ontological Dilemma: Epistemology and Methodology of Historical Journal of Biogeography 1996; 23 (3) 269-277. DOI: 10.1046/j.1365-2699.1996.00091.x

[13] Harold A S, Mooi R D. Areas of endemism: definition and recognition criteria. Systematic Biology 1994; 43 261-266. DOI: 10.1093/sysbio/43.2.261

[14] Hovenkamp P. Vicariance events, no areas, should be used in biogeographical analysis. Cladistics 1997; 13 67-79. DOI: 10.1111/j.1096-0031.1997.tb00241.x

[15] Morrone J J. On the identification of areas of endemism. Systematic Biology 1994; 43 438-441. DOI:10.1093/sysbio/43.3.438

[16] Linder H P. On areas of endemism, with an example from the African Restionaceae. Systematic Biology 2001; 50 892-912. DOI: 10.1080/106351501753462867

[17] Hausdorf B., Units in biogeography. Systematic Biology 2002; 51 4 648-651. DOI: 10.1080/10635150290102320

[18] Szumik C, Casagranda M D, Roig Juñent S. Manual NDM-VNDM: Programas para la identificación de áreas de endemismo. 2006 http://www.zmuc.dk/public/phylogeny/endemism/Manual_VNDM.pdf (accessed 11 september 2012)

[19] Szumik C, Goloboff P. Areas of endemism: improved optimality criteria. Systematic Biology 2004; 53 968-977. DOI: 10.1080/10635150490888859

[20] Casagranda M D, Taher L, Szumik C. Endemicity analysis, parsimony and biotic elements: a formal comparison using hypothetical distributions Cladistics 2012; 1 1-10. DOI: 10.1111/j.1096-0031.2012.00410.x

[21] Lomolino M V. Ecology´s most general, yet protean pattern: the species-area relationship. Journal of Biogeography 2000; 27 17-26. DOI: 10.1046/j.1365-2699.2000.00377.x

[22] Morrone J J. Homology, biogeography and areas of endemism. Diversity and Distributions 2001; 7 297–300. DOI: 10.1046/j.1366-9516.2001.00116.x

[23] 23 Crisp M D, Laffan S, Linder H P, Monro A. Endemism in the Australian flora. Journal of Biogeography, 2001; 28:183–198. DOI: 10.1046/j.1365-2699.2001.00524.x

[24] Hausdorf B, Hennig C, Biotic element analysis in biogeography. Systematic Biology 2003; 52 717-723. DOI: 10.1201/9781420007978.ch4

[25] Casagranda M.D., J.S. Arias, P.A. Goloboff, C.A. Szumik, L.M. Taher, T.Escalante & J.J. Morrone, (b). Proximity, Interpenetration, and Sympatry Networks: A Reply to Dos Santos et al. Systematic Biology 2009; 58(2) 271-276. DOI: 10.1093/sysbio/syp022.

[26] García-Barros E, Gurrea P, Lucañez M, Cano J, Munguira M, Moreno J, Sainz H, Sanz M, Simón J C Parsimony analysis of endemicity and its application to animal and plant geographical distributions in the Ibero-Balearic region (western Mediterranean). Journal of Biogeography 2002; 29, 109–124. DOI: 10.1046/j. 1365-2699.2002.00653.x.

[27] Cracraft, 1991; Patterns of diversification within continental biotas: hierarchical-Congruence among the areas of endemism of Australian vertebrates. Australian Systematic Botany 1991; 4 211-427. DOI: 10.1071/SB9910211

[28] Geraads D, Biogeography of circum-Mediterranean Miocene-Pliocene rodents; a revision using factor analysis and parsimonious analysis of endemicity. Palaeogeography. Palaeoclimatology Palaeoecology 1998; 137 273–288. DOI: 10.1016/ S0031-0182(97)00111-9

[29] De Grave S,.Biogeography of Indo-PacificPotoniinae (Crustacea,Decapoda): a PAE analysis. Journal of Biogeograhy 2001; 28, 1239–1254. DOI: 10.1046/j. 1365-2699.2001.00633.x

[30] Aguilar-Aguilar R, Contreras-Medina R, Salgado-Maldonado G. Parsimony analysis of endemicity (PAE) of Mexican hydrological basins based on helminth parasites of freshwater fishes. Journal of Biogeography 2003; 30, 1861-1872. doi/10.1111/j. 1365-2699.2003.00931.x

[31] Contreras-Medina R, Luna Vega I, Morrone J J. Application of parsimony analysis of endemicity to Mexican gymnosperm distributions: grid-cells, biogeographical provinces and track analysis. Biological Journal of the Linnean Society 2007; 92, 405–417. DOI: 10.1111/j.1095-8312.2007.00844.x

[32] Cabrero-Sañudo F J, Lobo J M, Biogeography of Aphodiinae dung beetles based on the regional composition and distribution patterns of genera. Journal of Biogeography 2009; 36, 1474-1492. DOI: 10.1111/j.1365-2699.2009.02093.x

[33] Aagesen L, Szumik C, Zuloaga F O, Morrone O. Biogeography of the South America highlands - recognizing the Altoandina, Puna, and Prepuna through the study of Poaceae. Cladistics 2009; 25 295-310. DOI: 10.1111/j.1096-0031.2009.00248.x

[34] Arias J S, Casagranda M D, Diaz Gómez J M. A comparison of NDM and PAE using real data. Cladistics2010; 26, 204.DOI: 10.1111/j.1469-0691.2009.00285.x

[35] Pizarro-Araya J, Jerez V. Distribución geográfica del género Gyriosomus Guérin-Méneville, 1834 (Coleoptera: Tenebrionidae): una aproximación biogeográfica. Revista Chilena de Historia Natural 2004; 77 491-500. DOI: 10.4067/S0716-078X2004000300008.

[36] Hennig C. Prabclus Package, test for clustering of presence absence data 2003; Available at: http://cran.r-project.org/src/contrib/Descriptions/prabclus/.html

[37] Shi G R. Multivariate data analysis in palaeoecology and palaeobiogeography–a review. Palaeogeography Palaeoclimatology Palaeoecology. 1993; 105 199–234.

[38] Kruskal J B. Multidimensional scaling by optimizing goodness of fit to a Nonmetric hypothesis. Psychometrika 1964; 29 1–27.

[39] Goloboff, P.A. 2004. NDM VNDM. Programs for identification of areas of endemism. Program and documentation. Available at: http://www.zmuc.dk/public/phylogeny/endemism/

[40] Casagranda M.D., S. Roig-Juñent & C.A. Szumik. Endemismo a diferentes escalas espaciales: un ejemplo con Carabidae (Coleoptera: Insecta) de América del Sur austral. Revista Chilena de Historia Natural 2009; 82 17-42. DOI: 10.4067/S0716-078X2009000100002

[41] Moline P M, Linder H P. Input data, analytical methods and biogeography of Elegia (Restionaceae) Journal of Biogeography 2006; 33 47–62. DOI: 10.1111/j.1365-2699.2005.01369.x

[42] Carine M A, Humphries C J, Guma I R, Reyes-Betancort J A, Santos Guerra A. Areas and algorithms: evaluating numerical approaches for the delimitation of areas of endemism in the Canary Islands archipelago. Journal of Biogeography 2009; 36, 593-611. DOI: 10.1111/j.1365-2699.2008.02016.x

[43] Casazza G, Minuto L. A critical evaluation of different methods for the determination of areas of endemism and biotic elements: an Alpine study. Journal of Biogeography 2009; 36 2056–2065. DOI: 10.1111/j.1365-2699.2009.02156.x

[44] Hortal J, Lobo J M, Jiménez-Valverde A. Limitations of biodiversity databases: case study on seed-plant diversity inTenerife, Canary Islands. Conservation Biology 2007; 21 853–863. DOI: 10.1111/j.1523-1739.2007.00686.x

[45] Olson D M, Dinerstein E, Wikramanayake E D, Burgess N.D, Powell G V N, Underwood E C, D'amico J A, Itoua I, Strand H E, Morrison J C, Loucks C J, Allnutt T F, Ricketts T H, Kura Y, Lamoreux J F, Wettengel W W, Hedao P, Kassem K R. Terrestrial ecoregions of the world: a new map of life on earth. Bioscience 2001; 51, 933–8. DOI: 10.1641/0006-3568(2001)051[0933:TEOTWA]2.0.CO;2

[46] Myers N, Mittermeier R A, Mittermeier C G, da Fonseca G A B, Kent G. Biodiversity hotspots for conservation priorities. Nature 2000; 403 853-858. DOI: 10.1038/35002501

[47] Lamoreux J F, Morrison J C, Ricketts T H et al. Global test of biodiversity concordance and the importance of endemism. Nature 2006; 440 212–14. DOI: 10.1038/nature04291

[48] Cabrera A L. Regiones fitogeográficas argentinas. In: Kugler W F (ed.), Enciclopedia Argentina de Agricultura y Jardinería, II, ACME, Buenos Aires; 1976. p. 1-85.

[49] Cabrera A L, Willink A. 1973. Biogeografía de América Latina. Monografía 13, Serie de Biología, OEA, Washington, D.C

[50] Cabrera A L, Willink A. Biogeografía de América Latina. Monografía 13, Serie de Biología, OEA, Washington, D.C. 2º Edic. Corregida. 1980.

[51] Willink A. Distribution patterns of Neotropical insects with special reference to the AculeateHymenoptera of southern South America.In: Heyer, W. R. y E. Vanzolini (eds.),Proceedings of a workshop on Neotropical distribution patterns Acad. Brasil. Ciencias, Rio de Janeiro, pp.205-221. 1988.

[52] Willink A. Contribución a la Zoogeografía de Insectos Argentinos. Boletín de la Academia Nacional de Ciencias, Córdoba 1991; 59 125-147.

[53] Cei J M. Amphibians of Argentina. Monitore Zoologico Italiano 1980; 2 1-609.

[54] Cei J M. Monographie lV: Reptiles del Centro, Centro-Oeste y Sur de la Argentina. Herpetofauna de las Zonas Áridas y Semiáridas. Museo Regionale di Scienze Naturali Torino 1986; Monogr. 4 1- 527

[55] Ringuelet R A. Rasgos fundamentales de la Zoogeografía de la Argentina. Physis 1961; 22 63 151-170

[56] Morrone J J. Biogeographic areas and transition zones of Latin America and the Caribbean Islands based on analyses of the entomofauna. Annual Review of Entomology 2006; 51 467-94. DOI: 10.1146/annurev.ento.50.071803.130447

[57] Stange L A, Teran A L, Willink A. Entomofauna de la provincia biogeográfica del Monte. Acta Zool. Lilloana 1976; 32 73–120.

[58] CONABIO http://www.conabio.gob.mx/

[59] GBIF http://www.gbif.org/

[60] SNDB http://www.sndb.mincyt.gob.ar/

[61] Jetz W, McPherson J M, Guralnick R P. Integrating biodiversity distribution knowledge: toward a global map of life. 2012; Trends in Ecology & Evolution

[62] Morrone J J. A new regional biogeography of the Amazonian subregion, based mainly on animal taxa. Anales del Instituto de Biología de Universidad Autónoma de México, Zoología 2000; 71 99-123.

[63] Domínguez C, Roig-Juñent S, Tassin J J, Ocampo F C, Flores G E.. Areas of endemism of the Patagonian steppe: an approach based on insect distributional patterns using endemicity analysis. Journal of Biogeography 2006; 33 (9) 1527-1537. DOI: 10.1111/j. 1365-2699.2006.01550.x.

[64] Szumik C, Aagesen L, Casagranda D, Arzamendia V, Baldo,D, Claps L, Cuezzo F, Díaz Gómez J, Giannini N, Goloboff P, Gramajo C, Kopuchian C, Kretzchsmar S, Lizarralde de Grosso M, Molina A, Mollerach M, Navarro F, Sandoval M, Pereyra V, Scrocchi G, Zuloaga F. Detecting areas of endemism with a taxonomically diverse data set: plants, mammals, reptiles, amphibians, birds and insects from Argentina. Cladistics 2012; 28 317-329. DOI: 10.1111/j.1096-0031.2011.00385.x

[65] Navarro F, Szumik C, Cuezzo F, Lizarralde de Grosso M, Goloboff P, Quintana M G. Can insect data be used to infer areas of endemism? An example from the Yungas of Argentina. Revista Chilena de Historia Natural 2009; 82 507-522. DOI: 10.4067/ S0716-078X2009000400006.

[66] Giraudo A, Matteucci S D, Alonso J, Herrera J, Abramson R R. Comparing bird assemblages in large and small fragments of the Atlantic Forest hotspots. Biodiversity and Conservation 2008; 17 5 1251–1265. DOI:10.1007/s10531-007-9309-9

[67] Arzamendia V, Giraudo A R. Influence of great South American Rivers of the Plata basin in distributional patterns of tropical snakes: a panbiogeographic analysis. Journal of Biogeography 2009; 36 1739–1749. DOI: 10.1111/j.1365-2699.2009.02116.x

[68] Barquez R M, Díaz M M. Bats of the Argentine Yungas: a systematic and distributional analysis. Acta Zoológica Mexicana 2001; 82 1–81.

[69] Straube F C, Di Giacomo A. A avifauna das regiões subtropical e temperada do Neotrópico: desafios biogeográficos. Ciência e Ambiente 2007; 35:137-166

[70] Collar N J, Gonzaga P L, Krabbe N, Madroño Nieto A, Naranjo L G, Parker T A. III, Wege, D.C. Threatened Birds of the Americas. The ICBP /IUCN Red Data Book. Smithsonian Institution Press, ICPB, Cambridge, UK; 1992.

[71] Díaz G B, Ojeda R A. Libro rojo de mamíferos amenazados de la Argentina. SAREM (Sociedad Argentina para el Estudio de los Mamíferos), Mendoza, Argentina. 2000.

[72] Lavilla E O, Richard E, Scrocchi G J. Categorización de los anfibios y reptiles de Argentina. Asociación Herpetológica Argentina, Tucumán, Argentina; 2000.

[73] Barquez R M, Díaz M M, Ojeda R A. (Eds). Mamíferos de Argentina. Sistemática y Distribución. Sociedad Argentina para el Estudio de los Mamíferos, Tucumán, Argentina; 2006. 359 pp

[74] López-Lanús, B., Grilli, P., Coconier, E., Di Giacomo, A., & Banchs, R. Categorización de las aves de la Argentina según su estado de conservación.*Informe de Aves Argentinas/AOP y Secretaría de Ambiente y Desarrollo Sustentable. Buenos Aires, Argentina*; 2008.

[75] Goloboff P A, Farris J S, Nixon K C. TNT, a free program for phylogenetic analysis. Cladistics 2008; 24 5 774-786. DOI: 10.1111/j.1096-0031.2008.00217.x

[76] Phillips S J, Anderson R P, Schapired R E. Maximum entropy modeling of species geographic distributions. Ecological Modelling 2006; 190 231-259. DOI 10.1016/j.ecolmodel.2005.03.026

[77] Arias S, Szumik C, Goloboff, P. Spatial Analysis of Vicariance: A method for using direct geographical information in historical biogeography. Cladistics 2011; 27: 617-628. DOI: 10.1111/j.1096-0031.2011.00353.x

[78] Catalano S, Goloboff P. Simultaneously Mapping and Superimposing Landmark Configurations with Parsimony as Optimality Criterion. Systematic Biology 2012; 613 392-400. DOI: 10.1093/sysbio/syr119

Chapter 2

Genomic Rearrangements and Evolution

Özlem Barış, Mehmet Karadayı, Derya Yanmış and
Medine Güllüce

Additional information is available at the end of the chapter

http://dx.doi.org/10.5772/55456

1. Introduction

All genomes in living organisms can change under influence of internal or external factors. That is why genomic materials are commonly defined as dynamic entities and it is believed that they have been repeatedly altered and rearranged since the beginning of the life on the planet [1-4]. Understanding this dynamism is a valuable key to unlock the chest of the mysterious existence story in an evolutionary manner. Therefore, a lot of studies have been conducted on the dynamism of genomic materials in organisms and the count of related researches has gradually risen by the day. An enormous data from these studies call attention to recombinational, tranpositional and mutational processes as three main sources of genomic changes [1,2,5-18].

Recombinational changes of genomes are mainly dependent on internal factors which are closely associated with a great many of intracellular and intercellular interactions. Enzyme catalyzed pathways and predetermined timing are the most descriptive properties for many types of recombination events. For instance, usual meiotic crossing over, the best known recombinational event, always occurs under control of specified enzymatic reactions at a certain time period in the cell cycle [2,4,19-22].

Transpositional events are also important sources for sequential rearrangements in genomes and induced by external or internal genomic material pieces that are described as mobile or transposable elements. In mechanism of transposition, a transposable element changes its relative position within the genome. "Copy and Paste" or "Cut and Paste" postulates work in this process. A transpositional event occurring with the copy and paste mechanism is called as replicative transposition that a transposable element is duplicated during the process and copied sequence transferred into the target genomic sequence, and the other one with the cut and paste mechanism is called as non-replicative transposition that duplication of the transposable element does not occur and the original sequence is transferred from one region into another [5,23-24]. In both cases, a transpositional event is commonly resulted in a mutational phenomenon and alteration in genomic sizes that makes them attractive for genomic evolution studies [6-7,23-26].

Mutations are described as sudden changes in genomic materials induced by internal and external factors [27]. They have importance in medicinal, agricultural and other related researches due to their deleterious, beneficial or functional effects on organisms [5,9,28]. Moreover, enormous potential for construction of novel genes and other types of genomic sequences, they are considered as the most attractive subject for genome evolution [2,29-32].

2. Recombinations

Genetic recombination is a process that is catalyzed by many different enzymes called as recombinases. It can take place in all living cells from bacteria to eukaryota as well as viral genomes. This process mainly results in DNA repair, genomic rearrangements, variations and evolutional forces. Genetic recombinations are assigned to one of two groups according to their mechanism, which can be described as either homologous or non-homologous recombination [2,4,20,22,33-35].

2.1. Homologous recombination

Homologous recombinational events are sequential changes that occur between similar or identical parts of genomic material. In the beginning of 20th century, initial descriptions of homologous recombinations were introduced by W. Bateson and R. Punnett to explain diversions from predicted Mendelian inheritance phenotypic ratios [4,36-37]. This process, which is commonly found in many organisms from bacteria to higher organized eukaryotes, plays a significant role in DNA repair mechanisms and genome evolution by producing variations [2,38-40].

In prokaryotic cellular organisms, the most known types of homologous recombinational events are transformation, conjugation and transduction [41]. All of these events are resulted in genomic variations that have great value for evolution [42].

Transformation was discovered by Frederick Griffith in the late 1920s. His transformation experiments are considered as the beginning mile stone of the molecular biology discipline [5]. In the mechanism of natural prokaryotic transformation, a naked DNA fragment released from a cell is taken up by another under appropriate conditions, thus an exogenous genetic material is introduced into a prokaryotic cell that result in genomic variation. Transformation occurs in several groups of Gram positive, Gram negative and Archaea. A healthy double strand DNA molecule with a homological property and specific size (mostly smaller than 1000 nucleotides) is the most fundamental requirement for transformation [2,41]. Figure 1 illustrates a summarized scheme for transformation.

http://dx.doi.org/10.5772/55456

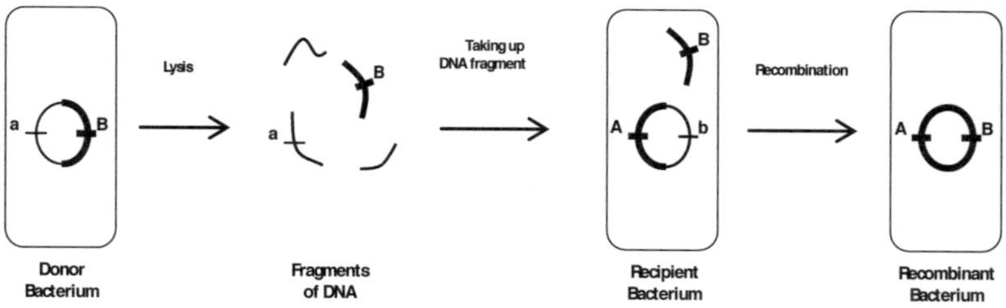

Figure 1. Simple mechanism of transformation

Bacterial conjugation, discovered in 1946 by Joshua Lederberg and Edward Tatum [43], is another process to transfer the genetic information in Prokaryotes. In its mechanism, the transfer of genetic material involves cell to cell contact and a plasmid encoded pathway. The process occurs between a donor cell, which includes a certain type of conjugative plasmid, and a recipient cell, which does not. In this process, the plasmid plays a key role by carrying all related genes on *tra* region. These genes encode the sex pilus (F pili) formation, which allow specific pairing to take place between the donor cell and the recipient cell. After generation of sex pilus mediated cell to cell contact, a copy of the plasmid is transferred to the recipient under control of various enzyme systems encoded by *tra* region. In most cases, this type of recombination does not cause genetic variation at high level because the transferred genetic information is restricted by sequential contents of the plasmid. However, in certain circumstances, conjugative plasmid may integrate into the main genomic material, resulting in the formation of Hfr (High Frequency Recombination) cells. These cells, commonly seen in Gram negative bacterial groups, have significant potential for recombination at higher levels due to leading transfer of genes from the host chromosome [2,41]. Figure 2 shows regular bacterial conjugation events and Hfr formation.

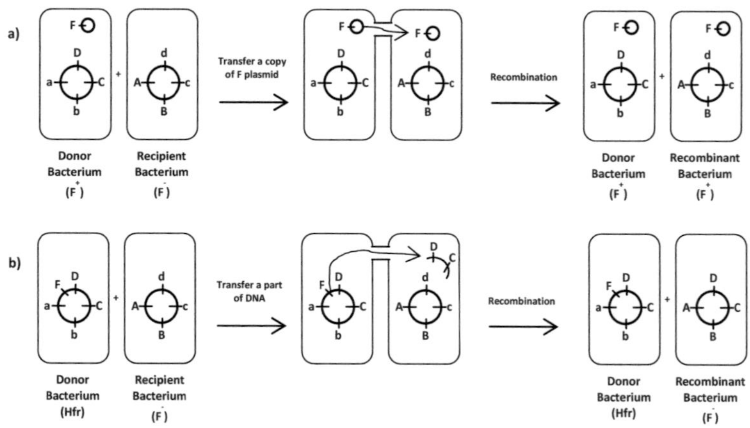

Figure 2. An illustrative scheme for bacterial conjugation of F^+ (a) and Hfr (b) cells

Transduction, initially discovered by Norton Zinder and Joshua Lederberg in 1951 [44], refers to virus-mediated transfers of genetic materials. There are two fundamental mechanisms as generalized and specialized transduction. In generalized transduction, any bacterial genomic sequence may be transferred to another bacterium via a modified bacteriophage that accidentally involves bacterial DNA instead of viral DNA. However, in specialized transduction, bacteriophage includes both bacterial and viral DNA at the same time [2,41]. Both types of transduction events are summarized at Figure 3.

In eukaryotic organisms, meiotic crossing over (chromosomal cross over) is the most well-known example for homologous recombination. This event occurs between homologous chromosomes at prophase I stage in meiosis and results in variation of genetic materials [2,5,45-46]. The scheme of meiotic crossing over is showed in Figure 4.

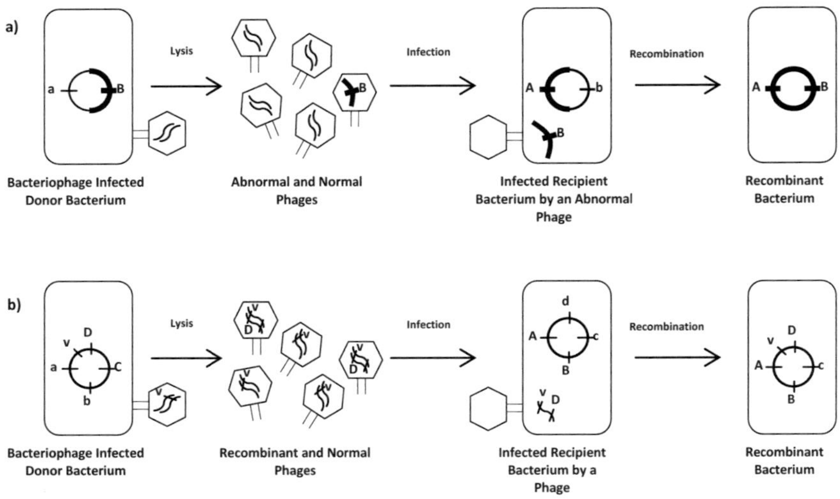

Figure 3. Mechanism of generalized (a) and specialized (b) transduction events

Homologous recombination also plays a significant role in DNA repair mechanisms in both prokaryotic and eukaryotic organisms. It is one of the major DNA repair processes in bacteria [2,46]. For example, double-strand breaks in bacteria are repaired by the RecBCD pathway of homologous recombination [42,47-49]. Moreover, it is well known that similar mechanisms work in eukaryotic organisms.

Homologous recombination also includes non-allelic ones that have been not well documented. These events occur between sequences arisen from duplications or deletions that show high homology, but are not alleles. It is believed that non-allelic homologous recombination has a great importance for evolution due to generating a decrease or an increase in copy number of sequences [50-52].

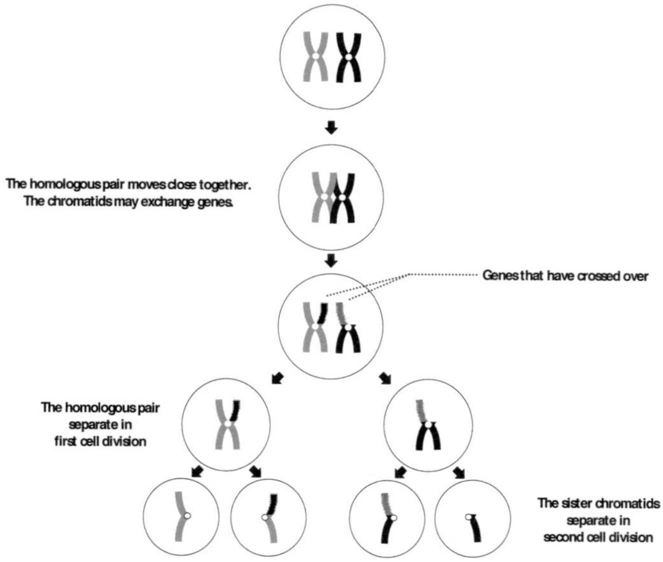

Figure 4. Mechanism of meiotic crossing over

2.2. Non-homologous recombination

Non-homologous recombination, also named as non-homologous end joining (NHEJ), is a pathway that mainly associated with DNA repair that especially works on double strand breaks. Contrary to the mechanisms of homologous recombination, it does not require sequential homology. However, this pathway has been identified in many groups of living organisms from bacteria to multicellular organisms, even in human being, recent studies have mainly focused on eukaryotes much more than bacteria. One reason for this is that prokaryotic DNA repair is heavily done by various processes of homologous recombination.

Nuclease, polymerase and ligase activities play the major role in NHEJ process. Despite its conservative mechanism, this process is generally resulting in variations of genetic materials [2,53-55].

3. Mobile genetic elements

Mobile genetic elements are described as DNA segments that can move within the genome. These include transposons, group II introns, plasmids and viral elements [56]. All these events result in genomic alterations that cause rising of evolutional forces [6,8,24-26,57-61].

3.1. Transposons

Transposons, also named as transposable elements, are major forces in the evolution and rearrangement of genomes [6,26,56]. Discovery of transposable elements was achieved in 1943 by Barbara McClintock who was awarded with a Nobel Prize after 40 years in 1983 [2,58]. Since that time, the importance of transposons has been well established and much more attention has been given to their formation and consequences [62]. To get more easily comprehensive information, they are divided into three main groups as retrotransposons, DNA transposons and insertion sequences.

3.1.1. Retrotransposons

Retrotransposons can be considered as the biggest group of transposable elements due to their abundance in many eukaryotic genomes (i.e. 49-78% of the total genome in maize and 42% in human) [63-64]. The term "retrotransposon" is attributed to the transposition mechanism that involves via RNA intermediates. In the mechanism, a retrotransposon is initially copied to RNA (transcription), then converted to DNA (reversetranscription) and finally inserted to the genome (integration), and this process is mainly under control of the gene region of retrotransposons encoding reverse transcriptase. These elements can increase genome size and induce mutational events by disturbing genes [2,24,26,56,59,62,65].

Retrotransposons are divided into three main groups according to the operation mechanisms: long terminal repeats (LTRs) encode reverse transcriptase, similar to retroviruses; long interspersed elements (LINEs) do not have LTRs and encode reverse transcriptase and small interspersed elements (SINEs) do not encode reverse transcriptase. LINEs and SINEs are transcripted by RNA polymerase II and III, respectively [66-68].

3.1.2. DNA transposons

DNA transposons are the first discovered ones of transposable elements, initially named as "jumping genes" by Barbara McClintock in 1943 [69]. These are also called as Class II transposons, operate with a "cut and paste" mechanism. In this mechanism, transposition event mainly requires to transposase enzymes. Under control of the enzymatic processes, a DNA transposon is cut out of its location and inserted into a new location on the genome. Some transposases require a specific sequence as their target site; others can insert the transposon anywhere in the genomic material [2,24,41,62].

3.1.3. Insertion sequences

These are also known as IS elements. They are short DNA sequences that act as a simple form of transposable elements. Characterized properties of IS elements are that they have shorter sizes than other types of transposable elements (approximately 700 – 2500 bp), and carry some specific genes such as antibiotic resistance. Insertion sequences are usually flanked by inverted repeats [23,24,70].

3.2. Group II introns

Group II introns were discovered by Alexandre de Lencastre and his teammates in 2005 [71]. These elements, an important group of self-catalytic ribozymes, are generated during RNA splicing, and may cause genetic alterations [71].

3.3. Plasmids

Plasmids are circular and extra chromosomal genomic materials naturally found in bacteria, but rarely in several yeasts as eukaryotic organisms [41]. These elements show intracellular or intercellular mobility (see section 2.1.) that result in genomic alterations and evolutional forces.

3.4. Viral elements

Viral elements are genomic materials transferring between living organisms via virus infections. According to the mechanism of infection, viruses are divided into two categories as lytic and lysogenic. Lytic ones complete their eclipse phase in the cell and cause lysis of the host. However, lysogenic ones integrate their genomic materials into the host genome and directly cause genomic alterations [41]. For example, some retroviruses are common type of lysogenic viral elements and their effect mechanism is similar to retrotransposons.

4. Mutations

The "Mutation" term was initially used by Hugo de Vries in 1905 to describe the phenotypic changes in evening-primrose plant (*Oenothera lamarckiana*). However, it commonly describes any sequential change in the genomic material of living organisms in the present day. Their various effects resulting in genotypic and phenotypic alterations that cause diseases, gaining or loss of advantageous or deleterious properties, attract the scientific attention on mutation focused investigations. In these researches, mutations are generally classified according to the effect mechanisms and size of effected genomic sequences to perform more apparent and comprehensive evaluations [1-3,5,29-31,34].

4.1. Classification of mutations

Effect size of mutations on genomes is one of the most widely-accepted criteria for classification. According to this, mutations can be divided into two groups named as gene mutations and chromosome mutations [5,27].

4.1.1. Gene mutations

Gene mutations are small-scale mutations that effect one or few bases in a genome. However, they can induce many important phenomenon depend on properties of effected genomic sequences. For example, a gene mutation in a protein coding region of genomic material can result in synthesis of a non-functional protein that mostly causes deleterious effects for the organism. Gene mutations are also divide subcategories as base substitution and insertion/deletion [2,5,27,34].

Base Substitutions: They are also called as point mutations. These types of mutations are characterized by taking place of a different base instead of original one in the genome. When a purine base replaces with another purine or a pyrimidine base with another pyrimidine ($A \leftrightarrow G$

or C↔T), it is called as transition. On the other hand, if a purine base replaces with a pyrimidine or a pyrimidine base with a purine (A↔C, A↔T, G↔C or G↔T), then it is called as transversion.

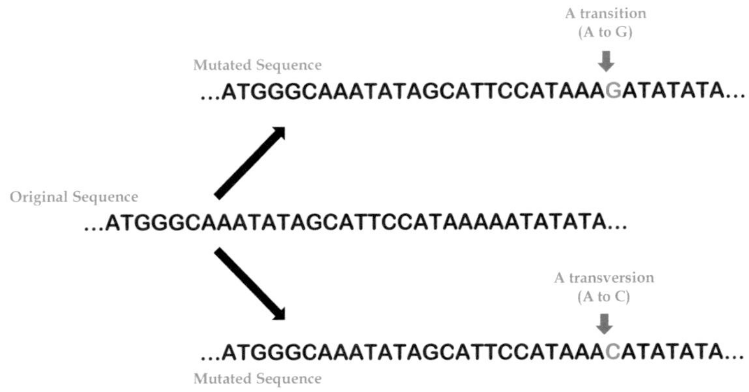

Figure 5. Base substitutions type of gene mutations

Insertions/Deletions: The insertion term means addition of one or few bases into a genomic material. Contrary to this, deletions are defined as removing of one or few bases from a genome.

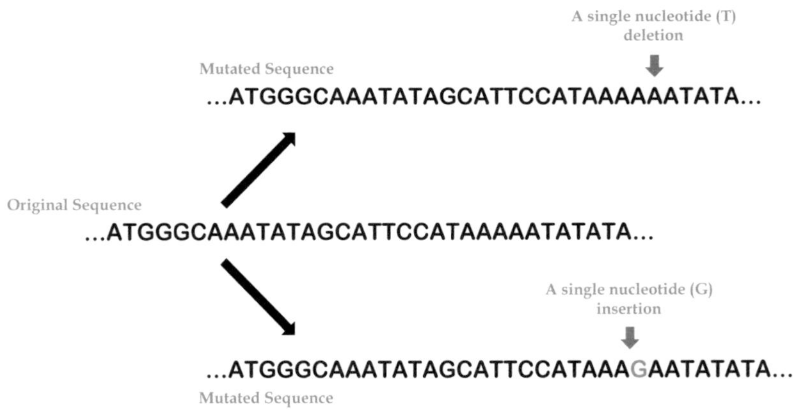

Figure 6. Insertion/Deletions type of gene mutations

4.1.2. Chromosome mutations

Chromosomal mutations are described as phenomenon that causes bigger sequence alterations than gene mutations. These are also called as macro-mutations due to their microscopically examination capabilities. There are two main subcategories as structural and numerical alterations in chromosomal mutations [5,9,27,34].

4.1.2.1. Numerical alterations

These types of mutations mainly cause alterations in chromosome numbers in the living cells. Euploidy and aneuploidy are two essential subgroups.

Euploidy: The word "euploidy" refers to cumulative alterations in chromosome numbers. For example, diploid (2n) chromosome number of an organism can be changed to tetraploid (4n) form after these kind of mutations.

Aneuploidy: The word "aneuploidy" refers to non-cumulative alterations in chromosome numbers. For example, diploid (2n) chromosome number of an organism can be changed to nullisomy (2n-2), monosomy (2n-1) or trisomy (2n+1) form after these kind of mutations.

4.1.2.2. Structural alterations

These types of mutations do not change chromosome numbers. However, their effects are mainly on chromosomal structure. According to their effect mechanisms, structural mutations are grouped in four subcategories including deletions, inversions, duplications and translocations [5,9,27,72].

Deletions: Chromosomal deletions include losing of chromosomal pieces resulting in gene losses from the genome.

Inversions: An inversion refers to a phenomenon in which a chromosome break following by 180° rotation and reattachment of the broken piece on the same chromosomal region. It does not cause gene losses, but results in an inverted genetic material.

Duplications: Duplication is a case having two or more copies of a chromosomal region.

Translocations: These types of alterations are arisen from non-homologues chromosomal piece exchanges.

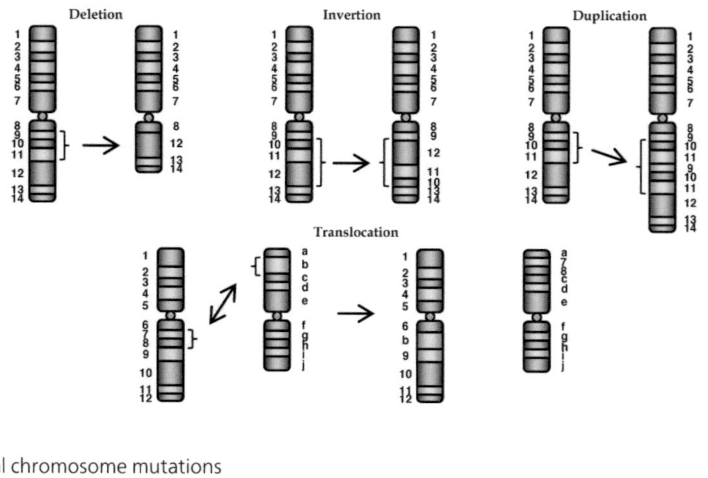

Figure 7. Structural chromosome mutations

5. Genome evolution

The origin of life on the earth has always been an attractive subject for all human beings. The question about formation of the first active biomolecule is one of the most important perspectives in this subject, and has been heavily researched for many years. Initial studies referred to proteins as first biomolecules due to their catalytic activities that operates various reactions for maintaining of life. Although this view was confirmed for a long time, their lack of potential to carry genetic information was the major handicap. In 1982, the commonly accepted thought about the first biomolecule was drastically changed by Thomas Cech and co-workers who published a paper that demonstrate the single intron of the large ribosomal RNA of *Tetrahymena thermophila* has self-splicing activity *in vitro*. This was the first report about catalytic RNA molecules. A year later, Sydney Altman and co-workers pointed out that the RNA component of ribonuclease P (RNase P) from *Escherichia coli* is able to carry out processing of pre-tRNA in the absence of its protein subunit *in vitro*. These studies lead to formation of "RNA world" perspective in genome evolution, and both scientists were awarded by Nobel Prize in 1989. In the recent view, the RNA world term means that ribonucleic acids have both the informational function of DNA and the catalytic function of proteins at the same time [2,12,73-78]. According to this concept, various types of RNAs can be proposed as initial genomes evolved on the planet. Major RNA types and their characteristic properties are given in Table 1.

Although the first genome has a potential to be ribonucleic acid form, instability and limited life of RNA molecules may have forced evolution of a more complex genomic material called as deoxyribonucleic acid (DNA). In this stage, there are several gaps and unanswered questions. However, the most discussed scenario about formation of DNA based genomes from initial RNA molecules (protogenome) proposes a phenomenon that is catalyzed by a reverse transcriptase [2,78,84].

Contrary to the high stability property, evolutional changes are continuously occurring in DNA based genomes that result in development of valuable features for adaptation. These changes have been mainly dependent on external forces since the beginning of the life on the planet (approximately 3.5 billion years ago) [2]. Understanding of this evolutional dynamism in genomic materials requires recognizing definitions of several important terms given in Table 2, prepared according to Eugene V. Koonin (2005) who is senior investigator at National Central of Biotechnology Information (NCBI) and studies on empirical comparative and evolutionary genomics [8].

Up to this point, all mentioned events cause changes in size and construction of genomic materials acting as evolutional forces. The genomic size is referred as "C value". Although the genomic size may reduce via deletions, it has generally intended to increase when compared to the first genome of universal common ancestor (UCA). This expansion is controlled by rearrangement forces, especially duplications and mobile genetic elements. There are two fundamental hypotheses for why genome sizes vary. According to the "Selfish-DNA hypothesis": genome size expansion is due to insertion and proliferation selfish genetic elements such as retrotransposons, and "Bulk-DNA hypothesis": having more genetic bulk can be adaptive because genome size effects nuclear volume, cell size, cell division rate in turn effecting developmental rate and size at maturity, thus it results in organisms with larger body size have larger cell sizes, and organisms with larger cells generally have larger genomes

[15,24-26,63,65,68,85-90]. In his paper, Zhang [88] underlined the positive correlation between duplicated gene amount and evolutional status of an organism. Table 3 represents prevalence of gene duplications in all three domains of life.

Type	Features	References
mRNA (Messenger RNA)	- responsible for coding - represents 4% of whole RNA amount in a cell - called as hnRNA or pre-mRNA before processing in eukaryotes	[2]
rRNA (Ribosomal RNA)	- composes ribosomes - the most abundant RNA in a cell (over 80%) - named as pre-rRNA before processing in all living organisms	[2]
tRNA (Transfer RNA)	- responsible for carrying amino acids to ribosomal complexes - specific for each amino acid - named as pre-tRNA before processing and modification in all living organisms	[2]
snRNA (Small Nuclear RNA)	- responsible for operation of splicing mechanism - found in nuclei of eukaryotes - also called as U-RNA - has a lot of sub-types with various catalytic activities	[2]
snoRNA (Small Nucleolar RNA)	- responsible for chemical modification of rRNA - found in nucleolar region of eukaryotic nuclei - shows catalytic activities	[2]
miRNA (MicroRNA)	responsible for regulation of gene expression double strand molecule intracellular origin (nucleus)	[2]
siRNA (Short Interfering RNA)	- responsible for regulation of gene expression - double strand molecule - extracellular origin (commonly synthetic) - called as small interfering or silencing RNA	[2]
piRNA (Piwi-interacting RNA)	- interacts with piwi proteins - the largest class of small non-coding RNA molecules	[76]
gRNA (Guide RNA)	- acts in mitochondrial mRNA processing - guides insertional or deletional events in mitochondrion	[77]
tmRNA (Transfer-messenger RNA)	- have tRNA and mRNA properties - also known as 10Sa RNA - found in bacterial genomes	[78]
shRNA (Small hairpin RNA)	- responsible for regulation of gene expression - makes a tight hairpin - extracellular origin	[79]
stRNA (Small Temporal RNA)	- regulates gene expression (down regulation)	[80]

Table 1. Major RNA types and their features

Homologs	**Genes sharing a common origin**
Orthologs	Genes originating from a single ancestral gene in the last common ancestor of the compared genomes.
Pseudoorthologs	Genes that actually are paralogs but appeared to be orthologous due to differential, linage-specific gene loss.
Xenologs	Homologous genes acquired via xenologous gene displacement (XGD) by one or both of the compared species but appearing to be orthologous in pairwise genome comparisons.
Co-orthologs	Two or more genes in one lineage that are, collectively, orthologous to one or more genes in another lineage due to a lineage-specific duplication(s). Members of a co-orthologous gene set are inparalogs relative to the respective speciation event.
Paralogs	**Genes related by duplication**
Inparalogs (Symparalogs)	Paralogs genes resulting from a lineage-specific duplication(s) subsequent to a given speciation event (defined only relative to a speciation event, no absolute meaning).
Outparalogs (Alloparalogs)	Paralogs genes resulting from a duplication(s) preceding a given speciation event (defined only relative to a speciation event, no absolute meaning)
Pseudoparalogs	Homologous genes that come out as paralogs in a single-genome analysis but actually ended up in the given genome as a result of a combination of vertical inheritance and horizontal gene transfer.

Table 2. Homology: terms and definitions from Koonin 2005 [8].

	Total number of genes	**Number of duplicate genes (% of duplicate genes)**
Bacteria		
Mycoplasma pneumoniae	677	298 (44)
Helicobacter pylori	1590	266 (17)
Haemophilus influenzae	1709	284 (17)
Archaea		
Archaeoglobus fulgidus	2436	719 (30)
Eukarya		
Saccharomyces cerevisiae	6241	1858 (30)
Caenorhabditis elegans	18424	8971 (49)
Drosophila melanogaster	13601	5536 (41)
Arabidopsis thaliana	25498	16574 (65)
Homo sapiens	40580[a]	15343 (38)

[a] The most recent estimate is ~30000.

[b] Use of different computational methods or criteria results in slightly different estimates of the number of duplicated genes.

Table 3. Prevalence of gene duplications in all three domains of life[b] from Zhang 2003 [88].

Besides, Xue et al. [91] laid emphasis on the roles of duplications in genomic size and compositional changes in their studies via exploring the evolution of segmental gene duplication in haploid and diploid populations by analytical and simulation approaches. The result of this study highlighted that duplications do not only cause alterations in genome size but they are also result in many recombinational events that closely related to formation of variations that have value in rising evolutional forces. In another paper, Force et al. [92] focused on the DDC (duplication-degeneration-complementation) model for the alternative fates (nonfunctionalization, neofuctionalization and subfuctionalization) of duplicate genes, and underlined their roles in genome evolution.

Mobile genetic elements also affect genome size. For example, horizontal transfer of transposable elements plays a key role in genome evolution. In their "copy-and-paste" operation mechanisms, retrotransposons, as common examples of mobile genetic elements that may cause horizontal gene transfer, transpose via an RNA-intermediated process, and this increases genomic material size [26,93-94]. Furthermore, all advanced biology sources covering microbial genetic title mention the role of other types of mobile genetic elements including plasmids and viral genomes in formation of variations in genomic size and structure [41].

On the other hand, reduction of genomic size in certain periods is an inevitable fact for genome evolution. In this manner, smaller genomes are more advantageous for selection than bigger ones due to their high replication potentials and metabolic inexpensiveness. Deletions can be given as the main force to diminish genomic size that causes gene losses [95-96]. In a recent paper, Pettersson and co-workers emphasized the role of deletions in regulation of genomic size and its coding density by using a mathematical model to determine the evolutionary fate [97].

A genomic material may accept deletions and reduce its size up to reach minimal genome limits that have the smallest number of genetic elements sufficient to build a modern-type free-living cellular organism. In addition, under some exceptional conditions, genomic materials of several endo-symbionts and co-symbionts carry much less genes than predicted minimal genome rates. For example, although *Pelagibacter ubique* (α-Proteobacteria) is known as a free-living organism with the smallest genome (only 1308 Kb in size and potentially contains 1354 genes), endo-symbiont *Hodgkinia cicadicola* (α-Proteobacteria) has the smallest genome (only 144 Kb in size and potentially contains 188 genes) among known-living organisms [98-102]. According to Juhas and co-workers' study [102], the extremely small genomes of endosymbionts usually encode only the most fundamental process, suggesting that some of their genes might have been transferred into the host cell genome. The endosymbiont *Wolbachia* strains that transfer ~1 Mb fragments of its genomic material to the host genome can be given as a good example for this phenomenon [98-102].

Contrary to the genomic material of *P. ubique* in which there is no pseudogenes, introns, transposons, or extrachromosomal elements, modern-type organism genomes need some or all of these differentiated genetic parts [97]. In this regard, genomic rearrangements have a critical potential via causing structural changes, especially new alleles and new regulatory regions in the genomes can be created by only mutations. There is a huge data giving information about the roles of mutations in evolution in the scientific literature

[1-3,5,8,9,11,12,29-33]. For instance, Halligan and Keightley [103] reviewed the relationship between mutagenesis and its role in genome evolution, and introduced mutational events as the ultimate source of genetic variation.

6. Conclusion

Recent attention of evolutionary studies has shifted to genetics, molecular and cellular biology as a result of finding out principles of genetics and DNA is the main molecule responsible for inheritance. Thus, the popularity of genome-wide studies has increased. In this regard, genomic rearrangement mechanisms (recombinations, mutations or mobility of several genetic elements) are major research topics for evolution of genomes because any change in the DNA molecule of the organisms may cause a valuable process for evolution when it has inheritable potential.

Thus, aim of the present study was conducted to emphasize potential value of genomic rearrangements for evolution, and therefore, basic rearrangement mechanisms were explained in detail, and their evolutionary effects on genomes were briefly discussed via giving important samples in this chapter.

Acknowledgements

The authors express their thanks to the Microbiology & Molecular Biology Research Team of Biology Department, Atatürk University. The author Mehmet Karadayı specially thanks to Biologist Alperen Tekin for his encouragement and support.

Author details

Özlem Barış, Mehmet Karadayı, Derya Yanmış and Medine Güllüce

Biology Department of Atatürk University, Erzurum, Turkey

References

[1] Watson JD and Berry A. DNA: The Secret of Life. New York: Alfred A. Knopf Inc.; 2003.

[2] Brown TA. Genomes 3 (3rd edition). New York: Garland Science; 2007.

[3] Lashin SA, Suslov VV and Matushkin YuG. Theories of Biological Evolution from the Viewpoint of the Modern Systemic Biology. Russian Journal of Genetics 2012;48(5) 481–496.

[4] Webster MT and Hurst LD. Direct and indirect consequences of meiotic recombination: implications for genome evolution. Trends in Genetics 2012;28(3) 101-109.

[5] Lewin B. Gene VIII (8th edition). New Jersey: Pearson Education; 2004.

[6] Frost LS, Leplae R, Summers AO, Toussaint A. Mobile Genetic Elements: The agents of open source evolution. Nature Reviews – Microbiology 2005;3: 722-732.

[7] Koonin EV. Comperative Genomics, Minimal Gene-Sets and Last Universal Common Ancestor. Nature Reviews – Microbiology 2003;1: 127-136.

[8] Koonin EV. Orthologs, Paralogs, and Evolutionary Genomics. Annual Review of Genetics 2005;39: 309–338.

[9] Lodish H, Berk A, Kaiser CA, Krieger M, Scott MP, Bretscher A, Ploegh H and Matsudaira P. Molecular Cell Biology (6th edition), New York: WH. Freeman Inc.; 2007.

[10] Gu W, Zhang F, Lupski JR. Mechanisms for human genomic rearrangements. PathoGenetics 2008;1: 4.

[11] Osborne LR. Genomic rearrangements in the spotlight. Nature Genetics 2008;40(1) 6-7.

[12] Futuyma DJ. Evolution (second edition). Massachusetts: Sinauer Associates; 2009.

[13] Koonin EV and Novozhilav AS. Origin and Evolution of the Genetic Code: The Universal Enigma. IUBMB Life 2009;61(2) 99–111.

[14] Mates LM, Chuah MKL, Belay E, Jerchow B, Manoj N, Acosta-Sanchez A, Grzela DP, Schmitt A, Becker K, Matrai J, Ma L, Samara-Kuko E, Gysemans C, Pryputniewicz D, Miskey C, Fletcher B, Driessche TV, Ivics Z and Izsvak Z. Molecular evolution of a novel hyperactive Sleeping Beauty transposase enables robust stable gene transfer in vertebrates. Nature Genetics 2009;41(6) 753–761.

[15] Krupovic M, Gribaldo S, Bamford DH and Forterre P. The Evolutionary History of Archaeal MCM Helicases: A Case Study of Vertical Evolution Combined with Hitchhiking of Mobile Genetic Elements. Molecular Biology Evolution 2010;27(12) 2716–2732.

[16] Nosil P and Schluter D. The genes underlying the process of speciation. Trends in Ecology and Evolution 2011;26(4) 160-167.

[17] Nosil P and Feder JL. Widespread yet heterogeneous genomic divergence. Molecular Ecology 2012;21: 2829–2832.

[18] Traulsen A and Reed FA. From genes to games: Cooperation and cyclic dominance in meiotic drive. Journal of Theoretical Biology 2012;299: 120–125.

[19] Eyre-Walker A. Evolutionary genomics. Trends in Ecology and Evolution 1993;14(5) 176.

[20] Gorbalenya AE and Koonin EV. Helicases: amino acid sequence comparisons and structure-function relationships. Current Opinion in Structural Biology 1993; 3(3) 419-429.

[21] Champoux JJ. A first view of the structure of a type IA topoisomerase with bound DNA. TRENDS in Pharmacological Sciences 2002;23(5) 199-201.

[22] Cutter AD and Moses AM. Polymorphism, Divergence, and the Role of Recombination in *Saccharomyces cerevisiae* Genome Evolution. Molecular Biology and Evolution 2011;28(5) 1745-1754.

[23] Kidwell MG. The Evolutionary History of The P-Family of Transpozable Elements. Journal of Heredity 1994; 85(5) 339-346.

[24] Kidwell MG and Lisch DR. Perspective: Transposable elements, parasitic DNA and genome evolution. Evolution 2001;55(1) 1-24.

[25] Federova L and Federov A. Introns in gene evolution. Genetica 2003;118: 123–131.

[26] Sabot F, Kalender R, Jaaskelainen M, Wei C, Tanskanen J, Schulman AH. Retrotransposons: Metaparasites and Agents of Genome Evolution. Israel Journal of Ecology and Evolution 2006;52(3-4) 319-320.

[27] Karadayı M, Barış Ö, Güllüce M. *Salmonella* as a unique tool for Genetic Toxicology. In Kumar Y (ed.) Salmonella – A Diversified Superbug. Rijeka: InTech; 2012.

[28] Hartl DL and Jones EW. Towards a theory of evolutionary adaptation. Massachusetts: Jones & Bartlett Pub.; 1998.

[29] Keightley PD and Eyre-Walker A. Deleterious Mutations and the Evolution of Sex. Science 2000;260: 331-333.

[30] Nei M. The new mutation theory of phenotypic evolution. Proceedings of the National Academy of Sciences 2007;104(30) 12235-12242.

[31] Lynch M. Evolution of the mutation rate. Trends in Genetics 2010;26: 345–352.

[32] Charlesworth B. The Effects of Deleterious Mutations on Evolution at Linked Sites. Genetics 2012;190: 5–22.

[33] Sobell HM. Molecular Mechanism for Genetic Recombination. Proceedings of the National Academy of Sciences 1972;69(9) 2483-2487.

[34] Tamarin RH. Principles of Genetics. Iowa: William C Brown Pub.; 2001.

[35] Lewis-Rogers N, Crandall KA and Posada D. Evolutionary analyses of genetic recombination. In Parisi V, De Fonzo V and Aluffi-Pentini F. (eds) Dynamical Genetics. Kerala: Research Signpost; 2004; p49-78.

[36] Bateson W, Sounders ER, Punnett RC. Experimental studies in the physiology of heredity. Reports to the Evolution Committee of the Royal Society 1904; pp154.

[37] Capecchi MR. Altering the genome by homologous recombination. Science 1989;244(4910) 1288-1292.

[38] O'Neil N and Rose A. DNA repair (January 13, 2006), *WormBook*, ed. The *C. elegans* Research Community, WormBook, http://www.wormbook.org.

[39] Li X and Heyer W-D. Homologous recombination in DNA repair and DNA damage tolerance. Cell Research 2008;18: 99-113.

[40] Holthausen JT, Wyman C, Kanaar R. Regulation of DNA strand exchange in homologous recombination. DNA Repair 2010;9: 1264–1272.

[41] Madigan MT and Martinko JM. Brock Biology of Microorganisms (eleventh edition). New Jersey: Pearson Education; 2006.

[42] Rocha EPC, Cornet E, Michel B. Comparative and Evolutionary Analysis of the Bacterial Homologous Recombination Systems. PLoS Genetics 2005;1(2) e15.

[43] Tatum EL and Gene Recombination in the Bacterium Escherichia coli. Journal of Bacteriology 1947;53(6) 673–684.

[44] Zinder ND and Lederberg J. Genetic Exchange in Salmonella. Journal of Bacteriology 1952;64(5) 679–699.

[45] Heyer W-D, Ehmsen KT and Liu J. Regulation of Homologous Recombination in Eukaryotes. Annual Review of Genetic 2010;44: 113–139.

[46] Greenwald E. Eukaryotic Homologous Recombination Repair: a Dynamic Cast of Characters. Master Thesis. Columbia University; 2012.

[47] Bianco PR and Kowalczykowski SC. The recombination hotspot Chi is recognized by the translocating RecBCD enzyme as the single strand of DNA containing the sequence 5′-GCTGGTGG-3′. Proceedings of the National Academy of Sciences 1997; 94, 6706-6711.

[48] Spies M and Kowalczykowski SC. Homologous Recombination by the RecBCD and RecF Pathways. In Higgins P. Bacterial Chromosomes. Washington, D.C: ASM Press; 2005; p389–403.

[49] Smith GR. How RecBCD Enzyme and Chi Promote DNA Break Repair and Recombination: a Molecular Biologist's View. Microbiology and Molecular Biology Reviews 2012;76(2) 217-228.

[50] Venturin M, Gervasini C, Orzan F, Bentivegna A, Corrado L, Colapietro P, Friso A, Tenconi R, Upadhyaya M, Larizza L, Riva P. Evidence for non-homologous end joining and non-allelic homologous recombination in atypical NF1 microdeletions. Human Genetic 2004;115: 69–80.

[51] Hurles ME and Lupski JR. Recombination Hotspots in Nonallelic Homologous Recombination. In Lupski JR and Stankiewicz P. (eds.) Genomic Disorders: The Genomic Basis of Disease. New Jersey: Humana Press; 2006; p341-355.

[52] Hermetz KE, Surti U, Cody JD and Rudd MK. A recurrent translocation is mediated by homologous recombination between HERV-H elements. Molecular Cytogenetics 2012;5: 6.

[53] Dai Y, Kysela B, Hanakahi LA, Manolis K, Riballo E, Stumm M, Harville TO, West SC, Oettinger MA and Jeggo PA. Nonhomologous end joining and V(D)J recombination require an additional factor. Proceedings of the National Academy of Sciences 2003;100(5) 2462–2467.

[54] Pastwa E and Blasiak J. Non-homologous DNA end joining. Acta Biochimica Polonica 2003;50(4) 891-908.

[55] Guerrero AA, Martinez-A C and van Wely KHM. Merotelic attachments and non-homologous end joining are the basis of chromosomal instability. Cell Division 2010;5: 13.

[56] Miller WJ and Capy P. Mobile Genetic Elements as Natural Tools for Genome Evolution. Methods in Molecular Biology 2004;260: 1-20.

[57] Petrov DA, Chao Y-C, Stephenson EC and Hartl DL. Pseudogene Evolution in *Drosophila* Suggests a High Rate of DNA Loss. Molecular Biology and Evolution 1998;15(11) 1562–1567.

[58] Hardison RC. Working with Molecular Genetics. Self published 2005. http://www.personal.psu.edu/rch8/workmg/workmolecgenethome.html.

[59] Xing J, Witherspoon DJ, Ray DA, Batzer MA and Jorde LB. Mobile DNA Elements in Primate and Human Evolution. Yearbook of Physical Anthropology 2007;50: 2–19.

[60] Cambray G, Guerout A-M and Mazel D. Integrons. Annual Review of Genetics 2010;44: 141–66.

[61] Mc Ginty SE, Rankin DJ, Brown SP. Horizontal gene transfer and the evolution of bacterial cooperation. Evolution 2010;65(1) 21-32.

[62] Wicker T, Sabot F, Hua-Van A, Bennetzen JL, Capy P, Chalhoub B, Flavell A, Leroy P, Morgante M, Panaud O, Paux E, SanMiguel P and Schulman AH. A unified classification system for eukaryotic transposable elements. Nature reviews – Genetics 2007;8: 973-982.

[63] SanMiguel P and Bennetzen JL. Evidence that a recent increase in maize genome size was caused by the massive amplification of intergene retrotranposons. Annals of Botany 1998;82(Suppl A) 37–44.

[64] International Human Genome Sequencing Consortium (Lander ES, Linton LM, Birren B. et al.). Initial sequencing and analysis of the human genome. Nature 2001; 409(6822) 860–921.

[65] Smit AFA. Interspersed repeats and other mementos of transposable elements in mammalian genomes. Current Opinion in Genetics and Development 1999; 9, 657–663.

[66] Singer MF. SINEs and LINEs: highly repeated short and long interspersed sequences in mammalian genomes. Cell 1982;28(3) 433–434.

[67] Ohshima K and Okada N. SINEs and LINEs: symbionts of eukaryotic genomes with a common tail. Cytogenetic and Genome Research 2005; 110(1–4) 475–90.

[68] Cordaux R and Batzer M. The impact of retrotransposons on human genome evolution. Nature Reviews - Genetics 2009; 10(10):691–703.

[69] McClintock B. Maize genetics. Carnegie Institution of Washington 1943 Year Book No. 42: 148–152.

[70] Kidwell MG. Horizontal transfer of P elements and other short inverted repeat transposons. Genetica 1992;86(1) 275–286.

[71] de Lencastre A, Hamill S, Pyle AM. A single active-site region for a group II intron. Natural Structure Mololecular Biology 2005;12(7) 626–627.

[72] Barton NH, Keightley PD. Understanding quantitative genetic variation. Nature reviews – Genetics 2002;3(1) 11–21.

[73] Wochner A, Attwater J, Coulson A, Holliger P. (April). Ribozyme-catalyzed transcription of an active ribozyme. Science 2011;332(6026) 209–212.

[74] Cech TR. Self-splicing and enzymatic activity of an intervening sequence RNA from tetrahymena. Nobel Lecture, 1989. http://www.nobelprize.org/nobel_prizes/chemistry/laureates/1989/cech-lecture.pdf

[75] Altman S. Enzymatic cleavage of RNA by RNA. Nobel Lecture, December 8, 1989. http://www.nobelprize.org/nobel_prizes/chemistry/laureates/1989/altman-lecture.pdf

[76] Dworkina JP, Lazcanob A, Miller SL. The roads to and from the RNAworld. Journal of Theoretical Biology 2003;222: 127–134.

[77] Copley SD, Smith E, Morowitz HJ. The origin of the RNA world: Co-evolution of genes and metabolism. Bioorganic Chemistry 2007;35: 430–443.

[78] Echols H The versatility of RNA. Operators and Promoters: The Story of Molecular Biology and Its Creators 2001;218.

[79] Klattenhoff C and Theurkauf W. Biogenesis and germline functions of piRNAs. Development 2008;135(1) 3-9.

[80] Connell GJ, Byrne EM and Simpson L. Guide RNA-independent and Guide RNA-dependent Uridine Insertion into Cytochrome b mRNA in a Mitochondrial Lysate from *Leishmania tarentolae*. The Journal of Biological Chemistry 1997;272(7) 4212–4218.

[81] Wower IK, Zwieb C and Wower J. Transfer-messenger RNA unfolds as it transits the ribosome. RNA 2005;11: 668-673.

[82] Sliva K, Schnierle BS. Selective gene silencing by viral delivery of short hairpin RNA. Virology Journal 2010;7: 248.

[83] Banerjee D, Slack F. Control of developmental timing by small temporal RNAs: a paradigm for RNA-mediated regulation of gene expression. BioEssays 2002;24, 119-129.

[84] Lazcano A, Guerrero R, Margulis L and Oró J. The evolutionary transition from RNA to DNA in early cells. Journal of Molecular Evolution 1988;27(4) 283-290.

[85] Miller WJ, Capy P. Mobile Genetic Elements as Natural Tools for Genome Evolution. Methods in Molecular Biology 2004;260: 1-20.

[86] Dimitri P, Junakovic N. Revising the selfish DNA hypothesis TRENDS in Genetic 1999;15(4) 123-124.

[87] Sabot F and Schulman AH. Parasitism and the retrotransposon life cycle in plants: a hitchhiker's guide to the genome. Heredity 2006;97: 381–388.

[88] Zhang J. Evolution by gene duplication: an update. TRENDS in Ecology and Evolution 2003;18(6) 293-298.

[89] Beaulieu JM, Leitch IJ and Knight CA. Genome Size Evolution in Relation to Leaf Strategy and Metabolic Rates Revisited. Annals of Botany 2007;99: 495–505.

[90] Petrov DA. Evolution of genome size: new approaches to an old problem. TRENDS in Genetics 2001;17(1) 23-28.

[91] Xue C, Huang R, Maxwell TJ and FuY-X. Genome Changes After Gene Duplication: Haploidy vs. Diploidy. Genetics 2010;186: 287–294.

[92] Force A, Lynch M, Pickett FB, Amores A, Yan YI and Postlethwait J. Preservation of Duplicate Genes by Complementary, Degenerative Mutations. Genetics 1999;151: 1531–1545.

[93] Vinogradov AE. Intron–Genome Size Relationship on a Large Evolutionary Scale. Journal of Molecular Evolution 1999;49: 376–384.

[94] Treangen TJ, Rocha EPC. Horizontal Transfer, Not Duplication, Drives the Expansion of Protein Families in Prokaryotes. PLoS Genetic 2011;7(1): e1001284.

[95] Nilsson AI, Koskiniemi S, Eriksson S, Kugelberg E, Hinton JCD and Andersson DI. Bacterial genome size reduction by experimental evolution. Proceedings of the National Academy of Sciences 2005;102(34) 12112–12116.

[96] Lin Y and Moret BME. A New Genomic Evolutionary Model for Rearrangements, Duplications, and Losses that Applies across Eukaryotes and Prokaryotes. Journal of Computational Biology 2011;18(9) 1055-1064.

[97] Pettersson ME, Kurland CG and Berg OG. Deletion Rate Evolution and Its Effect on Genome Size and Coding Density. Molecular Biology and Evolution 2009;26(6) 1421–1430.

[98] Giovannoni SJ, Tripp HJ, Givan S, Podar M, Vergin KL, Baptista D, Bibbs L, Eads J, Richardson TH, Noordewier M, Rappé MS, Short JM, Carrington JC, Mathur EJ. Genome Streamlining in a Cosmopolitan Oceanic Bacterium. Science 2005;19;309(5738): 1242-1245.

[99] Kent BN, Salichos L, Gibbons JG, Rokas A, Newton ILG, Clark ME and Bordenstein SR. Complete Bacteriophage Transfer in a Bacterial Endosymbiont (Wolbachia) Determined by Targeted Genome Capture. Genome Biology and Evolution 2011;3: 209–218.

[100] Glass JI, Assad-Garcia N, Alperovich N, Yooseph S, Lewis MR, Maruf M, Hutchison III CA, Smith HO and Venter JC. Essential genes of a minimal bacterium. Proceedings of the National Academy of Sciences 2006;103(2) 425–430.

[101] McCutcheon JP, McDonald BR and Moran NA. Convergent evolution of metabolic roles in bacterial co-symbionts of insects. Proceedings of the National Academy of Sciences 2009;106(36) 15394–15399.

[102] Juhas M, Eberl L and Glass JI. Essence of life: essential genes of minimal genomes. Trends in Cell Biology 2011;21(10) 562-568.

[103] Halligan DL and Keightley PD. Spontaneous Mutation Accumulation Studies in Evolutionary Genetics. Annual Review of Ecology and Evolutionary Systematics 2009;40: 151–72.

Chapter 3

Contribution to the Moss Flora of Kizildağ (Isparta) National Park in Turkey

Serhat Ursavaş and Barbaros Çetin

Additional information is available at the end of the chapter

http://dx.doi.org/10.5772/52937

1. Introduction

The Kızıl Mountain National Park chosen as the study area is in Dedegül Mountain range which is in the 122 important plant areas in Turkey [59]. As a reliable indication of its highly diversed flora. Although the National Park of Kızıl Mountain range was important plant area, was not studied for moss flora, up to now. So, we believed the necessity of studying the mosses of the Kızıl Mountain National Park in Turkey. It is located in a transitional zone of Mediterranean and continental climate. In accordance with its transitional location, Irano-Turanian and Mediterranean flora elements are dominant in the area (Figure 1).

Studies on the bryophyte flora of Turkey were carried out firstly in the 18th century by Müller [1829], Tchihatcheff [1860], Juratzka and Milde [1870], Wettstein [1889], Barbey [1890] and Schiffner [1896, 1897]. The available bryofloristic studies covering a number of localities in Turkey carried out by local and foreing botanists focus only on a small localized area. Especially from late 20th century up to date, many studies were published.

Mosses are important components of forest ecosystems. They have important contributions on biological diversity providing wet habitats for much type living organisms. The study on mosses in Turkey are not extensive as in many other contries, thus the moss flora of Turkey is still largely unknown.

According to the grid system adopted by Henderson [30], the reserch area is between B7 and C12 squares. While the total number of new records for these square grids is 63, new taxa records for B7 is 7, for C12 is 47, as well as both grid squares are 9, respectively.

To date, nearly studies have been deal with the bryophyte flora of southwest of Turkey. The new records belonging to the B7 mosses taxa were found out from the following literatures: Henderson and Muirhead [28], Henderson [27], Robinson and Godfrey [63], Walther [75],

Henderson and Prentice [29], Yücel and Tokur [80], Yücel and Magil [79], Erdağ et al. [23], Uyar and Ünal [76], Savaroğlu and Tokur [64], Kürschner and Erdağ [37]. On the other hand, the litratures followed up to obtain the new records belonging to the C12 mosses taxa were: Henderson and Prentice [29], Çetin [12-15, 17], Tonguç and Yayıntaş [67], Kürschner and Nestle [38], Erdağ et al. [21], Abay et al. [2], and Kırmacı and Özçelik [35].

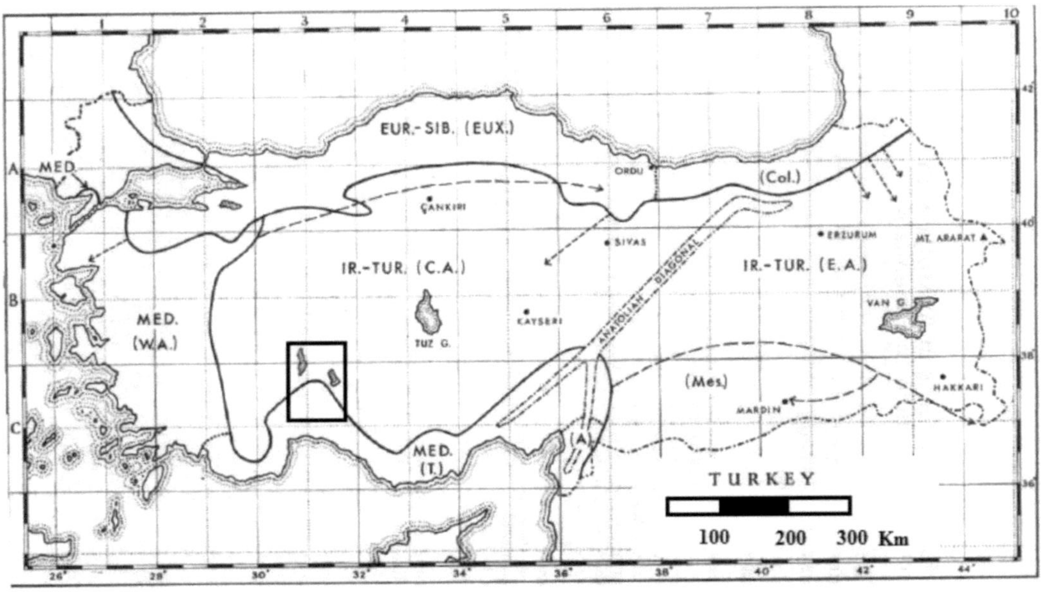

Figure 1. The flora areas of Turkey

This study was carried out between 2009 and 2011 in Kızıldağ National Park. The results obtained from a research on the bryophyte flora of Kızıldağ National Park (Isparta), Turkey) were reported in this paper. 156 taxa of bryophytes belonging to 66 genera and 29 families from the study area are recorded by the authors. Out of these, one species, *Seligeria donniana* (Sm.) Müll Hal. was a new record for Turkey. Also *Crossidium crassinerve* (De Not.) Jur. and one endemic species, *Cinclidotus vardaranus* Erdağ & Kürschner are reported for the second time from Turkey. Moreover, species such as *Plagiomnium cuspidatum* (Hedw.) T.J.Kop., *Pseudoleskea patens* (Lindb.) Kindb. *Isothecium holtii* Kindb. and *Racomitrium canescens* (Hedw.) Brid. reported many times for the northern part of Turkey, are reported for the first time for the southern part of Turkey.

The aim of this study was to explore the moss flora of Kızıldağ National Park. We hope that this study will serve as a valuable contribution to the knowledge of the bryophyte of Turkey and gives a base for future biodiversity and nature conservation surveys.

1.1. Description of the study area

Turkey contains a great variety of natural habitats, ranging from Mediterranean (e.g., Muğla, Antalya and Mersin cities), Aegean (e.g., Aydın and İzmir cities), and Black Sea beaches to towering coastal and interior mountains, (e.g., Zonguldak, Kastamonu, Sinop, Samsun, Ordu, Giresun, Trabzon, and Rize cities) from deeply incised valleys to expansive steppes (e.g., Altındere, Hatilla, Ihlara, Kelebek, Munzur valleys), and from fertile alluvial plains to arid, rocky hill slopes (e.g., Cihanbeyli, Haymana, Yazılıkaya and Bozok plains). Different community types (e.g., *Cedrus libani* with *Pinus nigra* subsp. *pallasiana; Abies cilicica* with *Quercus coccifera)* and habitat mosaics ocur (e.g., Beyşehir Lake and Dedegül Mountain), containing a rich mixture of plant and animal species, many of which are endemic [33, 54]. Endemic plants for Kızıl Mountain National Park is 201 some of them *Quercus vulcanica* (Boiss. Heldr. ex) Kotschy, *Abies cilicica* (Ant. & Kotschy) Carr. ssp. *isaurica* Coode & Cullen, *Consolida raveyi* (Boiss.) Raveyi, *Nigella lancifolia* Hub.-Mor. *Papaver apokrinomenon* Fedde, *Alyssum filiforme* Nyar, etc. Endemic animals for Kızıl Mountain National Park is 5, this is *Gobio gobio microlepidotus* Battalgil, *Pseudophoxinus battalgili* Bogutskaya, *Chondrostoma beysehirensis* Bogutskaya, *Alburnus akili* Battalgil, and *Cobitis bilseli* Battalgil [5]

The study areas' climate data were taken from the Yenişarbademli meteorological station (1150 m). According to the Anonymus [5], the annual average temperature is 20.9 ºC. The highest temperature is 25.4 ºC in July and the lowest is -7.2 ºC in February. The annual rain precipitation is 631.7 mm [5]. The annual temperature and rain rates recorded during the last 25 years (1980-2005) by the above mentioned meteorological observation station were considered also for a water balance graph according to Thornthwaite method was obtained (Figure 2). The climate type of the area is "moist and semi-humid" [5]. Thus, the components and the resource values such as biological diversity, wetlands, endemic species, medicinal and aromatic plants, natural ecosystems of the park are very diverge [5].

The Kızıldağ National Park was declared fist time as a national park in 1969 occupying 2316 hectares. Later, the area of the national park was expanded to 59400 hectares in 1993. The national park is situated in the Mediterranean region of Turkey. The geographical position of the park, encircling the north and east of Beyşehir Lake, lies between $37^{0}\ 38^{I}\ 32^{II}$ – $38^{0}\ 03^{I}\ 21^{II}$ Northern Latitudes and $31^{0}\ 14^{I}\ 59^{II}$ – $31^{0}\ 29^{I}\ 58^{II}$ East longitudes [5].

National Park district is surrounded by Şarkikaraağaç town and Beyköy province in the nort, Beyşehir Lake in the easth, Beyşehir town, Kurucuova village, Gavur hill, Tozan hill, Kuzgun hill, Yeropkunu hill, Karakaya hill, Dedegül hill, in the south, Üzümkarı hill, Melikler plateau, Dörtkardeşler hill, Mehmetkırı hill, Hacıbey plateau, Altınoluk hill, Höyük hill, Kızıldağ hill, Bozyamaç hill, Tuzlabeli hill, Çiçekli hill, Yoncalı hill, Büyükkaç hill in the west [5].

There are some high plateaus and hills such as; Büyükçeşan hill (2390 m), Alataş hill (2208 m), Küçükdağ hill (2302 m), Yumrutaş hill (2437 m), Karakaya hill (2384 m), Karagöl hill (2215 m), Üzüm karı hill (1978 m), Mehmetkir hill (1838 m), Zenit plateau (1755 m), Melikler plateau (1730 m), Saraycık plateau (1700 m),, Küçükseki plateau (1320 m), Küre plateau (1165 m) [5].

The chosen study area, Kızıldağ National Park, encloses very important plant areas (Endemic and Endangered) including the Dedegül Mountain (2996 m) range that is also among the 122 important plant areas in Turkey [59]. The study area is located in the Kızıldağ National Park that is in Isparta province. Its lies in the Beyşehir Lake range, which is running from north to south in the southern part of Turkey. The localities belong to B7 and C12 grid-square according to Henderson's [30] system (Figure 3).

The geological structure of the field is composed of formations consisting of limestone rocks. Vegetation from the National Park, tree species are: Cedrus libani A. Rich, *Pinus nigra* Arnold. subsp. *pallasiana* (Lamb.) Holmboe, *Abies cilicica* Car., and *Juniperus* species comprising the forest makes up. C. libani A. Rich, Şarkikaraağaç within the boundaries of the Kızıldağ National Park to the south of the town is 5 km north-facing slopes of the rising Kızıldağ shows the natural distributions of 1200-1700 meters. Shrub layer of the Cedrus libani A. Rich is *Quercus coccifera* L. [5].

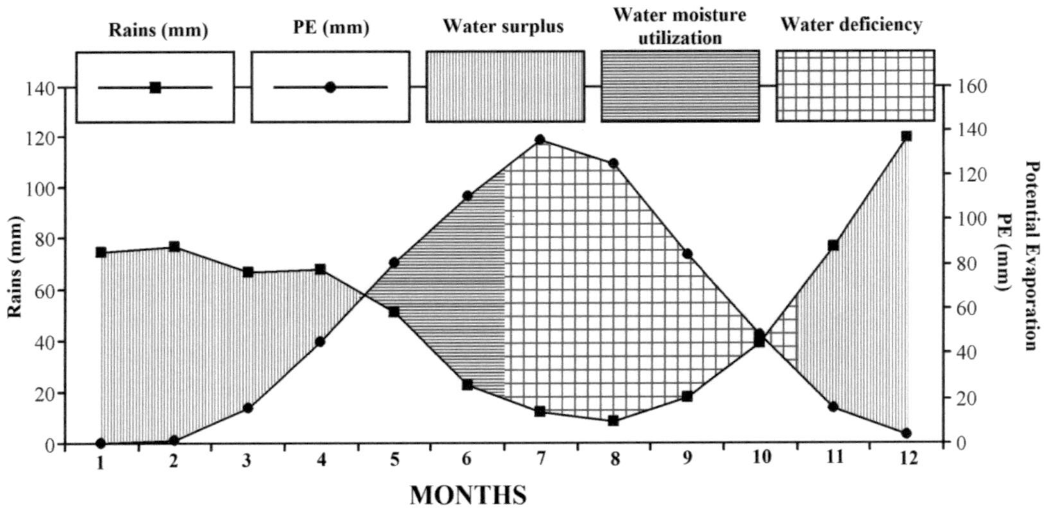

Figure 2. Graphic of the water balance according to Thornthwaite method [5]

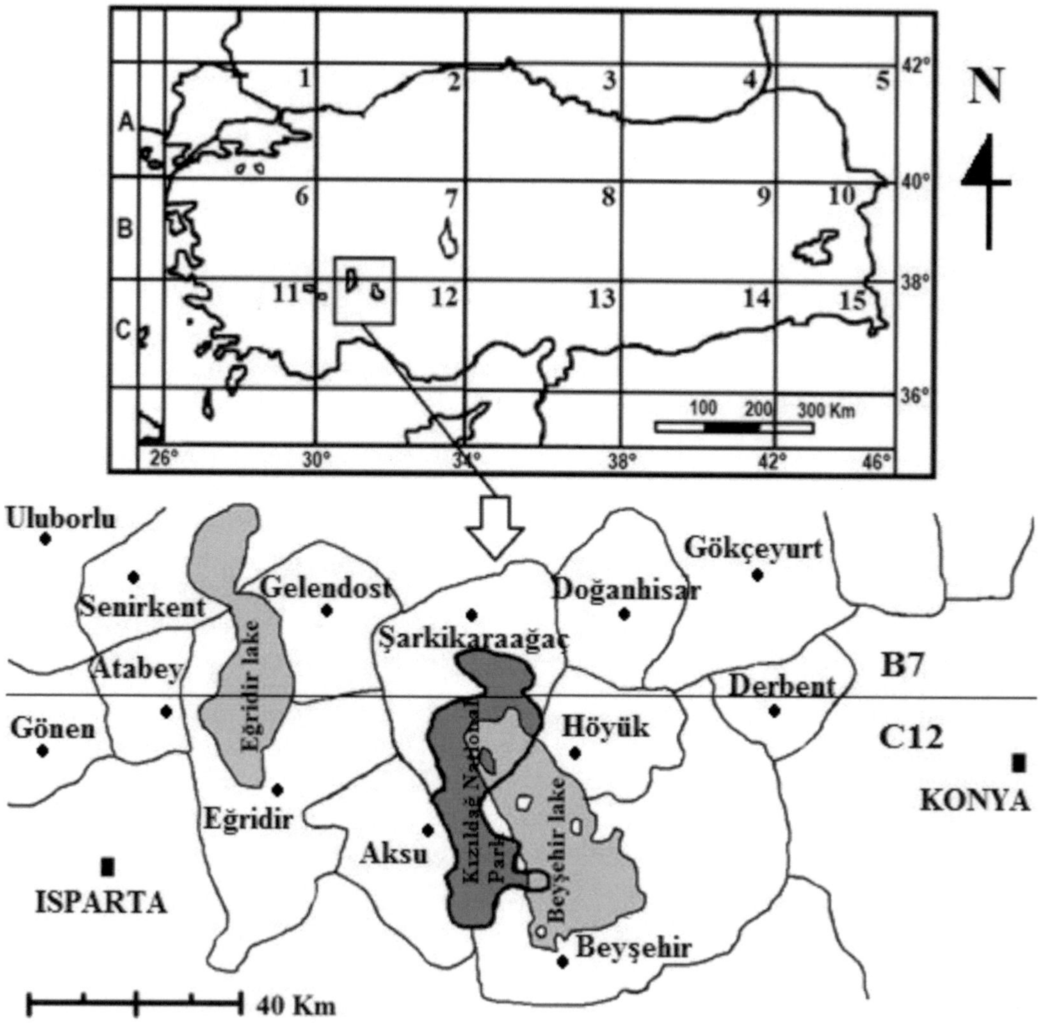

Figure 3. Location of Kızıldağ National Park in Turkey [5]

2. Materials and methods

The moss samples were collected from the study area during different vegetation periods between 2009 and 2011. The stations were selected according to different plant communities, and the geographical condition (Table 1).

The moss sample samples were incised by spatula from their habitats. After the samples were cleaned, they were preserved in plastic bags. Each plastic bag has a label providing the information about the habitat of the area. For example: Samples collecting number, moisture, exposure, substratum, the date of collecting, geographic coordinate, etc.

Identification of the specimens was based on Lawton [39], Crum [11], Smith [65-66], Nyholm [50-53], Gao Chien et al. [7], Cortini [9-10], Lu Xingjiang [41], Wu Peng-cheng et al. [62], Gao Chien [8], Greven [25], Herrnstadt and Heyn [31], Lüth [42-48]. Li Xing-Jiang et al. [40], Wang You-fang et al. [78] and Atherton et al. [6]. After the classificatrion was completed, specimens were placeed in the private collections of Serhat URSAVAŞ (Çankırı, Turkey).

Plants in the division Bryophyta have features that are considered to be rather primitive. These are plants with little specialization of tissue, which are not well-adapted to life in a relatively dry land environment. They also have comparatively simple reproductive processes, and are the only plants which have a dominant gametophyte generation. A study of the features of mosses will illustrate the major characteristics of this plant division [81].

In mosses, the gametophyte is small and at least partially erect, with very little specialization of cells and tissues, specifically, no true leaves, stems, or roots. The moss gametophyte has a shoot portion that appears leafy, and has rhizoids which emerge from its base to attach it to the substratum upon which it grows. The gametophyte is generally green and photosynthetic, and obtains water and other nutrients from the soil by direct absorption into its cells. It contains no cells specializing in the transport of water and/or nutrients (vascular tissue) and therefore cannot grow so large as to prevent contact between the soil and the majority of its cells [81].

At maturity, the moss gametophyte is capable of developing gametangia on its surface. Sperm-producing antheridia can arise amongst the leaf-like structures along the length of the thallus; egg-producing archegonia most often develop at the tip of the erect gametophyte. When fully developed, flagellated sperm are released from an antheridium and swim through a film of water to reach an egg-containing archegonium (Figure 4) [81].

Syngamy of the egg and sperm produce a zygote within the archegonium. This zygote undergoes mitosis to produce an embryo, again retained within the archegonium. Finally, the embryo matures into a sporophyte, consisting of a sporangium (capsule), a seta (stalk), and a foot which remains embedded in the gametophyte tissue. The continued attachment of the sporophyte to the gametophyte allows the sporophyte to absorb most of its needed nutrients from the gametophyte [81].

Meiosis occurring within the sporangium produces spores. Following spore production, the capsule opens up to release the spores, which germinate to produce new moss gametophytes [81].

The firstly recorded taxa from B7 were indicated by asteriks (*), from C12 by two asterisks (**) and from both of them (B7 and C12) by three asterisks (***). The status of the taxa for Turkey was determined by reviewing the related literature [36, 70]. The first record for the Turkish bryophyte flora was indicated by diamond (♦).

In the statements of specimens: The first number shows the Site no., the bold abbreviation shows the habitat, U abbreviations shows collector and identified (Serhat Ursavaş), and the last number shows the collection no.

Habitats in the study area: s: on soil, **r:** on rock: **src**: on soil in rock crevices, **rc:** rock crevices, **t:** on bark of tree trunk and branch, **dt:** on dead trunk, **ws:** wet soil, **wr:** wet rock.

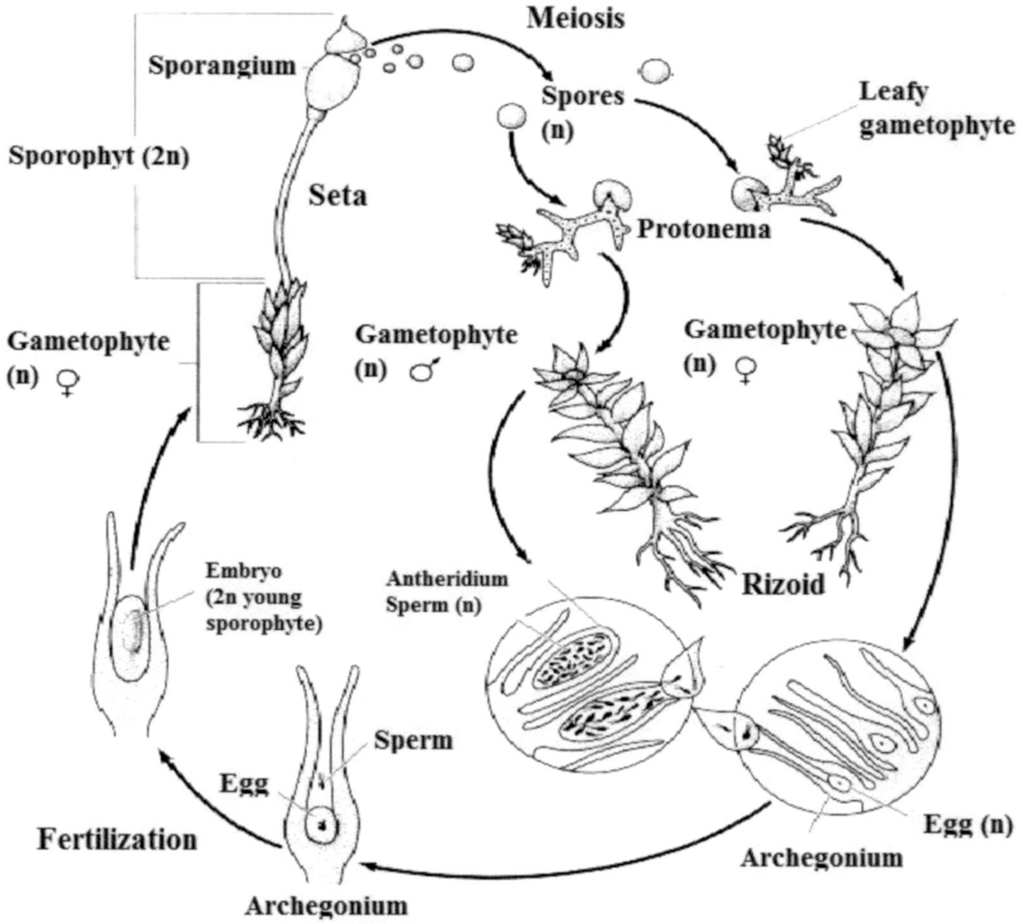

Figure 4. Life cycle of moss [81]

Table 1 provides a list of stations from the research area. Subsequently, the lists of taxa determined from the research area species are given.

Site No.	Date-Altitude(m)	Localites and geographic coordinate	Trees and some shrubs
1	29.08.2009-1410	Beş kardeşler, N 38° 22' 55.0" - E 31° 22' 48.7"	CL, JO, JE, JC, QC, MC
2	29.08.2009-1310	Ulusazlık pınarı, N 38° 17' 10.0" - E 31° 23' 04.7"	CL, JO, JE, JC, QC, MC
3	29.08.2009-1180	Kale, N 37° 59' 83.1" - E 31° 24' 32.4"	RP, AA, MC
4	29.08.2009-1140	Karayaka village, N 37° 58' 52.0" - E 31° 25' 20.5"	RB, G
5	30.08.2009-1308	Forest cottage, N 38° 02' 33.7" - E 31° 21' 40.1"	CL, QC, JE, JC
6	30.08.2009-1960	Büyük sivri hill., N 38° 13' 93.0" - E 31° 21' 84.7"	RP, O, JC
7	30.08.2009-1684	Küçük sivri hill., N 38° 02' 00.4" - E 31° 21' 69.4"	RP, O
8	31.08.2009-1540	Pınargözü cave, N 37° 41' 78.3" - E 31° 18' 46.1"	PN, PT, SA, JC, JE, CB
9	31.08.2009-1120	Pınarbaşı district, N 37° 45' 01.6" - E 31° 24' 95.3"	JO, JE, JC, RP
10	01.09.2009-1550	Ince oluk pınarı, N 37° 42' 90.1" - E 31° 19' 80.1"	PN, JE, JC, SA, RP
11	01.09.2009-1810	Vali Çeşmesi, N 37° 42' 93.4" - E 31° 17' 57.0"	PN, JC
12	15.06.2010-980	Kızıl hill, N 37° 53' 90.3" - E 31° 20' 39.2"	RP, O, LM
13	15.06.2010-1330	Gedikli village, N 37° 53' 38.0" - E 31° 19' 19.5"	JE, JC, JF, AN
14	15.06.2010-1490	Güzel sırt, N 37° 53' 38.0" - E 31° 19' 19.5"	CL, JF, JO
15	15.06.2010-1620	Akbel hill, N 37° 53' 17.0" - E 31° 17' 31.5"	CL, JF, JO, JC, QV
16	15.06.2010-1720	Katranbaşı hill, N 37° 51' 06.2" - E 31° 18' 52.7"	CL, JF, JO, QV, AP
17	15.06.2010-1700	Kaşıklı, N 35° 17' 84.0" - E 41° 90' 09.5"	CL, JF, JO, JE, QV, AP
18	15.06.2010-1610	Katran sivri hill, N 37° 50' 46.0" - E 31° 18' 55.4"	QV, CL, AP
19	15.06.2010-1440	İncebel hill, N 37° 50' 30.0" - E 31° 20' 39.9"	JO, JE
20	16.06.2010-1308	Bungalow, N 38° 02' 33.0" - E 31° 21' 40.3"	CL, PN, QC, PT, DO, JO, BI, QP
21	17.06.2010-1251	Pancar hill, N 37° 45' 06.0" - E 31° 22' 52.6"	QC, QI, JO, JF, AC
22	17.06.2010-1320	Küçükseki plateau, N 37° 44' 53.0" - E 31° 22' 19.4"	AC, JO, JF, JE
23	17.06.2010-1400	Körlük, N 37° 44' 53.0" - E 31° 21' 37.2"	AC, QC, QI, PN, JE
24	17.06.2010-1540	Pancar hill., N 37° 45' 09.9" - E 31° 20' 43.1"	AC, PN, JE, JF
25	17.06.2010-1555	Pınargözü cave, N 37° 41' 51.0" - E 31° 18' 30.7"	PN, PT, SA, JC, JE, CB
26	14.08.2010-1550	Pınargözü cave, N 37° 41' 42.6" - E 31° 18' 24.4"	PN, PT, JC, JE, CB
27	14.08.2010-1400	Hızar stream, N 37° 42' 34.0" - E 31° 19' 16.1"	PN, PT, SA, QC, QI
28	31.03.2011-1213	Konya road, N 38° 02' 40.89" - E 31° 26' 38.51"	PN, BV, CL, QC, JF, JO, PS
29	01.04.2011-1172	Fakılar village, N 38° 02' 19.03" - E 31° 18' 38.04"	AN, PS, O, AA
30	01.04.2011-1228	Çeltek village, N 38° 0' 35.52" - E 31° 21' 0.37"	CL, RP, O
31	01.04.2011-1148	Karayaka village, N 37° 58' 34.32" - E 31° 25' 27.94	JE, JO, RP
32	01.04.2011-1221	Yassıbel village, N 37° 58' 55.00" - E 31° 26' 31.87"	JE, JO, QC, RP
33	02.04.2011-1132	Sarıkaya village, N 37° 55' 23.19" - E 31° 18' 47.90"	JE, JO, AN, LM
34	02.04.2011-1137	Gedikli village, N 37° 55' 23.19" - E 31° 18' 47.90"	JE, JO, JF, RP, G
35	02.04.2011-1241	Mada valley, N 37° 51' 51.53" - E 31° 20' 28.53"	JE, JO, BV, AS, RP
36	31.05.2011-1736	Vali çeşmesi rooad, N 37° 42' 27.46" - E 31° 17' 47.24"	PN, PT
37	31.05.2011-1730	Melikler plateau, N 37° 42' 11.08" - E 31° 17' 41.08"	JE, JO, BV

http://dx.doi.org/10.5772/52937

Site No.	Date-Altitude(m)	Localites and geographic coordinate	Trees and some shrubs
38	31.05.2011-1555	Pınargözü cave, N 37° 41' 50.47" - E 31° 18' 34.27"	PN, PT, JC, JE, CB
39	31.05.2011-1571	Gedikli village, N 37° 50' 06.28" - E 31° 20' 16.98"	CL, JE, JO, JF, QC, QI
40	01.06.2011-1250	Mada island, N 37° 53' 24.40" - E 31° 22' 34.91"	JE, JO, JF, QC
41	01.06.2011-1165	Küre plateau, N 37° 51' 3.88" - E 31° 21' 31.63"	JE, JO, JF
42	02.06.2011-1387	Hızar stream, N 37° 42' 39.73" - E 31° 20' 13.20"	PN, JF
43	02.06.2011-1368	Hızar stream, N 37° 42' 26.35" - E 31° 20' 28.70"	PN, PT, SA, QI
44	02.06.2011-1754	Zenit plateau, N 37° 44' 2.58" - E 31° 19' 33.44"	G, RP, O
45	02.06.2011-1575	Kirazlı stream, N 37° 45' 01.77" - E 31° 20' 17.87"	AC, PN, JE, JO, JF
46	23.07.2011-1234	Küçükçal hill, N 37° 41' 34.88" - E 31° 21' 38.97"	PN, PT, SA
47	23.07.2011-1631	Malanda hill, N 37° 41' 12.41" - E 31° 20' 28.22"	PN, PT, SA
48	24.07.2011-1518	Fire tower, N 37° 41' 12.41" - E 31° 20' 28.22"	PN, JO, BV, AS
49	24.07.2011-1968	Üzüm karı hill, N 37° 41' 15.77" - E 31° 17' 6.22"	AS, V, E, O, RP
50	25.07.2011-1812	Mehmetkir hill, N 37° 43' 40.02" - E 31° 18' 46.81"	JE, JO, JF, BV, E, V
51	25.07.2011-1755	Zenit plateau, N 37° 43' 54.86" - E 31° 20' 12.46"	PN, JE, JF
52	25.07.2011-1775	Karnıccık area, N 37° 45' 42.56" - E 31° 18' 26.49"	JE, JO, JF, BV, E
53	25.07.2011-1802	Keşaphane hill, N 37° 46' 1.76" - E 31° 18' 53.60"	AC, PN, JE, BV
54	25.07.2011-1571	Dergül stream, N 37° 45' 33.94" - E 31° 20' 37.18"	AC, JE, BV
55	25.07.2011-1417	Canavar area, N 37° 46' 9.70" - E 31° 21' 7.48"	AC, JE, BV
56	25.07.2011-1154	Yenice district, N 37° 44' 16.14" - E 31° 24' 20.42"	RP, JO, BV
57	26.07.2011-1378	Karanlık stream, N 37° 39' 38.92" - E 31° 21' 18.01"	PN, JE, QI
58	26.07.2011-1565	Isılyurt hill, N 37° 39' 13.46"- E 31° 20' 23.03"	AC, PN, PT, V
59	26.07.2011-2000	Kara lake hill, N 37° 38' 47.80" - E 31° 19' 56.22"	RP, O, AS, V
60	26.07.2011-2215	Kara lake, N 37° 38' 18.23" - E 31° 18' 53.85"	RP, AS, V
61	27.07.2011-1150	Hamal hill, N 37° 58' 12.96" - E 31° 17' 46.72"	CL, AN, AS, V
62	27.07.2011-1138	Trout plant, N 37° 59' 59.14" - E 31° 18' 13.78"	SA, RP
63	27.07.2011-1242	Süzmedağ hill, N 37° 58' 39.35" - E 31° 21' 24.32"	QC, AS, V, RP
64	27.07.2011-1555	Pınargözü cave, N 38° 17' 10.00" - E 31° 23' 04.70"	PN, PT, SA, JC, JE, CB
65	28.07.2011-1850	Dedegül foothill, N 37° 41' 38.69" - E 31° 13' 41.05"	JO, BV, AS, E, RP
66	28.07.2011-2410	Dedegül foothill, N 37° 41' 16.76" - E 31° 18' 2.29"	AS, E, RP
67	28.07.2011-2885	Dedegül mountain, N 37° 40' 10.43" - E 31° 18' 8.62"	RP, O

AA: Agricultural area, **AC**: *Abies cilicica* (Antoine & Kotschy) Carrière, **AN**: *Amygdalus nana* L., **AP**: *Acer platanoides* L., **AS**: *Astragalus* sp., **BI**: *Berberis iberica* Steve. & Fisch. ex DC., **BV**: *Berberis vulgaris* L., **CB**: *Carpinus betulus* L., **CL**: *Cedrus libani* A. Rich., **DO**: *Daphne oleoides* Schreb., E: *Euphorbia* sp., G: Grass, **JO**: *Juniperus oxycedrus* L., **JF**: *Juniperus foetidissima* Willd., **JE**: *Juniperus excelsa* M. Bieb., **JC**: *Juniperus communis* L., **LM**: Lake margin, **MC**: *Myrtus communis* L., **O**: Opennes, **PN**: *Pinus nigra* Arnold subsp. *pallasiana* (Lamb.) Holmboe, **PS**: *Paliurus spina-christi* Mill., **PT**: *Populus tremula* L., **RB**: Rush bed, **RP**: Rock place, **QC**: *Quercus coccifera* L., **QI**: *Quercus infectoria* G. Olivier, **QP**: *Quercus pubescens* O. Schwarz, **QV**: *Quercus vulanica* Boiss. & Heldr. ex Kotschy, **SA**: *Salix alba* L., **V**: *Verbascum* sp.,

Table 1. Site no: Altitude in meters above sea level (m), Localities and geographic coordinates, Trees and some shrubs

3. Taxa list

Polytrichaceae Schwägr.

1. **Polytrichum juniperinum* Hedw. - 59:r, U545; 59:s, U546; 60:s, U547.

Timmiaceae Schimp.

2. **Timmia austriaca* Hedw. - 52:src, U540; 52:s, U541.

3. ***Timmia norvegica* J.E.Zetterst. - 15:rc, U542; 20:s, U543; 23:s, U544.

Encalyptaceae Schimp.

4. *Encalypta streptocarpa* Hedw. - 5:r, U854; 8:r, U856; 8:rc, U857; 10:r, U855; 13:r, U858; 16:r, U859; 20:s, U860; 25:wr, U861; 38:r, U862; 40:rc, U863; 41:r, U864; 45:r, U865; 46:s, U866; 49:r, U867; 51:r, U868; 52:r, U869; 53:r, U870; 65:r, U871; 66:r, U872.

5. *Encalypta rhaptocarpa* Schwägr. - 8:rc, U889; 20:s, U890.

6. *Encalypta vulgaris* Hedw. - 5:rc, U873; 13:r, U874; 16:r, U875; 30:s, U876; 32:r, U877; 34:r, U878; 39:rc, U879; 40:s, U880; 41:rc, U881; 48:t, U882; 49:r, U883; 52:r, U884; 60:r, 885; 63:r, U886; 65:r, U887; 67:s, U888.

7. *Encalypta ciliata* Hedw. - 58:r, U891.

Funariaceae Schwägr.

8. **Entosthodon muhlenbergii* (Turner) Fife - 41:s, U577; 61:r, U558; 62:src, U559.

9. **Entosthodon pulchellus* (H.Philib.) Brugue´s - 29:s, U560; 34:s, U561; 35:s, U562; 40:s, U563; 41:s, U564; 63:s, U565.

10. *Funaria hygrometrica* Hedw. - 5:s, U550; 33:r, U551; 35:s, U552; 38:r, U553; 44:dt, U554; 57:s, U555; 62:r, U556.

Grimmiaceae Arn.

11. *Grimmia anodon* Bruch & Schimp. - 1:r, U927; 3:r, U928; 4:r, U929; 15:r, U930; 28:r, U931; 29:r, U932; 49:r, U933; 63:r, U934; 66:r, U935.

12. **Grimmia caespiticia* (Brid.) Jur. - 59:r, U949.

13. ***Grimmia funalis* (Schwägr.) Bruch & Schimp. - 3:r, U941; 5:r, U942; 8:r, U943.

14. *Grimmia hartmanii* Schimp. - 41:r, U950.

15. *Grimmia laevigata* (Brid.) Brid. - 12:r, U946; 30:r, U947; 61:r, U948.

16. ***Grimmia montana* Bruch & Schimp. - 6:r, U944; 7:r, U946.

17. *Grimmia orbicularis* Bruch ex Wilson - 13:r, U951.

18. *Grimmia ovalis* (Hedw.) Lindb. - 6:r, U936; 7:r, U937; 12:r, U938; 37:r, U939; 58:r, U940.

19. *Grimmia pulvinata* (Hedw.) Sm. - 1:r, U910; 2:r, U911; 3:r, U912; 4:r, U913; 5:r, U914; 6:r, U915; 7:r, U916; 8:r, U917; 10:r, U918; 15:r, U919; 18:r, U920; 19:r, U921; 21:r, U922; 40:r, U923; 50:r, U924; 56:r, U925; 61:r, U926.

20. *Grimmia trichophylla* Grev. - 1:r, U892; 2:r, U893; 3:r, U894; 4:r, U895; 5:r, U896; 8:r, U897; 10:r, U898; 13:r, U899; 15:r, U900; 18:r, U901; 19:t, U902; 19:r, U903; 20:r, U904; 22:r, 905; 40:r, U906; 41:r, U907; 46:r, U908; 63:r, U909.

21. **Racomitrium canescens* (Hedw.) Brid. - 37:r, U952.

22. *Schistidium apocarpum* (Hedw.) Bruch & Schimp. - 5:r, U953; 8:r, U954; 16:r, U955; 23:r, U956; 34:r, U957; 42:r, U958; 43:r, U959; 45:r, U960.

23. *Schistidium atrofuscum* (Schimp.) Limpr. - 6:r, U970; 40:r, U971.

24. *Schistidium confertum* (Funck) Bruch & Schimp. - 1:r, U961; 5:r, U962; 6:r, U963; 8:r, U964; 47:r, U965; 49:r, U966; 59:r, U697; 65:r, U968.

25. *Schistidium flaccidum* (De Not.) Ochyra - 6:r, U1269.

26. *Schistidium helveticum* (Schkuhr) Deguchi - 49:r, U969.

27. ***Schistidium trichodon* (Brid.) Poelt - 8:r, U1270.

Seligeriaceae Schimp.

28. ◆ *Seligeria donniana* (Sm.) Müll.Hal. - 45:r, U1282.

Fissidentaceae Schimp.

29. ***Fissidens taxifolius* Hedw. - 47:ws, U549.

30. *Fissidens pusillus* (Wilson) Milde - 40:r, U1275; 40:s, U1276; 43:s, U1277; 45:r, U1278.

31. *Fissidens viridulus* (Sw. ex anon.) Wahlenb. - 43:ws, U548.

Ditrichaceae Limpr.

32. ****Ceratodon conicus* (Hampe) Lindb. - 6:r, U622; 8:src, U623, 47:s, U624; 60:s, 625.

33. *Ceratodon purpureus* (Hedw.) Brid. - 4:r, U609; 13:r, U610; 13:s, U611, 19:r, U612; 28:s, U613; 33:s, U614; 37:s, U615; 40:r, U616; 41:r, U617; 59:r, U618; 61:r, U619; 62:r, U620; 65:s, U621.

34. **Distichium capillaceum* (Hedw.) Bruch&Schimp - 8:rc, U601; 25:wr, U602; 40:r, U603; 47:r, U604; 49:r, U605; 52:r, U606; 67:s, U607.

35. ***Distichium inclinatum* (Hedw.) Bruch & Schimp. - 67:s, U599; 67:r, U600.

36. *Ditrichum flexicaule* (Schwägr.) Hampe - 1:r, U626; 5:r, U632; 8:r, U627; 8:rc, U628; 15:s, U629; 15:r, U630; 40:r, U631.

Rhabdoweisiaceae Limpr.

37. *Dicranoweisia cirrata* (Hedw.) Lindb. - 8:t, U633; 10:t, U634.

Dicranaceae Schimp.

38. ***Dicranum tauricum* Sapjegin - 8:dt, U635; 8:t, U636; 11:t, U637; 15:r, U638; 45:dt, U608; 59:t, U639.

Pottiaceae Schimp.

39. *Eucladium verticillatum* (With.) Bruch & Schimp. - 27:ws, U1092; 51:wr, U1093; 55:wr, U1094; 57:wr, U1095.

40. ***Gymnostomum aeruginosum* Sm. - 8:s, 1088.

41. *Gymnostomum calcareum* Nees & Hornsch. - 49:r, U1089.

42. ***Gyroweisia reflexa* (Brid.) Schimp. - 41:s, U1090; 44:s, U1091.

43. *Pleurochaete squarrosa* (Brid.) Lindb. - 13:s, U1059; 28:s, U1060; 30:rc, U1061; 34:r, U1062; 47:s, U1063; 63:src, U1064.

44. *Tortella fragilis* (Hook. & Wilson) Limpr. - 8:t, U1123.

45. ****Tortella inclinata* var. *densa* (Lorentz & Molendo) Limpr. - 1:r, U1126; 6:r, U1127; 7:r, U1128; 15:r, U1129; 17:r, U1130; 18:r, U1131; 66:r, U1132.

46.**Tortella nitida* (Lindb.) Broth. - 6:r, U1124; 8:r, 1125.

47. *Tortella tortuosa* (Hedw.) Limpr. - 1:r, U1133; 5:r, U1134; 7:r, U1135; 8:r, U1136; 15:r, U1137; 15:s, U1138; 16:r, U1157; 17:r, U1139; 19:r, U1140; 21:r, U1141; 23:r, U1142; 24:r, U1143; 39:r, U1144; 40:r, U1145; 43:s, U1146; 46:r, U1147; 48:r, U1148; 48:s, U1149; 49:r, U1150; 51:r, U1152; 60:r, U1153; 65:s, U1154; 66:r, U1155; 67:s, U1156.

48. ***Weissia brachycarpa* (Nees & Hornsch.) Jur. - 47:s, U1100.

49. *Weissia condensa* (Voit) Lindb. - 8:t, U1109; 49:r, U1110, 50:r, U1111; 65:r, U1112; 66:r, U1113; 67:r, U1114.

50. *Weissia controversa* Hedw. - 13:t, U1101; 41:t, U1102; 45:s, U1103; 45:t, U1104; 47:s, U1105; 53:t, U1106; 58:r, U1107; 60:r, U1108.

51. *Barbula convoluta* Hedw. - 51:src, U1065; 65:r, U1066.

52. ***Bryoerythrophyllum recurvirostrum* (Hedw.) P.C.Chen - 50:rc, U1280, 53:r, U1281.

53. *Cinclidotus fontinaloides* (Hedw.) P.Beauv. - 8:wr, 1118; 25:wr, U1119; 26:wr, U1120; 38:wr, U1121; 43:wr, U1122.

54. *Cinclidotus riparius* (Host ex Brid.) Arn. - 8:wr, U1115; 25:wr, U1116; 26:wr, U1117.

55. ***Cinclidotus vardaranus* Erdağ & Kürschner - 8:wr, U1274. (Not: The accuracy of this species were made by Michael Lüth.)

56. ***Crossidium crassinerve* (De Not.) Jur. - 28:r, U1098.

57. *Crossidium squamiferum* (Viv.) Jur. - 13:r, U1097, 31:r, U1097; 48:r, U1099.

58. *Didymodon fallax* (Hedw.) R.H.Zander - 45:r, U1069.

59. *Didymodon spadiceus* (Mitt.) Limpr. - 51:r, U1071; 57:wr, U1072.

60. *Didymodon tophaceus* (Brid.) Lisa - 48:r, U1070.

61. *Didymodon vinealis* (Brid.) R.H.Zander - 8:r, U1067; 45:r, U1068.

62. *Phascum cuspidatum* var. *cuspidatum* Hedw. - 29:s, U1078; 34:s, U1079; 63:s, U1080.

63. ***Phascum cuspidatum* var. *piliferum* (Hedw.) Hook. & Taylor - 29:t, U1081; 35:s, 1082.

64. ****Pseudocrossidium hornschuchianum* (Schultz) R.H.Zander - 1:r, U1073; 4:r, U1074.

65. *Pseudocrossidium revolutum* (Brid.) R.H.Zander - 13:r, U1075; 30:rc, U1076; 40:rc, U1077.

66. ***Pterygoneurum ovatum* (Hedw.) Dixon - 4:r, U1083; 13:r, U1084; 28:r, U1085; 29:s, U1086; 30:s, U1087.

67. *Syntrichia laevipila* Brid. - 1:s, U1235; 34:t, U1236.

68. *Syntrichia montana* Nees - 13:t, U1201; 15:r, U1002; 16:r, U1203; 17:r, U1204; 22:r, U1205; 24:r, U1206.

69. **Syntrichia norvegica* F.Weber - 1:r, U1207; 6:r, U1208; 28:s, U1209; 37:r, U1210; 49:r, U1211; 60:r, U1212; 65:r, U1213; 67:r, U1214.

70. *Syntrichia papillosissima* (Copp.) Loeske - 1:r, U1245.

71. *Syntrichia princeps* (De Not.) Mitt. - 40:t, U1215.

72. *Syntrichia ruralis* var. *ruraliformis* (Besch.) Delogne - 2:s, U1237; 2:r, U1244; 8:r, U1238; 10:r, U1239; 17:t, U1240; 18:r, U1241; 20:s, U1242; 22:r, U1243.

73. *Syntrichia ruralis* var. *ruralis* (Hedw.) F.Weber & D.Mohr - 1:r, U1246; 2:r, U1247; 3:r, U1248; 4:r, U1249; 5:r, U1250; 6:r, U1251; 7:r, U1252; 8:r, U1253; 8:t, U1254; 10:r, U1255; 10:s, U1256; 10:t, U1257; 18:r, U1258; 41:r, U1259; 47:rc, U1260; 48:r, U1261; 49:r, U1262; 50:r, U1263; 52:r, U1264; 60:s, U1265; 61:r, U1266; 63:s, U1267; 67:r, U1268.

74. ****Syntrichia virescens* (De Not.) Ochyra - 1:r, U1226; 5:r, U1227; 7:s, U1231; 8:r, U1232; 10:r, U1233; 21:t, U1228; 24:r, U1229; 25:r, U1234; 40:t, U1230.

75. ***Tortula atrovirens* (Sm.) Lindb. - 49:r, U1159; 62:r, U1160.

76. ***Tortula brevissima* Schiffn. - 4:r, U1161; 31:r, U1162; 33:r, U1163; 40:r, U1164; 41:r, U1165; 52:r, U1166; 60:r, U1167; 62:r, U1168.

77. *Tortula inermis* (Brid.) Mont. - 1:r, U1216; 4:r, U1217; 5:r, U1218; 8:r, U1219; 10:t, U1220; 10:r, U1221; 13:r, U1222; 15:r, U1223; 50:r, U1224; 60:r, U1225.

78. ****Tortula marginata* (Bruch & Schimp.) Spruce - 7:s, U1169; 43:rc, U1170; 65:r, U1171.

79. *Tortula muralis* Hedw. - 6:r, U1295; 10:r, U1191; 16:r, U1196; 28:r, U1197; 35:r, U1198; 53:r, U1199; 57:r, U1193; 62:r, U1194.

80. ***Tortula schimperi* M.J.Cano, O.Werner & J.Guerra - 47:s, U1200.

81. *Tortula subulata* Hedw. - 1:s, U1172; 6:s, U1173; 7:s, U1174; 8:s, U1175; 11:s, U1176; 18:s, U1177; 20:s, U1178; 28:s, U1179; 32:s, U1180; 40:r, U1181; 41:s, U1182; 44:s, U1183; 46:s, U1184; 57:s, U1185; 58:s, U1186; 59:s, U1187; 59:r, U1188; 60:r, U1189; 65:s, U1190.

Orthotrichaceae Arn.

82. **Orthotrichum anomalum* Hedw. - 1:r, U734; 5:r, U735; 8:r, U736; 10:r, U737; 17:r, U738; 20:r, U739; 21:r, U740; 56:r, U741; 61:r, U742.

83. *Orthotrichum cupulatum* Hoffm.exBrid. - 1:r, U682; 2:r, U683; 3:r, U684; 4:r, U685; 5:rc, U686; 5:r, U687; 6:r, U688; 8:r, U689; 10:r, U690; 13:r, U691; 16:r, U692; 18:r, U693; 19:r, U694; 20:r, U696; 22:r, U695; 24:r, U697; 25:r, U698; 26:r, U696; 33:r, U700; 38:r, U701; 40:r, U702; 41:r, U703; 43:r, U704; 44:r, U705; 52:r, U706.

84. *Orthotrichum urnigerum* Myrin - 6:r, U753; 8:rc, U754.

85. *Orthotrichum diaphanum* Schrad. ex Brid. - 40:t, U759.

86. *Orthotrichum rupestre* Schleich. ex Schwägr. - 6:r, U723; 7:r, U724; 8:r, U725; 10:t, U726; 19:r, U727; 25:r, U728; 27:r, U729; 46:r, U730; 47:r, U731; 49:r, U732; 58:r, U733.

87. *Orthotrichum affine* Schrad. ex Brid. - 1:t, U707; 5:t, U708; 6:t, U709; 10:t, U710; 15:t, U711; 16:t, U712; 17:t, U713; 20:t, U714; 21:t, U715; 22:t, U716; 23:t, U717; 24:t, U718; 27:t, U719; 50:t, U720; 54:t, U721; 55:t, U722.

88. *Orthotrichum lyellii* Hook. & Taylor - 16:t, U755; 20:t, U756; 21:t, U757; 22:t, U758.

89. *Orthotrichum speciosum* Nees - 5:t, U745; 10:t, U746; 16:t, U747; 17:t, U748; 20:t, U749; 27:rc, U750; 37:t, U751; 58:t, U752.

90. **Orthotrichum striatum* Hedw. - 5:t, U743; 7:r, U744.

91. ***Ulota crispa* (Hedw.) Brid. - 8:t, U760; 45:t, U761; 46:t, U762.

Bartramiaceae Schwägr.

92. *Bartramia pomiformis* Hedw. - 8:rc, U570; 38:s, U566; 38:s, U567.

93. ***Bartramia ithyphylla* Brid. - 8:rc, U568; 58:r, U569.

94. ***Philonotis marchica* (Hedw.) Brid. - 46:wr, U571.

95. ***Philonotis fontana* (Hedw.) Brid. - 10:rc, U572; 10:ws, U573; 27:ws, U574; 44:s, U575; 46:ws, U576; 57:ws, U577; 60:s, U577.

96. ***Philonotis tomentella* Molendo - 8:rc, U578.

Bryaceae Schwägr.

97. *Bryum alpinum* Huds. ex With. - 29:ws, U663; 42:s, U664; 44:ws, U665.

98. *Bryum argenteum* Hedw. - 6:r, U650; 28:r, U651; 60:r, U652; 62:r, U653.

99. *Bryum caespiticium* Hedw. - 5:rc, U666; 11:s, U667; 39:t, U669; 39:rc, U668; 40:s, U670; 63:s, U671.

100. *Bryum capillare* Hedw. - 1:r, U654; 5:r, U655; 8:r, U656; 10:s, U657; 20:s, U658; 40:r, U659; 41:rc, U660; 58:r, U661; 60:r, U662.

101. ***Bryum creberrimum* Taylor - 25:t, U677.

102. *Bryum moravicum* Podp. - 40:s, U672.

103. ***Bryum pallens* Sw. ex anon. - 8:src, U673; 28:wr, U674; 45:s, U675.

104. *Bryum pallescens* Schleich. ex Schwägr. - 44:s, U676.

105. *Bryum pseudotriquetrum* (Hedw.) P.Gaertn. et al. - 8:s, U678; 25:r, U679; 27:ws, U681; 58:ws, U680.

106.***Bryum schleicheri* DC. - 27:wr, U648; 60:ws, U649.

107. ***Bryum torquescens* Bruch & Schimp. - 1:s, U1279.

Mielichhoferiaceae Schimp.

108. *Pohlia cruda* (Hedw.) Lindb. - 25:wr, U640; 49:s, U641; 58:r, U642; 67:s, U643.

109. *Pohlia melanodon* (Brid.) A.J.Shaw - 47:ws, U647.

110. *Pohlia wahlenbergii* var. *wahlenbergii* (F.Weber&D.Mohr) A.L.Andrews - 10:s, U644; 42:s, U645; 47:ws, U646.

Mniaceae Schwägr.

111. ***Mnium marginatum* (Dicks.) P.Beauv. - 8:s, U763; 8:rc, U764.

Plagiomniaceae T.J.Kop.

112. ***Plagiomnium cuspidatum* (Hedw.) T.J.Kop. - 63:r, U767.

113. *Plagiomnium ellipticum* (Brid.) T.J.Kop. - 38:ws, U765.

114. ***Plagiomnium undulatum* (Hedw.) T.J.Kop. - 47:s, U768; 47:ws, U769; 58:ws, U770; 63:wr, U771.

115. *Plagiomnium* rostratum (Schrad.) T.J.Kop. - 25:wr, U766.

Aulacomniaceae Schimp.

116. ***Aulacomnium androgynum* (Hedw.) Schwägr. - 8:t, U533; 36:dt, U534; 38:t, U535; 42:dt, U536; 45:dt, U537; 47:t, U538; 53:t, U539.

Amblystegiaceae Kindb.

117. *Cratoneuron filicinum* (Hedw.) Spruce - 8:s, U841; 8:wr, U842; 25:wr, U843; 27:s, U844; 30:wr, U845; 38:wr, U846; 42:ws, U847; 42:r, U848; 44:s, U49; 47:wr, U850; 48:wr, U851.

118. ***Drepanocladus aduncus* (Hedw.) Warnst - 44:ws, 852.

119. *Hygroamblystegium tenax* (Hedw.) Jenn. - 10:s, U1272.

120. *Palustriella commutata* (Hedw.) Ochyra - 8:wr, U834; 10:rc, U835; 27:wr, U836; 27:s, U837; 46:ws, U839; 47:ws, U840; 48:wr, U838.

Leskeaceae Schimp.

121. *Pseudoleskea incurvata* (Hedw.) Loeske - 8:rc, U771; 49:r, U772; 67:r, U773.

122. ***Pseudoleskea patens* (Lindb.) Kindb. - 59:r, U774; 60:r, U775; 65:r, U776.

123. ***Pseudoleskeella catenulata* (Brid. ex Schrad.) Kindb. - 13:t, U777; 23:r, U778; 45:r, U779; 52:r, U780.

124. ***Pseudoleskeella tectorum* (Funck ex Brid.) Kindb. ex Broth. - 8:r, U781; 19:t, U782; 23:r, U783; 39:r, U784; 54:r, U785; 55:t, U786.

Brachytheciaceae Schimp.

125. *Eurhynchium striatum* (Hedw.) Schimp. - 1:r, U1028.

126. *Platyhypnidium riparioides* (Hedw.) Dixon - 8:t, U1049; 8:wr, U1050; 47:wr, U1051; 57:wr, U1052; 58:ws, U1053; 58:wr, U1054; 63:wr, U1055.

127. ***Rhynchostegium confertum* (Dicks.) Schimp. - 42:ws, U1056.

128. *Oxyrrhynchium hians* (Hedw.) Loeske - 47:wr, U1024; 47:ws, U1025.

129. ****Oxyrrhynchium schleicheri* (R.Hedw.) Röll - 8:r, U1026; 25:r, U1027.

130. ***Brachythecium albicans* (Hedw.) Schimp. - 8:rc, U1040; 10:s, U1041; 27:s, U1042;

131. ***Brachythecium erythrorrhizon* Schimp. - 7:s, U1043; 11:s, U1044; 45:s, U1045; 45:r, U1046; 46:r, U1047; 47:s, U1048.

132. *Brachythecium rivulare* Schimp. - 27:s, U1035; 38:wr, U1036; 47:wr, U1037; 59:ws, U1038; 63:r, U1039.

133. *Eurhynchiastrum pulchellum* (Hedw.) Ignatov & Huttunen - 7:s, U1029.

134. *Brachytheciastrum velutinum* (Hedw.) Ignatov & Huttunen - 10:s, U1030; 28:s, U1031; 45:t, U1032; 47:t, U1033; 53:t, U1034.

135. *Homalothecium aureum* (Spruce) H.Rob. - 2:s, U999; 34:s, U1000; 40:r, U1001; 40:s, U1002; 46:s, U1003; 47:t, U1004; 56:r, U1005.

136. *Homalothecium lutescens* (Hedw.) H.Rob. - 1:r, U977; 2:s, U972; 5:r, U973; 6:r, U974; 7:r, U975; 8:rc, U976; 10:r, U978; 10:t, U979; 15:r, U980; 16:r, U981; 19:s, U982; 20:t, U983; 22:r, U984; 45:s, U985; 54:r, U986.

137. *Homalothecium philippeanum* (Spruce) Schimp. - 13:r, U1006; 13:t, U1007; 15:r, U1008; 16:r, U1009; 17:r, U1010; 17:s, U1011; 20:r, U1012; 21:r, U1014; 21:t, U1014; 2:r, U1015; 23:r, U1016; 24:r, U1017; 34:r, U1018; 40:r, U1019; 45:r, U1020; 49:r, U1021; 51:r, U1022; 63:r, U1023.

138. *Homalothecium sericeum* (Hedw.) Schimp. - 1:r, U987; 7:r, U988; 8:r, U989; 11:t, U990; 13:s, U991; 15:r, U992; 17:r, U993; 18:r, U994; 19:r, U995; 20:s, U996; 21:t, U997; 49:r, U998.

Hypnaceae Schimp.

139. ***Calliergonella cuspidata* (Hedw.) Loeske - 8:s, U813.

140. *Ctenidium molluscum* (Hedw.) Mitt. - 8:rc, U814.

141. *Hypnum cupressiforme* var. *cupressiforme* Hedw. - 7:s, U802; 23:r, U803; 23:s, U804; 43:r, U805; 47:t, U806; 55:r, U807.

142. *Hypnum cupressiforme* var. *lacunosum* Brid. - 7:s, U808; 7:r, U809; 21:t, U810; 40:t, U811; 46:s, U812; 47:s, U813.

143. ***Hypnum cupressiforme* var. *resupinatum* (Taylor) Schimp. - 21:t, U800; 47:r, U801.

Pterigynandraceae Schimp.

144. *Habrodon perpusillus* (De Not.) Lindb. - 45:t, U799.

145. *Pterigynandrum filiforme* Hedw. - 8:t, U787; 13:t, U788; 16:t, U789; 17:s, U790; 18:t, U791; 19:t, U792; 21:t, U799; 37:r, U794; 40:t, U795; 53:t, U796; 57:t, U797; 58:r, U798.

Plagiotheciaceae (Broth.) M.Fleisch.

146. ***Plagiothecium laetum* Schimp. - 8:rc, U1271.

Pylaisiadelphaceae Goffinet & W.R.Buck

147. ***Platygyrium repens* (Brid.) Schimp. - 69:r, U815.

Leucodontaceae Schimp.

148. ***Leucodon immersus* Lindb. - 7:r, U1273.

149. *Leucodon sciuroides* var. *morensis* (Schwägr.) De Not. - 12:s, U590; 13:t, U591; 15:r, U592; 16:r, U593; 21:r, U594; 35:r, U595; 47:r, U596; 55:r, U597; 56:r, U598.

150. *Leucodon sciuroides* var. *sciuroides* (Hedw.) Schwägr. - 13:r, U579; 17:r, U580; 19:t, U581; 21:t, U582; 22:t, U583; 24:r, U584; 35:r, U585; 38:r, U586; 40:r, U587; 41:r, U588; 41:t, U589.

Neckeraceae Schimp.

151. **Homalia trichomanoides* (Hedw.) Brid. - 17:r, U830; 54:r, U831.

152. *Neckera besseri* (Lobarz.) Jur. - 52:r, U832.

153. *Neckera menziesii* Drumm. - 8:t, U816; 8:rc, U817; 8:r, U818; 17:r, U819; 18:r, U820; 23:r, U821; 23:rc, U822; 24:r, U823; 24:t, U824; 39:r, U825; 43:r, U828; 45:r, U826; 45:s, U827; 54:r, U829.

Leptodontaceae Schimp.

154. *Leptodon smithii* (Hedw.) F.Weber & D.Mohr - 23:r, U833.
Lembophyllaceae Broth.
155. *Isothecium alopecuroides* (Lam. ex Dubois) Isov. - 58:r, U1057.
156. ***Isothecium holtii* Kindb. - 63:r, U1058.

4. Synonyms

Subspecies and varieties are included; hybrids are omitted. The taxonomic hierarchy is based on one published by Goffinet & Buck in [24]. While it has been strongly influenced by results of modern molecular methods, there are still many remaining uncertainties, even at family level. Because of these uncertainties, taxonomic innovation has generally been avoided which was also interiorized in the Bryological Monograph related with the Mosses of Europe and Macaronesia prepared by Hill at al. in [32].

In this list, prepared according to the most recent nomenclatural changes in the mentioned monograph above, some species have been mentioned in different genus and some of them have been referred in different families. In accordance with that, taxonomic synonyms are given below.

Brachytheciumvelutinum (Hedw.) Bruch & Schimp. → *Brachytheciastrum velutinum* (Hedw.) Ignatov & Huttunen

*Bryum subelegans*Kindb. → *Bryum moravicum* Podp.

Eurhynchium hians (Hedw.) Sande Lac. → *Oxyrrhynchium hians* (Hedw.) Loeske.

Eurhynchium pulchellum (Hedw.) Jenn. → *Eurhynchiastrum pulchellum* (Hedw.) Ignatov & Huttunen

Eurhynchium schleicheri (R.Hedw.) Jur. → *Oxyrrhynchium schleicheri* (R.Hedw.) Röll

Funaria muehlenbergii Turner → *Entosthodon muhlenbergii* (Turner) Fife

Funaria pulchella H.H.Philib. → *Entosthodon pulchellus* (H.Philib.) Brugue´s

Homalia besseri Lobarz. → *Neckera besseri* (Lobarz.) Jur.

Hypnumlacunosum (Brid.) Hoffm.ex Brid. → *Hypnum cupressiforme* var. *lacunosum* Brid.

Hypnumresupinatum Taylor → *Hypnum cupressiforme* var. *resupinatum* (Taylor) Schimp.

Metaneckeramenziesii (Drumm.) Steere → *Neckera menziesii* Drumm.

Syntrichiaintermedia Brid. → *Syntrichia montana* Nees

Tortula subulata var. *angustata* (Schimp.) Limpr. → *Tortula schimperi* M.J.Cano, O.Werner & J.Guerra

http://dx.doi.org/10.5772/52937

5. Conclusions

A total number of 156 taxa belonging to 66 genera and 29 families were determined by evaluating 1.148 bryophytes collected from Kızıldağ National Park between 2009-2011 at different seasons and habitats. The number of taxa recorded from Pınargözü cave location was the highest (58 taxa) within all study area (Figure 5). The cracks on the rock which placed at the entrance and the surrounding area of a cave are suitable environments for the development of the mosses. In additional, Pınargözü cave streams and more rainfall has increased moss species diversity of this area. Among the 156 species determined in the research area, identified 63 species are new to the area for the mentioned grid squares. This means that approximately 40% of the records were determined as new records for the grid squares.

Seligeria donniana was recorded for the first time for Turkish bryophyte flora (Figure 6). This genus contains nineteen species in the European countries [32] and hitherto, six species; *Seligeria acutifolia* Lindb., *S. pusilla* (Hedw.) Bruch & Schimp., *S. recurvata* (Hedw.) Bruch & Schimp., *S. tristichoides* Kindb., *S. calycina* (*S. paucifolia* auct. non (With.) Carruth.), Mitt. ex Lindb. and *S. trifaria* (Brid.) Lindb. [54, 61, 70] have been recorded in Turkey.

In this study, an endemic taxon *Cinclidorus vardaranus* Erdağ and Kürschner was recorded for the second time for Turkish moss flora (Figure 7). This species was identified and reported by Adnan Erdağ and Harald Kürschner in [22] from B9 grid square (Kemaliye, Erzincan) for the first time. In addition, *Crossidium crassinerve* (De Not.) Jur. is an orther species reported for the second time from Turkey in this study (Figure 8). The first report of this species from Turkey was from Denizli Babadağ by Kırmacı et al. in [34].

Despite of being given several times in the northern part of Turkey's registration, species given for the first time for the southern Turkey's (C12) registration are:

Plagiomniumcuspidatum (Hedw.) T.J.Kop (Figure 9): The species was firstly identified from Turkey by Henderson [26], from a specimen collected from Artvin at 1500 a.s.l. In the following years, the records of this moss species were given by Henderson and Prentice [29]; Çetin [13]; Yayıntaş and Tonguç [77]; Yayıntaş et al. [76]; Özdemir [58]; Abay and Çetin [1]; Uyar [73]; Abay et al. [2]; Uyar and Çetin [71]; Özdemir and Koz [57]; Ursavaş and Abay [68]; Abay et al. [4]; and Abay et al. [3].

Pseudoleskeapatens (Lindb.) Kindb (Figure 10): According to Uyar and Çetin [70] "A new check-list of the moss flora of Turkey" was present. Subsequently, Özdemir and Batan [56], Ursavaş and Abay [68], and Abay et al. [4] records were given.

Isothecium holtii Kindb is not abundant in Turkey (Figure 11): first record was from Turkey of Balıkesir Kapıdağ peninsula (545 a.s.l.) by Uyar and Ören [72]. Afterwards, an other report from Kaçkar Mountains from Amlakit plateau (2000 a.s.l.) was given by Abay et al. [3].

Racomitrium canescens (Hedw.) Brid (Figure 12): The species was recorded for the first time from Artvin Çoruh Valley from Tiryal Mountain (2150 a.s.l.) on rock by Henderson [71] in Turkey. The later records of the species were given by Henderson [26]; Henderson and Prentice [29]; Çetin and Yurdakulol [19]; Çetin and Yurdakulol [20]; Çetin [16]; Özdemir and Çetin [55]; Çetin et al. [18]; Abay and Çetin [1]; Papp [60]; Uyar and Çetin [71]; Abay et al. [2]; Uyar et al. [69]; Natcheva et al. [49]; and Abay et al. [4].

New moss record for B7 square is Schistidium atrofuscum (Schimp.) Limpr., Distichium capillaceum (Hedw.) Bruch&Schimp., Tortella nitida (Lindb.) Broth., Syntrichia norvegica F.Weber, Orthotrichum anomalum Hedw., Orthotrichum striatum Hedw., Homalia trichomanoides (Hedw.) Brid.

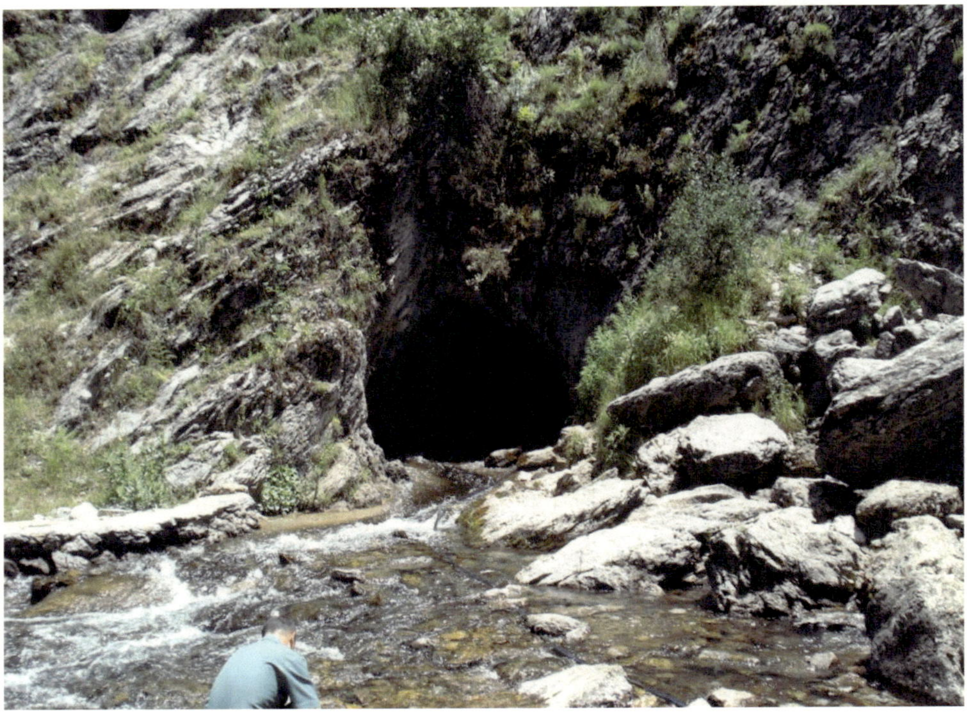

Figure 5. A view from the entrence of the Pınargözü cave (Image by Serhat URSAVAŞ)

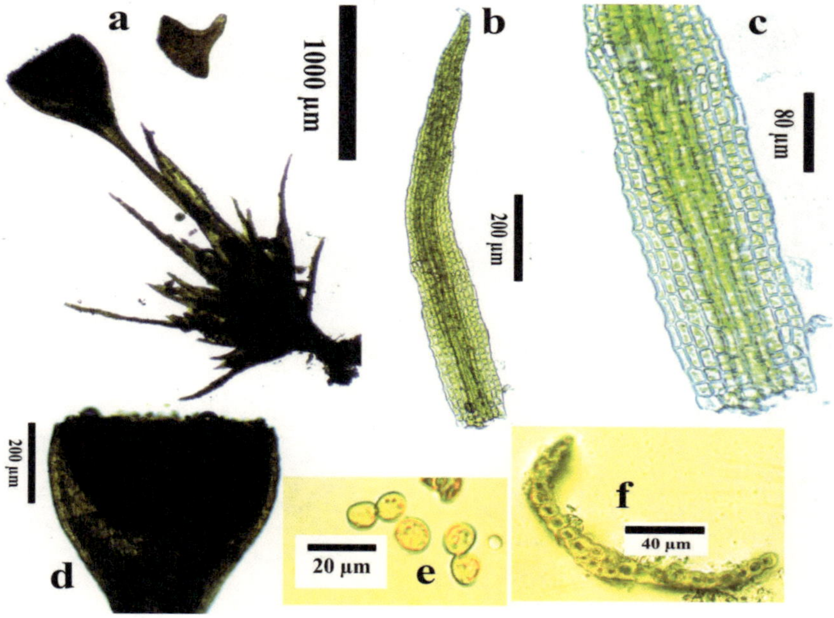

Figure 6. Characteristic features of *Seligeria donniana* (Image by Serhat URSAVAŞ) **a.** Plant, **b.** Leaf, **c.** Leaf base, **d.** Capsule, **e.** Spor, **f.** Transverse section

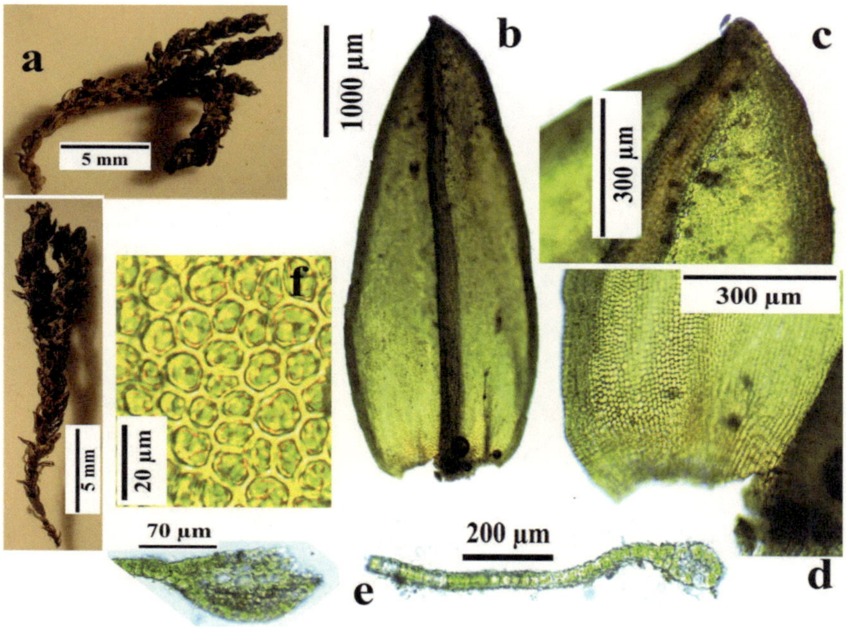

Figure 7. Characteristic features of *Cinclidotus vardaranus* (Image by Serhat URSAVAŞ) **a**. Plant, **b.** Leaf, **c.** Leaf apex, **d.** Leaf base, **e.** Transverse section, **f.** Middle cells

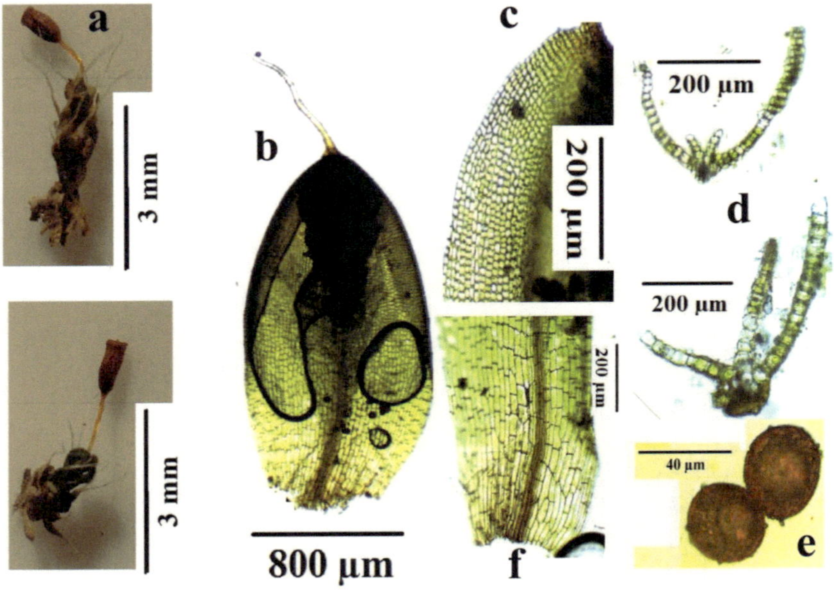

Figure 8. Characteristic features of *Crossidiumcrassinerve* (Image by Serhat URSAVAŞ) **a.** Plant, **b.** Leaf, **c.** Upper cells of leaf, **d.** Transverse section, **f.** Leaf base, **e.** Spore

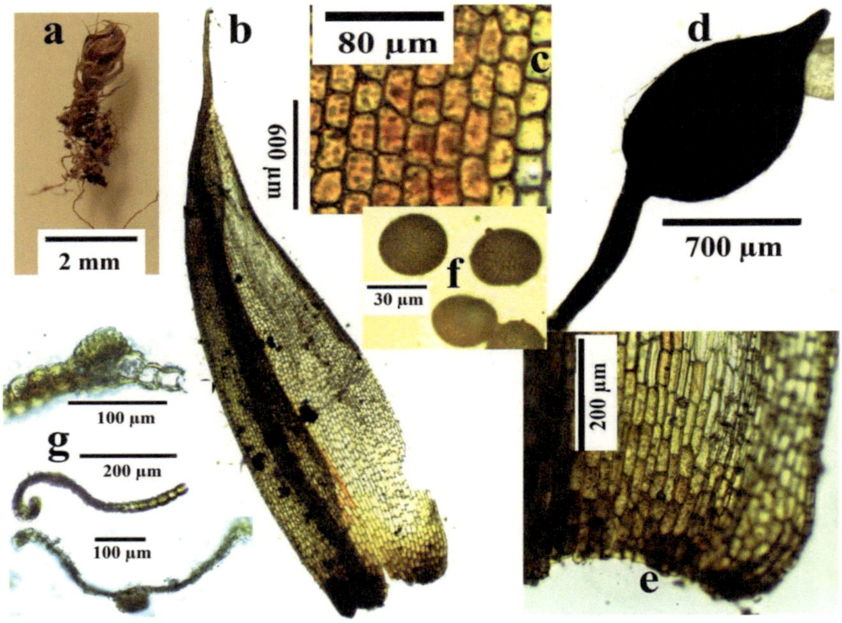

Figure 9. Characteristic features of *Phascum cuspidatum* (Image by Serhat URSAVAŞ) **a.** Plant, **b.** Leaf, **c.** Middle cells, **d.** Kapsule, **e.** Leaf base, **f.** Spore, **g.** Transverse section

http://dx.doi.org/10.5772/52937

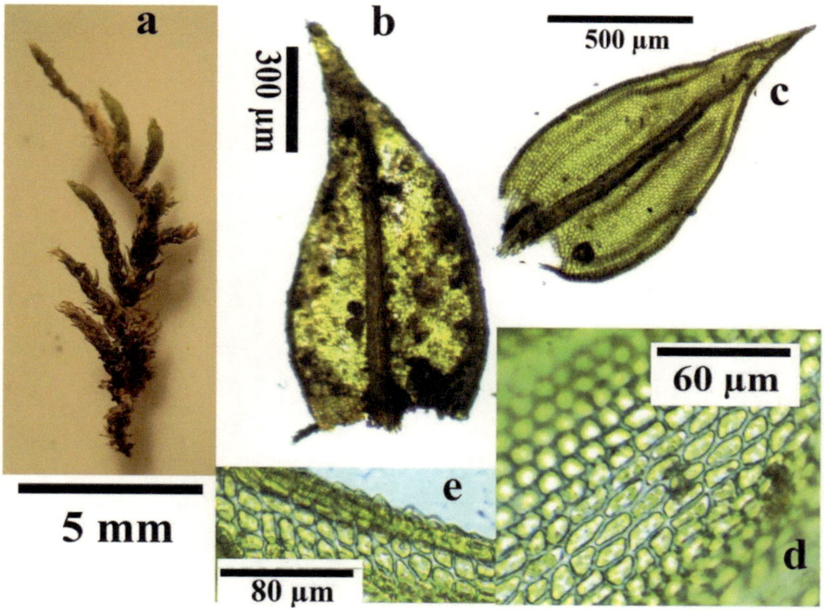

Figure 10. Characteristic features of *Pseudoleskea patens* (Image by Serhat URSAVAŞ) **a**. Plant, **b.** Stem leaf, **c.** Branch leaf, **d**. Middle cells, **e.** Leaf margine

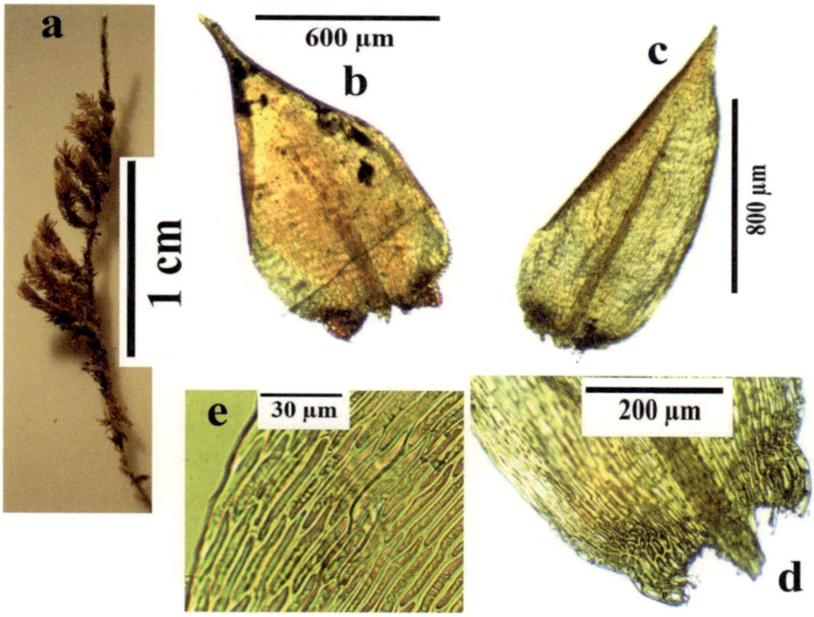

Figure 11. Characteristic features of *Isothecium holtii* (Image by Serhat URSAVAŞ) **a**. Plant, **b.** Stem leaf, **c.** Branch leaf, **d**. Leaf base, **e.** Middle cells

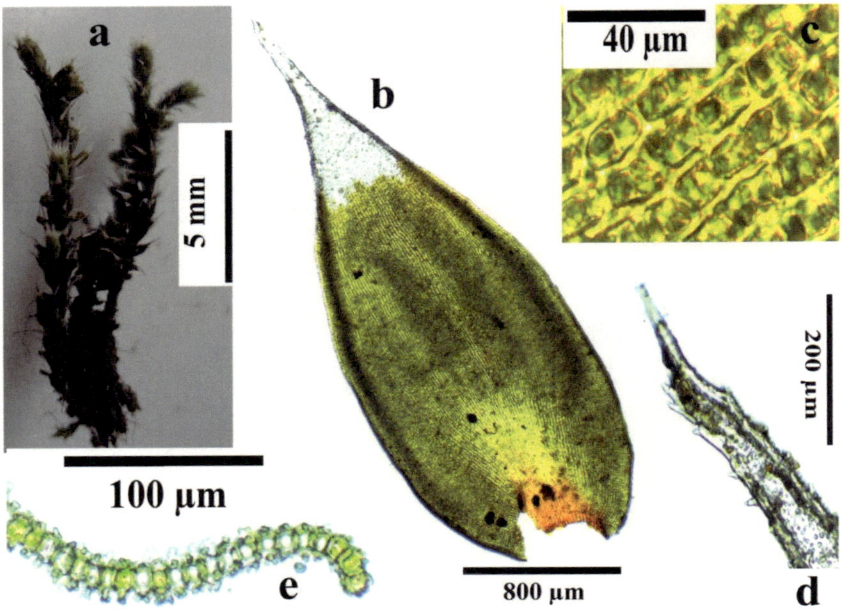

Figure 12. Characteristic features of *Racomitrium canescens* (Image by Serhat URSAVAŞ) **a.** Plant, **b.** Leaf, **c.** Middle cells, **d**. Leaf apex, **e.** Transverse section

New moss record for C12 square is *Polytrichum juniperinum* Hedw., Timmia austriaca Hedw., *Entosthodon muhlenbergii* (Turner) Fife, *Entosthodon pulchellus* (H.Philib.) Brugue´s, *Grimmia caespiticia* (Brid.) Jur., *Racomitrium canescens* (Hedw.) Brid., *Schistidium trichodon* (Brid.) Poelt, *Fissidens taxifolius* Hedw., *Distichium inclinatum* (Hedw.) Bruch & Schimp., *Dicranum tauricum* Sapjegin, *Gymnostomum aeruginosum* Sm., *Gyroweisia reflexa* (Brid.) Schimp., *Weissia brachycarpa* (Nees & Hornsch.) Jur., *Cinclidotus vardaranus* Erdağ & Kürschner, *Crossidium crassinerve* (De Not.) Jur., *Phascum cuspidatum var. piliferum* (Hedw.) Hook. & Taylor, *Pterygoneurum ovatum* (Hedw.) Dixon, *Tortula atrovirens* (Sm.) Lindb., *Tortula brevissima* Schiffn., *Tortula schimperi* M.J.Cano, O.Werner & J.Guerra, *Ulota crispa* (Hedw.) Brid., *Bartra-*

http://dx.doi.org/10.5772/52937

mia ithyphylla Brid., *Philonotis marchica* (Hedw.) Brid., *Philonotis fontana* (Hedw.) Brid., *Philonotis tomentella* Molendo, *Bryum creberrimum* Taylor, *Bryum pallens* Sw. ex anon., *Bryum torquescens* Bruch & Schimp., *Bryum schleicheri* DC., *Mnium marginatum* (Dicks.) P.Beauv., *Plagiomnium cuspidatum* (Hedw.) T.J.Kop., *Plagiomnium undulatum* (Hedw.) T.J.Kop., *Aulacomnium androgynum* (Hedw.) Schwägr., *Drepanocladus aduncus* (Hedw.) Warnst, *Pseudoleskea patens* (Lindb.) Kindb., *Pseudoleskeella catenulata* (Brid. ex Schrad.) Kindb., *Pseudoleskeella tectorum* (Funck ex Brid.) Kindb. ex Broth., *Rhynchostegium confertum* (Dicks.) Schimp., *Brachythecium albicans* (Hedw.) Schimp., *Brachythecium erythrorrhizon* Schimp., *Calliergonella cuspidata* (Hedw.) Loeske, *Hypnum cupressiforme var. resupinatum* Hedw., *Plagiothecium laetum* Schimp., *Platygyrium repens* (Brid.) Schimp., *Leucodon immersus* Lindb. *Neckera crispa* Hedw., *Isothecium holtii* Kindb.

New moss records for both of them (B7 and C12) are *Timmia norvegica* J.E.Zetterst., *Grimmia funalis* (Schwägr.) Bruch & Schimp., *Grimmia montana* Bruch & Schimp., *Ceratodon conicus* (Hampe) Lindb., *Tortella inclinata* var. *densa* (Lorentz & Molendo) Limpr., *Pseudocrossidium hornschuchianum* (Schultz) R.H.Zander, *Syntrichia virescens* (De Not.) Ochyra, *Tortula marginata* (Bruch & Schimp.) Spruce, *Oxyrrhynchium schleicheri* (R.Hedw.) Röll.

The revelation of the importance of Pınargözü Cave for the biodiversity of mosses comes out as another important finding of the study. Namely, the taxa detected from this locality constitutes alone approximately the one third (37%) of the overall taxa determined from the whole research area. This result indicates the value of the Pınargözü Cave in terms of its contribution to the bryophyte diversity. Unfortunately, human activities in and around the Pınargözü Cave either by using the site as a picnic area or as a hiking site on the Mount Dedegöl are certainly putting an enormous pressure on the local flora, which in turn, conceive a negative effect on the rich biodiversity of Pınargözü Cave.

According to the our findings, 4 families out of 29 in the study area detected from the research area constitute 55 % of the total taxa. These families are: Pottiaceae, Grimmiaceae, Brachytheciaceae and Bryaceae, which are also known to be the families containing the highest number of taxon of the Turkish Bryophyte Flora (Table 2).

While evaluating the table 2, the total number of taxon of each family was handled. According to this, it was inferred that the family containing the utmost number of taxa within the study area was Pottiaceae family with 43 taxa, constituting the 28 % of the total taxa.

This situation can be explained by the summer droughts (25.4 ºC and 8.2 mm) within the study area which takes place in the C12 square grid. Because, species showes acrocarp growth as the ones within the Pottiaceae family are relatively more resistant to the long term high temperatures and drought since they usually have hair like appendages that are called "hair-point" on the tip of their leaves and show a dense, cushion like growth. Also, the existence of a great number of taxa belonging to the drought resistant families such as Grimmiaceae, Brachytheciaceae and Bryaceae in the study area can be seen as a result arising from the long lasting drought period at C12 square.

Families	Number of Taxa	Percentage of taxa according to total number of taxa (%)
Pottiaceae	43	28.0
Grimmiaceae	17	11.0
Brachytheciaceae	14	9.0
Bryaceae	11	7.0
Orthotrichaceae	10	6.5
Bartramiaceae	5	3.2
Ditrichaceae	5	3.2
Hypnaceae	5	3.2
Encalyptaceae	4	2.6
Plagiomniaceae	4	2.6
Amblystegiaceae	4	2.6
Leskeaceae	4	2.6
Neckeraceae	3	1.9
Funariaceae	3	1.9
Fissidentaceae	3	1.9
Mielichhoferiaceae	3	1.9
Leucodontaceae	3	1.9
Timmiaceae	2	1.2
Pterigynandraceae	2	1.2
Lembophyllaceae	2	1.2
Polytrichaceae	1	0.6
Rhabdoweisiaceae	1	0.6
Dicranaceae	1	0.6
Mniaceae	1	0.6
Aulacomniaceae	1	0.6
Plagiotheciaceae	1	0.6
Pylaisiadelphaceae	1	0.6
Leptodontaceae	1	0.6
Seligeriaceae	1	0.6
Total	156	100

Table 2. The distributions of the taxa according to the families

Acknowledgements

Many thanks to Funda OSKAY and Üstüner BİRBEN for the linguistic corrections of the manuscript and also thanks a lot to Türk Eğitim Vakfı (TEV) which I was provided scholarships by. Special thanks to Richard H. Zander for confirming the determination of *Seligeria donniana* (Sm.) Müll. Hal. and Michael Lüthe for confirming the determination of *Cinclidotus vardaranus* Erdağ and Kürschner.

Author details

Serhat Ursavaş[1*] and Barbaros Çetin[2]

*Address all correspondence to: serhatursavas@gmail.com

1 Çankırı Karatekin University, Faculty of Forestry, Department of Forest Engineering, Çankırı, Turkey

2 Dokuz Eylül University, Faculty of Science, Department of Biology, İzmir, Turkey

References

[1] Abay G. Çetin B. The moss flora (Musci) of Ilgaz mountain national park. Turkish Journal of Botany. 2003; 27: 321-332.

[2] Abay G. Ursavaş S. Kadıoğlu N.B. Tarhan İ. Artvin (A4) ve Antalya (C12)'dan bazı karayosunu (musci) kayıtları. Tabiat ve İnsan. 2006; 4: 19-32.

[3] Abay G. Uyar G. Keçeli T. Çetin B. Contributions to the bryoflora of the Kaçkar Mts. (NE Anatolia, Turkey). Phytologia Balcanica. 2009b; 15(3): 317-329.

[4] Abay G. Uyar G. Keçeli T. Çetin B. Sphagnum centrale and other remarkable bryophyte records from the Kaçkar Mountains (Nothern-Turkey). Cryptogamie, Bryolagie. 2009a; 30(3): 399-407.

[5] Anonim. Kızıldağ Milli Parkı Uzun Devreli Gelişme Planı (UDGP) Analitik Etüt ve Sentez Raporu. Ankara; 2005.

[6] Atherton I. Bosanquet S. Lawley M. Mosses and Liverworts of Britain and Ireland a field guide. British Bryological Society. United Kingdom; 2010.

[7] Chien G. Marshall R.C. Si H. Moss Flora of China, English version, Volume 1. Sphagnaceae-Leucobryaceae. Missouri Botanical Garden. USA; 1999.

[8] Chien G. Moss Flora of China, English version, Volume 3: Grimmiaceae-Tetraphidaceae. Missouri Botanical Garden. USA; 2003.

[9] Cortini P.C. Flora dei muschi d'Italia (Sphagnopsida, Andreaeopsida, Bryopsida. I parte). Roma: Antonio Delpfino Editore; 2001.

[10] Cortini P.C. Flora dei muschi d'Italia (Sphagnopsida, Andreaeopsida, Bryopsida. I parte). Roma: Antonio Delpfino Editore; 2006.

[11] Crum H. Mosses of the Great Lakes forest. Üniversity of Michigan. Michigan. USA; 1973.

[12] Çetin B. Antalya Çevresi (Köprülü Kanyon ve Güllük Dağı (Termessos) Milli Parkları ve Kurşunlu Şelalesi) Karayosunları (Musci). Doğa Türk Botanik Dergisi. 1989a; 13(3): 456-469.

[13] Çetin B. Checklist of the mosses of Turkey. Lındbergia. 1988a; 14: 15-23.

[14] Çetin B. Cinclidotus nyholmiae, a new species from Köprülü Canyon National Park (Antalya) in Turkey. Journal of Bryology. 1988b; 15: 269-273.

[15] Çetin B. Köprülü Kanyon. Fauna och Flora. 1989b; 84: 97-105.

[16] Çetin B. The moss flora of the Uludağ national park (Bursa/Turkey). Turkish Journal of Botany. 1999; 23: 187-193.

[17] Çetin B. Türkiye için yeni bir karayosunu (Musci). Doğa Turk Botanik Dergisi. 1989c; 13(2): 139-142.

[18] Çetin B. Unç E. Uyar G. The moss flora of Ankara-Kızılcahamam-Çamkoru and Çamlıdere districts. Turkish Journal of Botany. 2002; 26: 91-101.

[19] Çetin B. Yurdakulol E. Gerede-Aktaş (Bolu) ormanlarının karayosunları (musci) florası. Doğa Bilimleri Dergisi. 1985; 9(1): 29-39.

[20] Çetin B. Yurdakulol E. Yedigöller Milli Parkı'nın Karayosunu Florası. Doğa Türk Botanik Dergisi. 1988; 12(2): 128-145.

[21] Erdağ A. Kırmacı M. Kürschner H. The Hedwigia ciliata (Hedw.) Ehr. ex P.Beauv. Complex in Turkey, with a New Record, H. ciliata var. leucophaea Bruch & Schimp. (Hedwigiaceae, Bryopsida). Turk Journal of Botany. 2004; 27: 349-356.

[22] Erdağ A. Kürschner H. Cinclidotus vardaranus Erdağ and Kürschner (Bryopsida, Pottiaceae) sp. nov. from Eastern Turkey, with some remarks on the speciation centre of the genus. Nova Hedwigia. 2009; 88(1-2): 183-188.

[23] Erdağ A. Kürschner H. Parolly G. Three new records to the bryphyte flora of Turkey. Nova Hedwigia. 2001; 73(1-2): 239-246.

[24] Goffinet B. Buck WR. Systematics of the bryophyta (mosses): from molecules to a revised classification., In: Goffinet B, Hollowell VC, Magill RE, eds. Molecular systematics of bryophytes. St. Louis: Missouri Botanical Garden Press, 2004; p205–239,.

[25] Greven H.C. Grimmias of The World. Leiden: Backhuys Publishers. The Netherlands; 2003.

[26] Henderson D.M. Contributions to the bryophyte flora of Turkey VI. Notes from the Royal Botanic Garden Edinburgh. 1963; 25(3): 279-291.

[27] Henderson D.M. Contributions to the Bryophyte Flora of Turkey: III. Notes from the Royal Botanic Garden Edinburgh. 1958; 22: 611-620.

[28] Henderson D.M. Muirhead C.W. Contributions to the bryophyte flora of Turkey. Notes from the Royal Botanic Garden Edinburgh. 1955; 22: 29-43.

[29] Henderson D.M. Prentice H.D. Contributions to the bryophyte flora of Turkey: VIII. Notes from the Royal Botanic Garden Edinburgh. 1969; 29: 235-262.

[30] Henderson D.M.. Contributions to the Bryophyte Flora of Turkey: IV. Notes from the Royal Botanic Garden Edinburgh. 1961; 23: 263-278.

[31] Herrnstadt I. Heyn C.C. The Bryophyte Flora of Israel and Adjacent Regions. The Israel Academy of Sciences and Humanities. Jerusalem; 2004.

[32] Hill MO. Bell N. Buruggeman-Nannenga MA. Brugues M. Cano MJ. Enroth Flatberg KI. Fraham J-P. Gallego MT. Garilleti R. Guerra J. Hedenäs L. Holyoak DT. Hyvönen J. Ignatov MS. Lara F. Mazimpaka V. Munoz J. Söderström L. An annotated checklist of the mosses of Europe and Macronesia. Journal of Bryology. 2006; 28: 198–267.

[33] Kaya Z. Raynal D.J. Biodiversity and conservation of Turkish forests. Biological Conservation. 2001; 97: 131-141.

[34] Kırmacı M. Erdağ A. Çetin M. Two new records to the bryophyte flora of Turkey: Crossidium crassinerve (De Not.) Jur. and C. laxefilamentosum Frey et Kürschner (Pottiaceae, Bryophyta). Cryptogamie Bryologie. 2009; 30(3): 383-388.

[35] Kırmacı M. Özçelik H. Köprülü Kanyon Milli Parkı (Antalya) Karayosunu Florasına Katkılar. Süleyman Demirel Üniversitesi Orman Fakültesi Dergisi. 2010; 2: 59-73.

[36] Kürschner H. Erdağ A. Bryophytes of Turkey: An Annotated Reference List of the Species with Synonyms from the Recent Literature and an Annontated List of Turkish Bryological Literature. Turkish Journal of Botany. 2005; 29: 95-154.

[37] Kürschner H. Erdağ A. The Grimmietum commutato-campestris in Turkey. Ecology and Life syndromes of a saxicolours bryophyte community with the description of two new subassociations. Nova Hedwigia. 2009; 88(3-4): 441-463.

[38] Kürschner H. Nestle R.L. Cinclidotus bistratosus (Cinclidotaceae, Musci), a new species to the hygrophytic moss flora of Turkey. Nova Hedwigia. 2000; 70(3-4): 471-478.

[39] Lawton E. Moss Flora of Pasific Northwest. Journal of Hattori Botanical Garden Laboratory, Nichinan. USA; 1971.

[40] Li Xing-Jiang Marshall R.C. Si H. Moss Flora of China, English version, Volume 4: Bryaceae to Timmiaceae. Missouri Botanical Garden. USA; 2007.

[41] Lu Xing-Jiang. Moss Flora of China, English version, Volume 2: Fissidentaceae-Ptychomitriaceae. Missouri Botanical Garden. USA; 2001.

[42] Lüth M. Bildatlas der Moose Deutschlands, Faszikel 1, Grimmiaceae, Freiburg; 2006.

[43] Lüth M. Bildatlas der Moose Deutschlands, Faszikel 2, Dicranaceae-Mniaceae-Politrichaceae, Freiburg; 2006.

[44] Lüth M. Bildatlas der Moose Deutschlands, Faszikel 3, Pottiaceae, Freiburg; 2006.

[45] Lüth M. Bildatlas der Moose Deutschlands, Faszikel 4, Bryaceae-Funariales, Freiburg; 2007.

[46] Lüth M. Bildatlas der Moose Deutschlands, Faszikel 5, Andreaeaceae-Timmiaceae, Freiburg; 2008.

[47] Lüth M. Bildatlas der Moose Deutschlands, Faszikel 6, Amblystegiaceae-Thuidiaceae, Freiburg; 2009.

[48] Lüth M. Bildatlas der Moose Deutschlands, Faszikel 7, Brachytheciaceae-Sematophyllaceae, Freiburg; 2010.

[49] Natcheva R. Coşkun M. Çayır A. Contribution to the bryophyte flora of European Turkey. Phytologia Balcanica. 2008; 14(3): 335-341.

[50] Nyholm E. Illustrated Flora of Nordic Mosses, Fasc. 1. Fissidentaceae - Seligeriaceae, Nordic Bryological Society. Stockholm; 1987.

[51] Nyholm E. Illustrated Flora of Nordic Mosses, Fasc. 2. Pottiaceae-Sphagnaceae - Schistostegaceae, Nordic Bryological Society. Stockholm. 1989; p73-142.

[52] Nyholm E. Illustrated Flora of Nordic Mosses, Fasc. 3. Bryaceae - Rhodobryaceae - Mniaceae - Cinclidiaceae - Plagiomniaceae, Nordic Bryological Society. Stockholm. 1993; p143-244.

[53] Nyholm E. Illustrated Flora of Nordic Mosses, Fasc. 4. Aulacomniaceae - Meesiaceae - Catoscopiaceae - Bartramiaceae - Timmiaceae - Encalyptaceae - Grimmiaceae - Ptychomitraceae - Hedwigiaceae - Orthotrichaceae, Nordic Bryological Society. Stockholm. 1998; p245-406.

[54] Ören M. Uyar G. Keçeli T. The bryophyte flora of the western part of the Küre Mountains (Bartın, Kastamonu), Turkey. Turk J. Bot. 2012; 36, 1-20.

[55] Özdemir T. Çetin B. The moss flora of Trabzon and Environs. Turkish Journal of Botany. 1999; 23: 391-404.

[56] Özdemir T. Batan N. Contributions to the Moss Flora of Gümüşhane Province (Torul and Kürtün Districts, Turkey). Pakistan Journal of Biological Sciences. 2009; 12(4): 346-352.

[57] Özdemir T. Koz B. Contribution to the Moss Flora of Dereli, Giresun District (Turkey). Acta Botanica Hungarica. 2008; 50(1-2): 171-180.

[58] Özdemir T. Some Taxa of Bryophyta Spreaded in Eynesil district (Giresun-Turkey). Enegy, Education, Science and Technology. 1999; 4(1): 30-41.

[59] Özhatay N. Byfield, A. Atay, S. Türkiye'nin 122 Önemli Bitki Alanı. WWF-Türkiye, DHKD, Fauna & Flora International and İ.Ü. Eczacılık Fakültesi. İstanbul; 2005.

[60] Papp B. Contributions to the bryoflora of the Pontic Mts., North Anatolia, Turkey. Studia botanica hungarica. 2004; 35: 81-89.

[61] Papp B. Sabovljević M. Contribution to the bryophyte flora of Turkish thrace. Studia botanica hungarica. 2003; 34: 43-54.

[62] Peng-cheng W. Bang-juan L. Chien G. Tong C. Zhi-hua L. Tan B.C. He S. Yu J. Mei-zhi W. Xing F. Jun S. Ben-gu Z. Moss Flora of China, English version, Volume 6: Hookeriaceae-Tuhuidiaceae. Missouri Botanical Garden. USA; 2002.

[63] Robinson H. Godfrey R.K. Contribution to the bryophyte flora of Turkey. Revue Bryologique et Lichènologique. 1960; 29: 244-253.

[64] Savaroğlu F. Tokur S. The moss flora (musci) of The Sündiken mountains. Turkish Journal of Botany. 2006; 30: 137-148.

[65] Smit A.J.E. The Moss Flora of Britain an Ireland. Cambridge University Press; 2004.

[66] Smith A.J.E. The Moss Flora of Britain and Ireland. Cambridge University Press; 1980.

[67] Tonguç Ö. Yayıntaş A. Çal dağı (Manisa) karayosunları. Turkish Journal of Botany. 1996; 20: 59-63.

[68] Ursavaş S. Abay G. Contributions to the bryoflora of Ilgaz Mountains, Yenice Forests, Turkey. Biological Diverity and Conversation. 2009; 2(3): 112-121.

[69] Uyar G. Alataş M. Ören M. Keçeli T. The Bryophyte Flora of Yenice Forests (Karabük, Turkey). International Journal of Botany. 2007; 3(2): 129-146.

[70] Uyar G. Çetin B. A new check-list of the mosses of Turkey. Journal of Bryology. 2004; 26: 203-220.

[71] Uyar G. Çetin B. Contributions to the moss flora of Turkey: Western Black Sea Region (Bolu, Kastamonu, Karabük, Bartın and Zonguldak). Iternational Journal of Botany. 2006; 2(3): 229-241.

[72] Uyar G. Ören M. Isothecium holtii Kindb. (Brachytheciaceae, Bryopsida), new to the moss flora of Turkey. Cryptogamie, Bryologie. 2005; 26(4): 425-429.

[73] Uyar G. The moss flora of Akçakoca mountains (Düzce). Ot Sistematik Botanik Dergisi. 2003; 10(1): 77-95.

[74] Uyar G. Ünal M. A note on Grimmia capillata De Not. (Grimmiaceae, Musci) in Turkey. Turk Journal of Botany. 2005; 29: 467-470.

[75] Walther V.K. Bieträge zur Moosflora Westanatoliens I. Mitteilungen des Staatsinstitut für Allgemeine Botanik in Hamburg. 1967; 12: 129-186.

[76] Yayıntaş A. Higuchi M. Tonguç Ö. The moss flora of Istıranca (Kırklareli) mountains in Turkey. Journal of Faculty of Science Ege University. 1996; 19(2): 33-45.

[77] Yayıntaş A. Tonguç Ö. New Moss Records From Thrace for A1. Journal of Faculty of Science Ege University. 1994; 16(1): 51-61.

[78] You-fang W. Ren-liang H. Yu-huan W. Chien G. Deng-ke L. Wei L. He S. Irelend R.R. Moss Flora of China, English version, Volume 7: Amblystegiaceae-Plagiotheciaceae, Missouri Botanical Garden. USA; 2008.

[79] Yücel E. Magil R.E. Eskişehir Bölgesi karayosunları (musci) üzerine bir araştırma. Anadolu Üniversitesi Fen Fakültesi Dergisi. 1997; 3: 47-54.

[80] Yücel E. Tokur S. Eskişehir Yöresi Bazı Brydae Alt Sınıfı Türleri Üzerine Floristik Çalışmalar I. Fen Edebiyat Dergisi. 1989; 2(1): 9-16.

[81] http://www.esu.edu/~milewski/intro_biol_two/lab_2_moss_ferns/Mossand-Fern_Diversity.html (accessed 08 October 2012).

Chapter 4

Twenty Years of Molecular Biogeography in the West Mediterranean Islands of Corsica and Sardinia: Lessons Learnt and Future Prospects

Valerio Ketmaier and Adalgisa Caccone

Additional information is available at the end of the chapter

http://dx.doi.org/10.5772/55458

1. Introduction

The Mediterranean Sea comprises a wide array of insular systems. Sardinia and Corsica are respectively the second and forth-largest islands of the Mediterranean Sea and they are environmentally complex due to their topography and orography. Owing to their central position in the Tyrrhenian Sea (Figure 1) humans started settling on the islands relatively early, during the Mesolithic. Pliny and Ptolemy were among the first to briefly mention the islands' fauna. More systematic surveys of their biodiversity started around 300 years ago, when Sardinia became part of the Kingdom of Sardinia ruled by the House of Savoy and Corsica was incorporated into France [1]. Our current knowledge of the islands' biological diversity can be considered quite accurate; the fauna is relatively species-poor compared to the surrounding continental areas, still rate of endemism is high, approaching about 7% for Sardinia [2]. Most of the Corsican-Sardinian endemisms show clear affinity with species distributed across that part of Southern Europe that embraces Northern Spain and Southern France. Some of these elements are also closely related to species occurring in Central insular and peninsular Italy (Tuscan Archipelago and coastal areas of Tuscany; Figure 1). These concordant, yet disjunct, distributions (peri-Tyrrhenian hereinto) are shared among a variety of unrelated organisms, from plants to invertebrates and vertebrates (see [3] for a synthesis) all having very low (if any) potential for long distance, over-sea dispersal.

Recurrent patterns in geographical ranges of unrelated species have traditionally attracted the interest of biogeographers because they can be reasonably related to the same underlying event(s). In the case of the Corsica-Sardinia system, the presence of a pre-Miocene land bridge connecting the different landmasses had been initially hypothesized [4]; affinities of nowadays allopatrically distributed lineages were consequently interpreted under a dispersal scenario. The advent of the theory of plate tectonics allowed a detailed reconstruction of the geological history of the islands [5,6] (see Figure 1 and next chapter for details) and induced many authors to favour vicariance over dispersal as the main process that originated the islands' biodiversity [1,3].

The uniqueness of a biogeographic situation with several co-distributed, yet unrelated, species all presumably sharing the same history did not escape the attention of molecular evolutionary biologists. The Corsican-Sardinian system offers the opportunity to test explicit biogeographic hypotheses in light of a well-known geological background; the available geological time estimates can be used to test for the clocklike nature of genetic divergence and eventually calibrate rates of molecular evolution. In 1990 the first molecular data ever on a Corsican-Sardinian endemism with Iberian affinities (newts of the genus *Euproctus*) were included as part of a review on molecular island biogeography [7]. Since then a good wealth of molecular work has been done on a variety of terrestrial and freshwater species (both invertebrates and vertebrates) based on different molecular markers (Table 1). The molecular and analytical tools employed in those studies reflect the unparalleled technological and analytical development that the field has witnessed in the last two decades.

In light of the central importance that insular settings have had in the development of the evolutionary thinking, we assembled this review with the aim to specifically address the following points. First, we will present a synthesis of the most representative molecular studies (i.e. explicitly centred on Corsica-Sardinian endemisms and not part of larger phylogenetic studies) conducted on animal groups whose distribution is limited to the Corsica-Sardinia system and surrounding continental landmasses involved in the past geological evolution of the islands. Second, we want to test for each of these groups whether phylogenetic relationships fit those expected if cladogenetic events were due to vicariance only. Third, we will summarize the available molecular estimates of divergence times to discuss how they relate to current views on the geological evolution of the landmasses. Fourth, we will summarize whether for each group substitution rates accumulate linearly over time or not (if this was tested in original study) and compare rates based on the same markers and calibrated using the very same geological event(s) across taxonomically unrelated groups. Finally, to place this review in a larger context and to ultimately suggest future avenues in the study of the evolution of insular biota we will explore how molecular evidence on the Corsica-Sardinia system relates to comparative phylogeographies available for other insular systems.

2. Geographical setting

Corsica is located in the Tyrrhenian Sea south of France, west of Italy and north of the island of Sardinia. Its surface totals about 8700 km^2 extending for 183 km; the island is 83 km wide and it is about 90 km away from Italy (Tuscany), 170 km from Southern France and it is separated from Sardinia by the Strait of Bonifacio (minimum width 11 km). Mountains comprise about two-third of the island forming a single chain that runs in a north-south direction.

Sardinia, with an area of about 24000 km^2, is the second largest island of the Mediterranean Sea. The island is 270 km long and 145 km wide and is almost equally distant from peninsular Italy on the east (187 km) and North Africa (Tunisia) on the south (184 km). Many small islands and islets surround Sardinia, the largest being the island of Sant'Antioco (109 km^2) situated at its southwest tip. Most of its territory is mountainous (about 80%) and a number of mountain chains can be identified separated by intervening alluvial plains and flatlands, the largest being the Campidano plain in the southwest part of the island.

3. Geological history

Corsica and Sardinia are old continental islands and their geological evolution has been reconstructed in good details. A consensus on the overall process of formation of the two islands exists. Some questions are still open, though, regarding the timing of final detachment of two islands from the continent and pattern and timing of contacts between them. Traditionally, the split of Corsica and Sardinia from the Iberian Peninsula as a single microplate had been dated at about 29 million years (Myrs) ago; the rotation of the microplate and the disjunction of the two islands started 15 Myrs ago and was completed by 9 Myrs ago [5,6,8,9,10,11,12]. Recently, new geological data challenged this scenario. According to [13,14] the beginning of the split of the microplate should be dated at 24-20 Myrs. The maps presented in [15] support these views but also suggest that the microplate remained connected to the southern edge of Palaeo-Europe during its anti-clock wise rotation through a land bridge that will constitute the future Maritime Alps and the Ligurian Apennines (Italy). The final detachment of the microplate from the continent was contemporary with the onset of the uplift of Tuscany in continental Italy and occurred in the Pliocene (around 5 Myrs ago). The interaction between the Corsica-Sardinia microplate and the Apennines, which were then being formed, caused the emergence of the Tuscan Archipelago, including the islands that later became incorporated in the mainland (the so- called "fossil islands") [11]. Further connections between the Corsica-Sardinia microplate and the continent were probably established during the Messinian Salinity Crisis (5.7-5.3 Myrs) [10,12]. Finally, sea-level oscillations, which occurred repeatedly in the Quaternary at each ice age (from 2 to 0.5 Myr ago), led to connect northern Corsica to Tuscany and southern Corsica to northern Sardinia [16-19]. It is worth noting that all the connections of the two islands to the continent after the initial detachment of the microplate were short-lived, regardless of how many times they happened and when [20,21]. A schematic representation of the alternative views on the geological evolution of the area is given in Figure 1.

In spite of the temporal vagaries outlined in the previous paragraph, the geological cladogram of the area, that is the representation of relationships among areas based on their geological history, can be summarized as follows. The Iberian Peninsula is basal in the cladogram and the two islands are each other's sister areas. When also Balearic Islands, Tuscan Archipelago and continental Italy are considered, then Balearic Islands would be sister to the Iberian Peninsula while Corsica and Sardinia would no longer be sister areas but Sardinia would be basal to a clade formed by Corsica, Tuscan Archipelago and coastal areas of Central Italy. The two geological area cladograms are depicted in Figure 2.

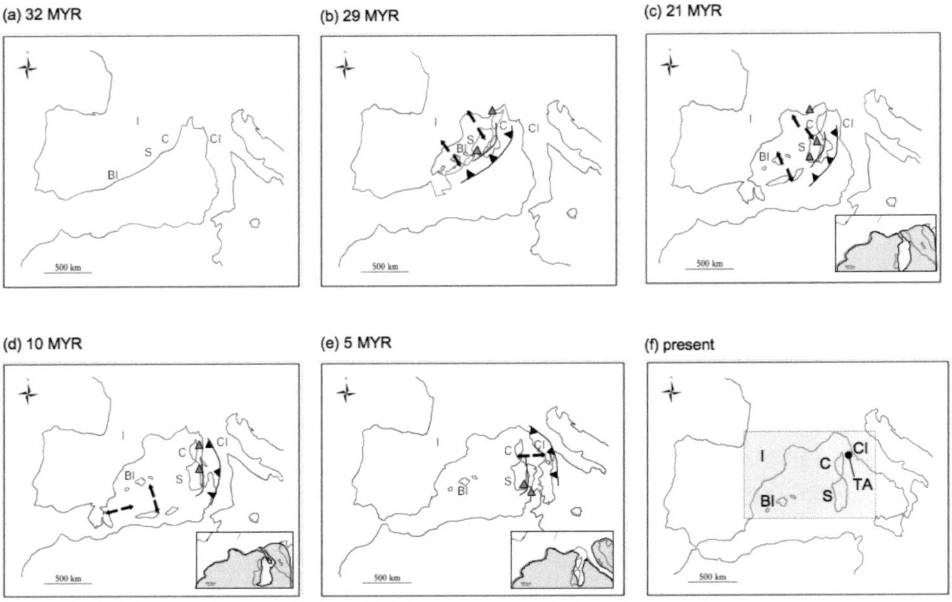

Figure 1. Geological evolution of the peri-Tyrrhenian area. Panels (a) to (e) show reconstructions of the split of the Corsica-Sardinia microplate from the Iberian Peninsula, its subsequent rotation and interaction with the still extant Tuscan Archipelago and the current coastal area of Tuscany (fossil islands; see text). Approximate age of each geological phase is also given. Bottom right inlets in panels (c), (d), and (e) show the interactions between Corsica-Sardinia and Continental Italy between 21 and 5 Myr proposed by [15] as alternative to the classical scenarios shown in the larger panels (grey and white shaded areas correspond to sea and land, respectively). Black and grey triangles indicate oceanic subduction and thrusting. Panel (f) shows the present geographic location of main areas considered in the study: the Iberian Peninsula (I), Balearic Islands (BI), Sardinia (S), Corsica (C), Tuscan Archipelago (TA) and Continental Italy (CI). Maps were drawn on the basis of present geography.

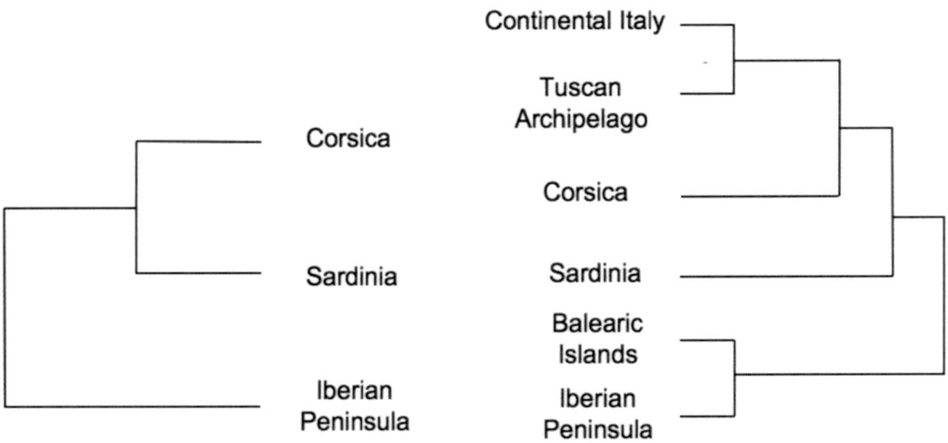

Figure 2. Geological area cladograms of the peri-Tyrrhenian area. The cladogram on the left depicts relationships only when the three major landmasses are considered while on the right are expected relationships when additional areas are also included (see text for details).

4. Ecology and endemism

Corsica and Sardinia have a Mediterranean climate characterized by hot and dry summers and mild and wet winters. Rainfalls are concentrated in autumn and winter with sporadic showers in spring. Owing to the presence of numerous mountains, the Mediterranean climate of the coastal zone (between the sea level and 600 m of altitude) changes into a milder, cooler and wetter climate in the temperate mountain zone comprised between 600 and 1800 m above the sea level. In Corsica, where elevation reaches 2700 m of altitude, it is possible to identify a high alpine zone (between 1800 and 2700 m) where snow-caps and small glaciers are not infrequent.

The vegetation of the islands reflects the climate altitudinal zones. In the coastal areas Mediterranean forests, woodlands, and shrubs predominate with evergreen sclerophylls. Much of the coastal lowlands have been cleared for agriculture, grazing and logging, activities that have considerably reduced the forest cover. Maritime Pines interspersed with forests of deciduous trees are typical of middle elevations. Above 1800 m of altitude (Corsica only), sub alpine shrub lands progressively substitute forests of Corsican Pine, Silver Fir and European Beech. Endemic plant species are chiefly restricted to high altitudes in Corsica and to coastal areas in Sardinia [3].

Corsica and Sardinia are faunistically impoverished as compared to potential surrounding continental sources. Based on taxonomic and faunistic considerations a three-phase model of colonization of the islands (pre-Miocene, Messinian and Quaternary; a fourth phase considers species introduced by humans) has been proposed [3]. The first phase would correspond to the detachment of the microplate from the Iberian Peninsula. Most of the endemic species that are nowadays distributed in Sardinia and Corsica (either in common between the two islands or unique to each of them) have differentiated from ancestors that were supposedly co-distributed on the microplate and the Iberian Peninsula when these were still forming a single landmass. Thus, the origin of these lineages is at least 29 Myrs old, even thought we cannot exclude that cladogenesis predated geological splits. Invertebrates are particularly well represented. Freshwater planarians of the genus *Dugesia* belong to this stock along with multiple endemic lineages of terrestrial gastropods (genera *Rupestrella, Solatopupa, Hypnophila* and *Tacheocampylaea*). Similarly, examples are found among earthworms (genus *Hormogaster*), crustaceans isopods (both epigean and hypogean, aquatic and terrestrial with the genera *Proasellus, Stenasellus, Helleria, Nesiotoniscus, Tiroloscia* and *Lucasius*), arachnids (harvestmen of the genera *Parasiro* and *Scotolemon*, the Acari genera *Damaeus* and *Oribatella* and at least five lineages of pseudoscorpions) and centipedes. Insects are present with different orders. Among others, stoneflies and beetles are very interesting biogeographically. The stonefly genus *Tyrrhenoleuctra* includes three endemic lineages; cave Bathysciine beetles are rich in endemism with at least 11 species (genera *Ovobathysciola, Patriziella* and *Speonomus*) likewise are scarab beetles with the genera *Elaphocerida, Triodonta, Cetonia, Thorectes* and *Typhoeus*. Amphibians and Reptiles also contributed to this early phase of colonization. Urodela share no species with any of the adjacent continental landmasses and include at least six endemic species (two genera; newt *Euproctus* and salamander *Speleomantes*). The endemic lineages of the lizard genera *Archeolacerta, Algyroides* and *Podarcis* also belong to this early stock of colonizers. No mammalian representatives of this ancient stock are still extant; known from fossil records are the perissodactyls *Atalodon* and *Lophiodon* and the ruminant *Amphytragulus boulengeri*.

During the Messinian Salinity Crisis (MSC; 5.7-5.3 Myrs) the Mediterranean Sea almost completely dried up. The MSC was short-lived; nonetheless it allowed a number of species to reach the islands. These constitute most of the extant Corsican-Sardinian fauna, although none of them had diversified on the islands into endemic species. The only endemic subspecies is the colubrid snake *Natrix natrix cettii*. Species that reached the islands during the MSC are typical of a warm to hot climate because they had to withstand the harsh conditions of the drained and hyper saline Mediterranean basin. Colonization proceeded along two major paths from south and east. Sardinia and Corsica thus share earthworms, arachnids, insects, reptiles and many fossil mammals with North Africa and Sicily. An eastern wave of colonization from continental Italy carried to the islands land snails, amphibians, reptiles and mammals (the last three groups left representatives almost exclusively in the fossil records).

The last connection(s) between our insular system and the adjacent continent (Central Italy) took place during the Quaternary ice ages. These connections were relatively short-lived, allowed dispersal of species adapted to a temperate to cold climate and have originated no extant endemism. Particular abundant is the mammalian fossil record, which includes extinct species of deer, wild boars, dwarf elephants, giant water voles and macaques. The endemic Sardinia pika (*Prolagus sardus*), a primitive lagomorph of Quaternary origin, went extinct in the late 1700s or early1800s, probably due to a combination of habitat loss, predation and competition with introduced alien species [22].

Humans have started introducing species on the islands intentionally or accidentally since historical times. The extinction of much of the pre-Quaternary fauna is due to human activities (hunting above all), competition with alien introduced species or a combination of both. The Barbary partridge (*Alectoris barbara*) is an example of an introduced bird. Among mammals, rats, mice, hedgehogs, martens, weasels, wild cats and boars, follow deer, red deer and mouflons are all introduced. Some of them have been on the islands long enough to acquire unique morphological features that granted them a sub specific rank (the red deer *Cervus elaphus corsicanus* and the mouflon *Ovis orientalis musimon*).

5. The data set

Available molecular data on Corsica-Sardinia endemisms, on their continental Iberian counterparts (and/or insular and continental Central Italian when existing) are summarized in Table 1. They cover four classes of invertebrates and two classes of vertebrates. While a few studies employed simultaneously markers of different origin (mitochondrial and nuclear), the vast majority is based upon mitochondrial DNA (mtDNA) only; *Cytochrome Oxidase subunit I* (*COI*), the large (*16S*) and small (*12S*) ribosomal subunits are the most frequently used genes. Regardless of the type of marker used, number of lineages discovered molecularly exceeds those assumed on the basis of morphology alone (i.e. nominal taxa). Exceptions to this otherwise generalized pattern are cave beetles and newts but for both groups a one-species one-population sampling strategy was used [23-25]. In two circumstances (the terrestrial isopod *Helleria brevicornis* and the Bediagra rock lizard) the same lineage is distributed across predicted phylogeographic breaks [26,27]. For *Helleria brevicornis* the same mtDNA haplotype has been found in Southern France, Central Italy and on three islands of the Tuscan Archipelago. One mtDNA lineage of the Bediagra rock lizard is in common between Sardinia and Corsica. Conversely, no haplotype sharing was detected for any of the other analyzed taxa.

Class	Taxa	N of nominal species	N of lineages[1]	Distribution (N of lineages)[2]	Molecular marker	Molecular clock[3]	Source
Oligochaeta	Earthworms *Hormogaster*	2	4	I (2)/S (1)/TA (1)	Allozymes (26 loci)	No	[35]
Gastropoda	Land snails *Solatopupa*	6	8	I (4)/S (1)/C (2)/TA (1)	mt- (*12S*, *16S*, *COI*)/ nucDNA (*H3*)	Yes	[37,39]
Malacostraca	Aquatic cave Isopods *Stenasellus*	2	6	I (2)/S (2)/C (1)/ CI (1)	Allozymes (15 loci) mtDNA (*COI*)	Yes	[33,40,56]
	Terrestrial Isopods *Helleria*	1	6	I (1*)/S (3)/C (2)/TA (1*)/CI (1*) * same lineage	mtDNA (*12S*, *16S*, *COI*)	Yes	[26]
Insecta	Stoneflies *Tyrrhenoleuctra*	3	5	I (2)/BI (1)/C (1)/ S (1)	Allozymes (11 loci) mtDNA (*12S*, *COI*)	Yes	[34,41]
	Cave beetles *Ovobathysciola* *Patriziella* *Anillochlamys* *Speonomus*	11	11	I (4)/ S (7)	mtDNA (*COI*)	Yes	[25]
Amphibia	European newts *Euproctus*	2	2	S (1)/ C (1)	mtDNA (*12S*, *16S*, *Cytb*)	Yes	[23,24]
Reptilia	Bediagra rock lizard *Archaeolacerta*	1	2	S (1)/C (2*) *one lineage is shared with S	mtDNA (*ND4*, $tRNA^{SER, LEU, HIS}$)	Yes	[27]

[1] Following the criteria in [65]; [2] I= Southern France + Iberian Peninsula; BI = Balearic Islands; S = Sardinia; C = Corsica; TA = Tuscan Archipelago (extant islands); CI = Continental Italy (mostly fossil islands; see Introduction and Figure1); [3] Linearity of rates tested and/or calibration given in the study source.

Table 1. Summary of taxa with a Corsica- Sardinia- Iberian Peninsula distribution studied molecularly. For each group we give the nominal number of species, the number of lineages identified molecularly, the geographical distribution of such lineages, the markers employed, whether linearity of substitution rates has been tested and whether an explicit calibration of the molecular clock has been proposed in the original study.

When more than one conspecific population per geographical area was considered, molecules often revealed multiple lineages that are more closely related to one another than they are to any of those distributed on the other landmasses. This suggests that within-area diversification took place after the geological splits.

6. Hypothesis testing and TreeMap analysis

Was vicariance hence predominant over dispersal in promoting speciation in Corsica-Sardinia-Iberian taxa, as expected given the low dispersal capability of the groups listed in Table 1? If so, relationships within groups should mirror the geological area cladogram of the landmasses they occupy (see the Geological history section and Figure 1 for details). In other words, a vicariance scenario would be supported if the phylogeny of a given group were congruent with the known sequence of vicariant events as determined by geology [28]. To test this hypothesis, we used an approach initially developed to detect co-speciation in host-parasite systems and later on applied to biogeography [29,30]. It should be noted here that we had no access to raw datasets for any of the study cases based on allozymes included in this review. Furthermore, papers based on retrievable sequence data considered, with the sole exceptions of land snails and rock lizards, few populations and individuals (often just a single population per species). All this hampered applicability of the recently developed Approximate Bayesian Computation (ABC) approaches. ABC integrates the many parameters typical of any population genetics study into a Bayesian framework and takes advantage of the flexibility of the Bayesian statistics to derive inferences. ABC, however, arose primarily in the field of population genetics to investigate the demographic history of populations and implicitly assumes a dense sampling in terms of both individuals/populations and loci [31]. We hence limited ourselves to compare branching patterns of molecular phylogenies (as presented in the original papers; Table 1) to the area cladogram to reconstruct the alleged "host-parasite" associations (where the hosts are the geographic areas and the parasites are lineages of a given group). Associations between the molecular phylogenies and the area cladograms as well as all the subsequent statistical analyses were carried out in TreeMap 1.0 [32]. We used the heuristic option to reconcile the area and the group trees and to find a single optimal reconstruction. We tested the significance of the fit between the host and parasite trees by generating 10000 random "parasite" trees with the same number of taxa and "host-parasite" associations. We then measured how the random parasite trees fit the observed parasite trees in comparison with the area cladogram. The proportion of random gene trees that have the same (or greater) number of speciation-separation events as the observed tree is the probability of obtaining the observed value by chance alone. The null hypothesis is that the area cladogram and molecular phylogenetic trees are independent. TreeMap distinguishes and counts the following events: speciation by area, speciation within area, migratory and sorting events. The latter are assumed due to extinction and/or sampling errors; they hence reflect instances where "parasites" were expected to occur but do not.

Results of these analyses are summarized in Table 2. No migratory events were detected for any of the associations tested. The analysis was significant at the 0.05 level or below for the subterranean aquatic isopod *Stenasellus* (allozymes and mtDNA), stoneflies (*Tyrrhenoleuctra*) and European newts (*Euproctus*). For these groups we have thus to reject the null hypothesis of no association between molecular relationships and the area cladogram. This implies that vicariance has been the main force driving their diversification.

	Events				
Taxa	**Speciation by area**	**Speciation within an area**	**Migratory**	**Sorting**	***P*** *
Earthworms *Hormogaster*	3	2	0	1	0.071
Land snails *Solatopupa*	2	5	0	4	0.610
Aquatic cave Isopods *Stenasellus* (Allozymes)	4	2	0	1	<<0.001
Aquatic cave Isopods *Stenasellus* (mtDNA)	4	1	0	1	<0.001
Terrestrial Isopods *Helleria*	1	8	0	9	0.985
Stoneflies *Tyrrhenoleuctra*	4	1	0	0	<<0.001
Cave beetles *Ovobathysciola Patriziella Anillochlamys*	2	4	0	0	0.410
Cave beetles *Speonomus*	2	2	0	0	0.288
European newts *Euproctus*	2	0	0	0	<<0.001
Bediagra rock lizard *Archaeolacerta*	2	7	0	3	0.866

* based on 10.000 random permutations; *P* is significant when ≤ 0.05

Table 2. Summary of the reconstruction of lineage-area assemblage performed in TreeMap [32]. For each group TreeMap sorts the total number of scored events into four categories (columns 2-5; see text for details). The last column reports the significance of the observed fit between the area cladogram (see Figure1) and the molecular phylogenies; the null hypothesis is that there is no association between them.

Aquatic isopods of the genus *Stenasellus* are highly adapted to subterranean life, they spend their whole life cycle in subsurface freshwaters and active dispersal can only happen when such a habitat is continuous [33]. Given these characteristics, it was not unexpected to find molecular relationships (regardless of the markers employed) to be remarkably in agreement with the palaeogeography of the area. Stoneflies are very poor fliers and spend most of their life cycle as nymphs in running freshwaters [34]. The terrestrial winged adults are short-lived and tend to stay close to the water edge to reproduce. Considerable oversea dispersal is difficult to hypothesize. Likewise unrealistic would be to invoke between islands sea dispersal for European newts, given the strict intolerance of amphibians to salt water [23,24].

TreeMap analyses were not significant for earthworms, land snails, terrestrial isopods, cave beetles and rock lizards, groups where the potential for dispersal is also low. For none of these groups TreeMap suggested multiple colonization events of the islands. Genetic relationships in the earthworm genus *Hormogaster* do not match the area cladogram, because the lineage from the Elba Island is basal to the Sardinian ones [35], contrary to what expected on the basis of geological considerations alone (Figure 2). These results are likely due to the lack of resolution of the markers employed (allozymes) coupled with an incomplete taxon sampling [35]. Relationships within the genus and the family (Hormogastridae) are problematic and still in need of additional work based on as exhaustive taxon coverage as possible [36]. For land snails of the genus *Solatopupa* we found a relatively high number of within-area speciation and sorting events (Table 2). In particular, *S.guidoni* has diversified within the Sardinia-Corsica-Tuscan Archipelago area into mtDNA lineages that maintained a substantial morphological uniformity in shell and genital traits [37]. These insular lineages are not reciprocally monophyletic as expected if vicariance had been the only cause of divergence; haplogroups found on Sardinia and Elba Island are embedded within some of those distributed in Corsica. The sorting events detected are likely due to episodes of extinction because the species is nowadays absent from ecologically suitable areas where it has been reported in the past [37,38,39]. The high number of speciation within an area and sorting events as opposed to the very few speciation by area episodes justify the lack of fit between the phylogeographies of both the terrestrial isopod *Helleria brevicornis* and the Bediagra rock lizard and a purely vicariant model of divergence [26,27]. In either case, diversification started in the Pliocene, much later than the completion of the detachment of the Corsica-Sardinia microplate from the Iberian Peninsula. Mitochondrial DNA genealogies support relatively recent between-islands dispersal as demonstrated by the intermingling of haplotypes originating from the two islands. For the isopod, historic human-mediated transport has been also postulated [26]. None of these explanations applies to cave beetles, owing to their strict association with the subterranean environment [25]. In this case, the TreeMap analyses might have been partially distorted by the fact that the lineages considered in [25] are absent from Corsica (hence only two areas could be included in the analyses) and by the strong bias in number of species included in the study in favour of Sardinia. Consequently, speciation-by-area events are either the same or half of those detected within areas.

7. Divergence times and molecular rates

The peri-Tyrrhenian area offers at least two independent geological time estimates for calibrating rates of gene evolution (the split of the microplate from the Iberian Peninsula and the split between the two islands) within the same geographical setting across a variety of unrelated taxonomic groups. All the studies centred on this system but one took indeed advantage of this opportunity (Table 1). With the sole exceptions of [40,41], where calibration of sets of allozymic loci was attempted, all other studies exclusively considered mtDNA. Table 3 summarizes the main results. Linearity (i.e. acceptance of the molecular clock hypothesis) of rates was rejected on the whole for stoneflies only [34], while at least some (if not all) of the gene partitions tested in the other studies passed the molecular clock test. A remarkable slowdown in rates was detected for the stonefly *Tyrrhenoleuctra* [34,41]; younger lineages accumulate substitutions at a relatively faster pace (yet slower than that of other insect orders). In the only case where nuclear DNA sequences were used (land snails *Solatopupa*, histone *H3* gene; [39]), these were not evolving in a clock-like manner.

Taxa[1]	**Linearity**	**Gene partition**	**Rates**
Land snails *Solatopupa*	Yes	*12S*, *COI* 1st codon pos.*	0.131, 0.025
Aquatic cave Isopods *Stenasells*	Yes	15 allozymic loci	2-2.1
Aquatic cave Isopods *Stenasellus*	Yes	*COI* all pos., *COI* Tv+Ti 3rd codon pos.; *COI* Tv3rd codon pos.	1.25, 0.1, 0.46
Terrestrial Isopods *Helleria*	Yes	*COI* all codon pos.**	N/A
Stoneflies *Tyrrhenoleuctra*	Yes	11 allozymic loci	0.8
Stoneflies *Tyrrhenoleuctra*	No	*12S*, *COI* all codon pos.	0.01-0.25, 0.09-0.79
Cave beetles *Ovobathysciola* *Patriziella* *Anillochlamys*	Yes	*COI* all codon pos., *COI* 3rd codon pos., *COI* Tv3rd codon pos.	1.3, 0.86, 0.5
Cave beetles *Speonomus*	Yes	*COI* all codon pos., *COI* 3rd codon pos., *COI* Tv3rd codon pos.	1.2, 0.98, 0.9
European newts *Euproctus*	Yes	*12S* + *16S* all sub., *12S* + *16S* Tv, *Cytb* all codon pos., *Cytb* Tv all codon pos., *Cytb* Tv3rd codon pos.	0.22, 0.04, 0.38, 0.08, 0.22
Bediagra rock lizard *Archaeolacerta*	No	*ND4*, *tRNA*$^{SER, LEU, HIS}$	2.74, 1.78

[1] Earthworms are not shown here because [35] did not test the molecular clock hypothesis.

***16S,COI* 2nd and 3rd codon positions and *H3* did not pass the molecular clock test. ** *12S* and *16S* not tested for linearity of rates.

Table 3. Summary of molecular rates for Corsica- Sardinia- Iberian Peninsula lineages. The first column shows whether substitution rates passed a molecular clock test; the second and third columns give the data as partitioned in the original study and the relative rates of substitutions. Rates are given as percentages of substitutions per site per lineage per million years for all partitions but for allozymes where rates are in percentages of genetic divergence *D* [66] per lineage per million years.

Even though *COI* rates are relatively similar in our dataset, we are by no means implying that these rates could be carelessly applied to other organisms and/or geographic contexts. There are at least two aspects that we think deserve attention; the time-slice we are looking at and the geographic setting. Deep nodes of a phylogeny often suffer from saturation of sequences; choosing the appropriate model of sequence evolution is then crucial to incorporate saturation in the estimates [42]. If sequences are not behaving in a clock-like manner, methods should be used to accommodate acceleration and deceleration of rates along the branches of a given phylogenetic tree without the need to clear the data set of the non-clock data [43,44]. As we move closer in time, the problem of the discrepancy between times of gene and population divergence arises. This is because prior to species divergence, a degree of gene divergence has already accrued in the ancestral species gene pool. This ancestral species divergence can be a large fraction of the total species divergence if the ancestral species was highly structured and, depending on the size of the ancestral population, could impact the first several million of years after divergence [42]. A way to get around this problem is to adopt a genealogical coalescent- based approach in the data analysis because this can robustly take into account the stochastic genealogical component to divergence [45]. Insularity is usually seen as a simplification when it comes to estimate divergence times. Species divergence, however, might precede isolation due to insularity. In other words, species age might be older than island age. If so and the island age is still used as calibration point, we would end up with biased estimates of molecular rates. Galàpagos and Barbados are examples of insular settings harbouring lineages older than the extant islands [46,47].

Figure 3 shows the molecular age estimates for the peri-Tyrrhenian groups considered in the present study arranged by the major geological events that affected the area.

It should be noted that those groups with a significant TreeMap analysis (aquatic subterranean isopods, stoneflies and newts) have ages consistently closer to the older geological estimates of splits of landmasses than groups with a non-significant TreeMap analysis have. The implication is that gene flow within these groups was discontinued at the geological onset of geographical barriers (detachment between the microplate from the Iberian Peninsula and split between the two islands, respectively). For those groups whose distribution includes the Tuscan Archipelago and/or coastal areas of Central Italy, divergence is relatively young in agreement with the recent interaction between those areas and Corsica. The only exception to this otherwise generalized pattern is *Hormogaster* (earthworms). For this group, allozymes indicate the split between Sardinian and Iberian lineages as coeval with the split between Sardinia and Tuscan Archipelago/Central Italy (17.5-13 Myr). If this hypothesis were true, this would imply that gene flow among these lineages ceased sometimes in the Middle Miocene. At the time, Corsica and Sardinia were either completely detached from the continent (classic scenario Figure 1) or connected through a land bridge to the emerging Italian peninsula (alternative scenario; inlets in Figure 1). Since we have to exclude both oversea dispersal for evident ecological reasons and human-mediated transport (genetic divergent would be much lower in that case) we should give credit to the land bridge hypothesis. Alternatively, and perhaps more parsimoniously, we think that the lack of any Corsican population in the data set is responsible [35]. The island is likely to host lineages phylogenetically intermediate between Sardinia and the Tuscan Archipelago/ Central Italy [48].

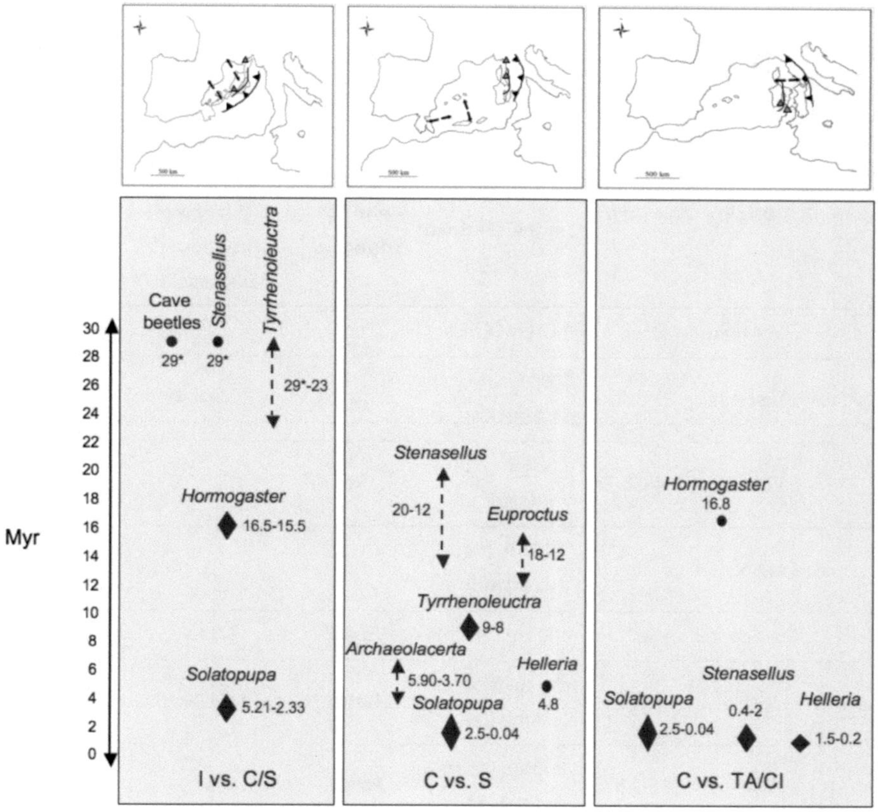

Figure 3. Within taxonomical group molecular age estimates of cladogenetic splits. Splits are sorted according to the three major geological events in the area (I vs. C/S: detachment of the microplate; C vs. S: separation of the two islands; C vs. TA/CI interaction between Corsica and coastal Tuscany). Age ranges (when available in the original source) are shown; asterisks indicate that a particular dating was used to calibrate substitution rates. The three uppermost panels illustrate the geological settings of the three events and are simplified versions of panels (b), (d), and (e) of Figure 1.

Comparisons between Corsican and Tuscan (both insular and continental) populations of *Helleria brevicornis* gave very young age estimates and a pattern of relationships without a visible geographic component [26]. MtDNA genealogy, coalescence inferences and distribution pattern (the species occurs spottily in Tuscany regardless of the abundance of suitable habitats) suggest historic, human-mediated transport as responsible, possibly due to the intense commercial trades existing in the area when the Tyrrhenian Sea was under Etruscan control [26].

8. Comparisons to other insular systems

All the molecular studies reviewed here consistently support a monophyletic origin for the Corsican-Sardinian lineages, regardless of what the relationships within the system are. Table

4 summarizes the main findings deduced from the evolutionary literature available for both continental and oceanic islands.

Island system	Origin	Age (Myr)	Minimum distance from the continent	Connection with the continent	Colonization Single (S)/ Multiple (M) Process Vicariance (V)/ Dispersal (D)	Radiation/ Adaptive radiation
Canary Islands[1]	Volcanic	21-1	110 km (Africa)	No	S/M-D	Yes/?
Hawaiian Islands[2]	Volcanic	29-0.40	3000 km (North America)	No	S/M-D	Yes/Yes
Galàpagos Islands[3]	Volcanic	4-0.5	960 km (South America)	No	S/M-D	Yes/Yes
Chatham Islands[4]	Continental	70	800 km (New Zealand)	No	S-V	Yes/?
Madagascar[5]	Continental	88	400 km (Africa)	Yes	S/M-V/D	Yes/Yes
West Indies[6]	Mixed*	48-20	81 km (North America)	Partial	S/M-D/V(?)	Yes/Yes
Philippine Islands[7,8]	Mixed*	28-2.5	800 km (Asian mainland)	Partial	M-D	Yes/Yes

* West Indies are of continental origin but Lesser Antilles are mostly volcanic. Philippines are the result of tectonic and volcanic activity and progressive uplift.

References: [1][52]; [2][53]; [3][47]; [4][51]; [5][28]; [6][55]; [7][54]; [8][67].

Table 4. Summary of phylogeographic reviews available on other insular systems. For each of them information on the origin, age (extant islands only), minimum distance from and past connection to the continent are given. The two last columns indicate whether insular lineages originated through single or multiple events, via vicariance or dispersal and whether there is evidence of within-system radiation and/or adaptive radiation.

We are aware that a crude comparison between islands of different origin would be meaningless, because intimately different are the ancestry and evolution of the respective biota. Remote oceanic islands can only be colonised through dispersal while both vicariance and dispersal play a role in determining the biological diversity of continental islands [49,50]. The contribution of either factor is related to a large extent to the dispersal ability of organisms. Vicariance is expected to be predominant in poor dispersers (as also shown for the Corsica-Sardinia system) while such a force would be less relevant (if not negligible) in those lineages with a strong vagility. Comparing the studies listed in Table 4 requires additional caution because the molecular data sets they are based upon are quite unbalanced in terms of taxonomic coverage. Hawaii, Galàpagos, Madagascar and West Indies have been covered from a

http://dx.doi.org/10.5772/55458

fair to a deep extent. This is not the case for the Chathams where only a few taxa have been considered.

Keeping in mind the above considerations, these studies show that a vicariant, monophyletic origin can be assumed only in the case of the four genera of large flightless insects from the old continental Chatham Islands (cockroaches, crickets and beetles) analyzed by [51]. About 60% of the invertebrates and 20% of the vertebrates Madagascar harbours have an ancient (i.e. Gondwanian; about 80 Myrs old) vicariant origin. On all the oceanic systems, lineages derived from multiple colonization events co-exist with lineages originated through single founding episodes. Multiple lineages of Canarian reptiles were established via independent episodes of colonization, while darkling beetles, brimstone butterflies and fruit flies reached the archipelago only once [52]. Some representatives of the extant terrestrial fauna of the remote archipelagos of Hawaii and Galàpagos, perhaps the best studied oceanic insular settings, derives from single colonizing episodes while for others molecular data do not justify such an assumption [47,53]. Groups with a monophyletic origin include some evolutionary paradigms such as the Hawaiian drosophilids and honeycreepers and the Galàpagos giant tortoises and Darwin's finches. The past physical connection, although partial, with the mainland of both West Indies and Philippine Islands facilitated colonization [54,55]. Intriguingly, West Indies have been identified also as source of colonization for the surrounding continents and not only as a sink [55].

Frequently lineages diversify on islands. Local lineage production can be repeated many times resulting in a radiation; radiation is sometimes associated with adaptation (adaptive radiation; Table 4). Table 1 shows that Corsica and Sardinia generally host lineages that have diversified locally. It shouldn't be overlooked, however, that only a few studies are based on a dense sampling of populations. We hence suspect the true number of genetic lineages to be underestimated. Keeping in mind the limitations in terms of sampled populations of the studies listed in Table 1, it should be noted that the highest number of detected lineages within either Corsica or Sardinia is seven (cave beetles; [25]). This figure is well below the estimates reported in Table 4, which in some cases exceed 50 (i.e. Hawaiian honeycreepers). Diversification on Corsica and Sardinia was certainly triggered when they became detached from the continent. Subsequent within-island evolution has been documented molecularly but very often it did not produce appreciable morphological differences. Illustrative is the case of the subterranean isopod *Stenasellus* [33,40,56]. The few known populations of this crustacean are virtually indistinguishable morphologically and yet they are deeply divergent from one another at both mitochondrial and nuclear loci.

Given the available data it is impossible to argue in favour of a Corsica-Sardinia radiation, let alone adaptive radiation. Corsica and Sardinia are not as isolated as the majority of the other insular systems listed in Table 4. Also, they are considerably younger than Madagascar and the Chathams, continental islands that witnessed radiation (with adaptation for Madagascar). Finally, it is not unrealistic to think that when the two islands started moving away from the continent they were not as species-poor as typically are young oceanic islands, which provide plenty of ecological opportunities for immigrants. The number of fossil and extant taxa that can be brought back to the initial phases of insularity of Corsica and Sardinia (see the Ecology and Endemism section) do not depict these islands as blank slates available for colonization and subsequent diversification but rather like hosting already structured biota.

9. Conclusions

Studies conducted so far on organisms with a peri-Tyrrhenian distribution have confirmed the area as one of primary interest for evolutionary research. It offers, in fact, the opportunity to test hypotheses in a well-defined biogeographical context due to the uniqueness of its fauna and the detailed knowledge of its past geological evolution. Available molecular data, along with the analyses carried out *de novo* for this review, suggest that diversification was predominantly driven by vicariance. Allopatry can be safely assumed for organisms strictly bound to freshwaters (both superficial and subterranean; crustacean isopods, stoneflies and newts). Nonetheless, we do believe that these researches have only started scraping the surface of a scenario that is emerging as more complex than previously thought.

The studies reviewed here were meant to unveil relationships at the species or even at the genus level; therefore sampling designs were rarely conceived to disentangle processes below those levels. The few studies designed at the population level failed in retrieving one-landmass one-monophyletic-lineage associations (land snail *Solatopupa guidoni*, terrestrial isopod *Helleria brevicornis*, Bediagra rock lizard *Archaeolacerta bediagrae*) [26,27,37]. This suggests that dispersal could dim the historical signal even in taxa that are apparently not well equipped for substantial movements over long distances. The number and kind of molecular markers used in relation to the evolutionary timescale they are trying to target is yet another critical issue. Most of the studies reviewed here are based on a single locus (often mtDNA). Such an approach works well to resolve old splits, but as one moves towards more recent events the information content of a single locus (which provides us with a gene tree) is rapidly blurred by the random noise typically associated with stochastic population processes. Hence, the discordance between what we have in hands (a gene tree) and what we should aim to (the species tree) is maximized.

From what emerges from this and other reviews (Table 4), it is evident that an accurate understanding of evolutionary processes on islands could be better attained when co-distributed taxonomically independent taxa are investigated in a comparative manner. For the Corsica-Sardinia system we are already in a good position because the work done so far in the area has already identified a number of species that could be used for the scope and for which we have fairly accurate phylogenetic reconstructions. We would now need samplings at the population level to maximize the likelihood to retrieve an accurate representation of their evolutionary histories. Studies conducted on insular endemisms (i.e. Galápagos tortoises, *Anolis* lizard) [47,55] have taught us that size of the island and within-island potential barriers to gene flow correlates positively with number of evolutionary independent lineages. In the case of Sardinia, the phylogeographic structure of the endemic carabid beetle *Percus strictus* [57] was found to accurately reflect the subdivision of the island into three separated landmasses at the beginning of the Pliocene. This potential source of genetic regionalism shouldn't be overlooked when planning further genetic studies. Ideally, samplings should include multiple populations to contrast genetic structuring on either side of the putative barriers to that across them.

Accurate sampling at the population level should then be coupled with a thorough screen of multiple molecular markers to minimize the gap between gene and species trees. This is being made easier by the escalating availability at reduced costs of high-throughput second-generation sequencing. Only until a few years ago, avoiding the limitations idiosyncratic to the single locus approach (as that applied to most of the peri-Tyrrhenian organisms reviewed here) would have required considerable investments in terms of both working time and financial resources. Nowadays, we are in the position to easily isolate batteries of highly polymorphic nuclear markers (microsatellites) [58]. Multi-locus Single Nucleotide Polymorphisms (SNPs) are emerging as even more powerful tools than microsatellites to infer structure of natural populations [59] and they are becoming increasingly popular as the technical challenges associated with their optimization subside. Thousands of SNPs can be identified in a relatively easy manner by using high-throughput sequencing of restriction-site-associated DNA tags (RAD tags); these markers have proved able to supply resolution sufficient to infer patterns of population relatedness [60]. For Corsica-Sardinia organisms we could take advantage of the molecular phylogenies already available. These could be used as guidelines to develop SNPs that are fixed or nearly fixed within populations but variable among them [61]. The genome-wide sample of genotype data is likely to overwhelm most of the sampling error (if any) and, hence, to produce better estimates of phylogeographic relationships without any prior investment in genomic resources being necessary.

The flourishing of new methods to harness large numbers of tailored-to-the-scope molecular markers has proceeded in parallel with (and partially stimulated) the development of sophisticated phylogeographic analytical tools [62]. At the same time, the rise of the coalescence theory is causing a shift in the treatment of phylogeographic data from exploratory to model-driven [62,63]. In an exploratory framework, phylogeographic inferences are based on qualitative interpretations of (often) single-locus gene genealogies. Molecular data, coupled with external information such as species ecology and landscape context, are used directly to infer the demographic history of taxa. This approach is necessary when an *a priori* phylogeographic hypothesis for the taxon (or the area) of interest is not available and has to be generated anew. In the fortunate circumstance that such *a priori* hypotheses exist, alternative scenarios could be discriminated statistically and the one that fits the data best be chosen [64]. In doing that we obviously restrict ourselves to a subset of the whole possible scenarios but with the advantage to accurately estimate key components of the species demography and history of divergence ([62] and references therein). Under a model-driven approach, gene genealogies are not anymore central to the phylogeographic analysis but they rather represent variables for connecting data to demographic parameters under an explicit statistical coalescent model [63]. The peri-Tyrrhenian area offers a unique opportunity to use the model-driven approach and to test its strengths and weaknesses because its geological history is well understood and relatively simple, thus restricting considerably the number of possible alternative phylogeographic scenarios, granted that the appropriate taxon is chosen (i.e. poor disperser). A further advantage is that the insular condition is per definition simpler than any continental one and, hence, complexity of models could be reduced at limited costs in terms of model misspecification risk.

About twenty years of molecular work on these fascinating Mediterranean islands have unveiled their potential as yet another natural laboratories for the study of evolutionary processes. This review, besides summing up what has already been done, wants to stimulate further research in the area. With both the methodological and analytical progresses that evolutionary biology has witnessed in recent years, it is not difficult to envision the Corsica-Sardinia system as an exceptional playground to investigate phylogeographic patterns at an unprecedented level.

Acknowledgements

We wish to thank Francesca Pavesi for producing the maps inFigures 1 and 3.

Author details

Valerio Ketmaier[1,2] and Adalgisa Caccone[3]

*Address all correspondence to: ketmaier@uni-potsdam.de

1 Institute of Biochemistry and Biology, University of Potsdam, Potsdam, Germany

2 Department of Biology and Biotechnology "Charles Darwin", University of Rome "La Sapienza", Rome, Italy

3 Department of Ecology & Evolutionary Biology, Yale University, New Haven, USA

References

[1] Baccetti B. Per una storia dell'esplorazione biogeografica delle isole che circondano la Sardegna. Biogeographia 1995; 18: 1-26.

[2] Minelli S, Ruffo S, Stoch F. Endemism in Italy. In: Ruffo S, Stoch F (eds.) Checklist and distribution of the Italian fauna. Memorie del Museo Civico di Storia Naturale di Verona. Verona; 2006. p29-31.

[3] Baccetti B. Biogeografia sarda venti anni dopo. Biogeographia 1980; 8: 859-870.

[4] Jeannel R. Les Psélaphides de l'Afrique du Nord. Essai de Biogéographie berbère. Memoirs du Museum d'Histoire Naturelle 1956; 14: 1-233.

[5] Alvarez W. Rotation of the Corsica- Sardinia microplate. Nature 1972; 235: 103-105.

[6] Alvarez W. Sardinia and Corsica, one microplate or two? Rendiconti del Seminario della Facoltà di Scienze dell'Università di Cagliari. Cagliari: Libreria Cocco; 1972.

[7] Sbordoni V, Caccone A, Allegrucci G, Cesaroni D. Molecular island biogeography. In: Azzaroli A (ed.) Biogeographical aspects of insularity, Atti dei Convegni Lincei, Volume 85. Accademia Nazionale dei Lincei. Roma; 1990. p55-83.

[8] Bellon H, Coulon C, Edel JB. Le déplacement de la Sardigne: synthèse des donnees géochronologiques, magmatiques et paléomagnétiques. Bulletin de la Societe Géologique de France 1977; 7: 825-831.

[9] Bonin B, Chotin P, Giret A, Orsini JB. Etude du bloc corso-sarde sur documents satellites: Le problème des mouvements différentiels entre les deux iles. Revue de Geographie Physique et de Geologie Dynamique 1979; 21: 147-154.

[10] Esu D, Kotsakis T. Les vertebres et les mollusques continentaux du Tertiarire de la Sardaigne: Palaeobiogeographie et biostratigraphie. Geologica Romana 1983; 22: 177-206.

[11] Lanza B: Sul significato biogeografico delle isole fossili, con particolare riferimento all'Arcipelago pliocenico della Toscana. Atti della Societa' Italiana di Scienze naturali 1984; 125: 145- 158.

[12] Boccaletti M, Ciaranfi N, Cosentino D, Deiana G, Gelati R, Lentini F, Massari F, Moratti G, Pescatore T, Lucchi FR, Tortorici L. Palinspatic restoration and palaeogeographic reconstruction of the peri-Tyrrhenian area during the Neogene. Palaeogeography Palaeoclimatology Palaeoecology 1990; 77: 41-50.

[13] Carmignani L, Decandia FA, Disperati L, Fantozzi PL, Lazzarotto A, Liotta D, Oggiano G. Relationships between the Tertiary structural evolution of the Sardinia-Corsica-Provencal Domain and the Northern Apennines. Terra Nova 1995; 7: 128-137.

[14] Robertson AHF, Grasso M. Overview of the late Tertiary-Recent tectonic and palaeoenvironmental development of the Mediterranean region. Terra Nova 1995; 7: 114-127.

[15] Meulenkamp JE, Sissingh W. Tertiary palaeogeography and tectonostratigraphic evolution of the Northern and Southern Peri-Tethys platforms and the intermediate domains of the African-Eurasian convergent plate boundary zone. Palaeogeography Palaeoclimatology Palaeoecology 2003; 196: 209-228.

[16] Lipparini T. Per la storia del popolamento delle isole dell'Arcipelago Toscano (contributo geo-paleontologico). Lavori della Societa' Italiana di Biogeografia 1976; 5: 13-25.

[17] Cherchi A, Montadert L. Oligo- Miocene rift of Sardinia and the early history of the western Mediterranean basin. Nature 1982; 298: 736- 739.

[18] Burgassi PD, Decandia FA, Lazzarotto A. Elementi di stratigrafia e paleogeografia nelle colline metallifere (Toscana) dal Trias al Quaternario. Memorie della Societa' Geologica Italiana 1983; 25: 27-50.

[19] La Greca M. The insect biogeography of west Mediterranean islands. Atti dei Convegni Lincei 1990; 85: 459-468.

[20] Duggen S, Hoernle K, van den Bogaard P, Rupke L, Morgan JP. Deep roots of the Messinian salinity crisis. Nature 2003; 422: 602–606.

[21] Lambeck K, Antonioli F, Purcell A, Silenzi S. Sea-level change along the Italian coast for the past 10,000 year. Quaternary Science Reviews 2004; 23: 1567–1598.

[22] Smith AT, Johnston CH. Prolagus sardus. IUCN Red List of Threatened Species. Version 2011.2 [www.iucnredlist.org]

[23] Caccone A, Milinkovitch MC, Sbordoni V, Powell JR. Molecular biogeography: using the Corsica- Sardinia microplate disjunction to calibrate mitochondrial rDNA evolutionary rates in mountain newts (*Euproctus*). Journal of Evolutionary Biology 1994; 7: 227- 245.

[24] Caccone A, Milinkovitch MC, Sbordoni V, Powell JR. Mitochondrial DNA rates and biogeography in European newts (genus *Euproctus*). Systematic Biology 1997; 46: 126-144.

[25] Caccone A, Sbordoni V. Molecular biogeography of cave life: a study using mitochondrial DNA from Bathysciine beetles. Evolution 2001; 55: 122-130.

[26] Gentile G, Campanaro A, Carosi M, Sbordoni V, Argano R. Phylogeography of Helleria brevicornis Ebner 1868 (Crustacea: Isopoda): old and recent differentiations of an ancient lineage. Molecular Phylogenetics and Evolution 2010; 54: 640-646.

[27] Salvi D, Harris DJ, Bombi P, Carretero MA, Bologna MA. Mitochondrial phylogeography of the Bedriaga's rock lizard, *Archaeolacerta bedriagae* (Reptilia: Lacertidae) endemic to Corsica and Sardinia. Molecular Phylogenetics and Evolution 2010; 56: 690-697.

[28] Yoder AD, Nowak MD. Has vicariance or dispersal been the predominant biogeographic force in Madagascar? Only time will tell. Annual Revue of Ecology Evolution Systematics 2006; 37: 405-431.

[29] Durand JD, Bianco PG, Laroche J, Gilles A. Insight into the origin of endemic mediterranean ichthyofauna: Phylogeography of *Chondrostoma* genus (Teleostei, Cyprinidae). Journal of Heredity 2003; 94: 315-328.

[30] Ketmaier V, Bianco PG, Durand JD. Molecular systematics, phylogeny and biogeography of roaches (*Rutilus*, Teleostei, Cyprinidae). Molecular Phylogenetics and Evolution 2008; 49: 362-367.

[31] Csilléry K, Blum MGB, Gaggiotti OE, François O. Approximate Bayesian Computation (ABC) in practice. Trends in Ecology and Evolution2010; 25: 410-418.

[32] Page RDM. Parallel phylogenies: reconstructing the history of host-parasite assemblages. Cladistics 1994; 10: 155-173.

[33] Ketmaier V, Argano R, Caccone A. Phylogeography and molecular rates of subterranean aquatic Stenasellid Isopod with a peri-Tyrrhenian distribution. Molecular Ecology 2003; 12: 547-555.

[34] Fochetti R, Sezzi E, Tierno de Figueroa JM, Modica MV, Oliverio M. Molecular systematics and biogeography of the Western Mediterranean stonefly genus *Tyrrhenoleuctra* (Insecta, Plecoptera). Journal of Zoological Systematics and Evolutionary Research 2009; 47: 328-336.

[35] Cobolli Sbordoni M, De Matthaeis E, Alonzi A, Mattoccia M, Omodeo P, Rota E. Speciation, genetic divergence and palaeogeography in the Hormogastridae. Soil Biology and Biochemistry 1992; 24: 1213-1221.

[36] Novo M, Almodóvar A, Fernández R, Giribet G, Díaz Cosín DJ. Understanding the biogeography of a group of earthworms in the Mediterranean basin- The phylogenetic puzzle of Hormogastridae (Clitellata: Oligochaeta). Molecular Phylogenetics and Evolution 2011; 61: 125-135.

[37] Ketmaier V, Manganelli G, Tiedemann R, Giusti F. Peri-Tyrrhenian phylogeography in the land snail *Solatopupa guidoni* (Pulmonata). Malacologia 2010; 52: 81-96.

[38] Giusti F. Biogeographical data on the malacofauna of Sardinia. Malacologia 1977; 16: 125-129.

[39] Ketmaier V, Giusti F, Caccone A. Molecular phylogeny and historical biogeography of the land snail genus *Solatopupa* (Pulmonata) in the peri-Tyrrhenian area. Molecular Phylogenetics and Evolution 2006; 39: 439 – 451.

[40] Ketmaier V, Argano R, Cobolli M, De Matthaeis E. Genetic divergence and evolutionary times: calibrating a protein clock for South- European *Stenasellus* species (Crustacea, Isopoda). International Journal of Speleology 1999; 26: 63-74.

[41] Fochetti R, Ketmaier V, Oliverio M, Tierno de Figueroa JM, Sezzi E. Biochemical systematics and biogeography of the Mediterranean genus *Tyrrhenoleuctra* (Plecoptera, Insecta). *Insect Systematics and Evolution* 2004; 35: 299-306.

[42] Arbogast BS., Edwards SV, Wakeley J, Beerli P, Slowinski JB. Estimating divergence times from molecular data on population genetic and phylogenetic time scales. Annual Review of Ecology Evolution and Systematics 2002; 33: 707–740.

[43] Sanderson MJ. A non-parametric approach to estimating divergence times in the absence of rate constancy. Molecular Biology and Evolution 1997; 14: 1218-1231.

[44] Sanderson MJ. Estimating absolute rates of molecular evolution and divergence times: A penalized likelihood approach. Molecular Biology and Evolution 2002; 19: 101-109.

[45] Rosenberg NA, Feldman MW. The relationship between coalescence times and population divergence times. In Slatkin M, Veuille M. (eds.) Modern developments in theoretical population genetics. Oxford: Oxford University Press; 2002. p130-164.

[46] Thorpe RS, Reardon JT, Malhotra A. Common garden and natural selection experiments support ecotypic differentiation in the Dominican anole (*Anolis oculatus*). American Naturalist 2005; 165: 495-504.

[47] Parent CF, Caccone A, Petren K. Colonization and diversification of Galàpagos terrestrial fauna: a phylogenetic and biogeographical synthesis. *Philosophical Transactions of the Royal Society B* 2008; 363: 3347-3361.

[48] Omodeo P, Rota E. Earthworm diversity and land evolution in three Mediterranean districts. Proceedings of the California Academy of Sciences 2008; 59: 65-83.

[49] Poulakakis N, Russello M, Geist D, Caccone A. Unravelling the peculiarities of island life: vicariance, dispersal and the diversification of the extinct and extant Galàpagos giant tortoises. Molecular Ecology 2011; 21: 160-173.

[50] Sequeira AS, Stepien CC, Sijapati M, Roque Albelo L. Comparative genetic structure and demographic history in endemic Galàpagos weevils. *Journal of Heredity* 2012; 103: 206-220.

[51] Trewick SA. Molecular evidence for dispersal rather than vicariance as the origin of flightless insect species on the Chatham Islands, New Zeland. Journal of Biogeography 2000; 27: 1189-1200.

[52] Juan C, Emerson BC, Oromí P, Hewitt GM. Colonization and diversification: towards a phylogeographic synthesis for the Canary Islands. Trends in Ecology and Evolution 2000; 15: 104-109.

[53] Cowie RH, Holland BS. Molecular biogeography and diversification of the endemic terrestrial fauna of the Hawaiian Islands. Philosophical Transactions of the Royal Society B 2008; 363: 3363-3376.

[54] Jones AW, Kennedy RS. Evolution in a tropical archipelago: comparative phylogeography of Philippine fauna and flora reveals complex patterns of colonization and diversification. Biological Journal of the Linnean Society 2008; 95: 620-639.

[55] Ricklefs R, Bermingham E. The West Indies as a laboratory of biogeography and evolution. Philosophical Transactions of the Royal Society B 2008; 363: 2393-2413.

[56] Ketmaier V, Messana G, Cobolli M, De Matthaeis E, Argano R. Biochemical biogeography and evolutionary relationships among the six known populations of *Stenasel-*

lus racovitzai (Crustacea, Isopoda) from Corsica, Tuscany and Sardinia. Archiv fuer Hydrobiologie 2000; 147: 297-309.

[57] Ketmaier V, Casale A, Cobolli M, De Matthaeis E, Vigna Taglianti A. Biochemical systematics and phylogeography of the *Percus strictus* subspecies (Coleoptera, Carabidae), endemic to Sardinia. The Italian Journal of Zoology 2003; 70: 339-346.

[58] Santana QC, Coetzee MPA., Steenkamp ET, Mlonyeni OX, Hammond GNA, Wingfield MJ, Wingfield BD. Microsatellite discovery by deep sequencing of enriched genomic libraries. BioTechnique 2009; 46: 217-223.

[59] Glover KA, Hansen MM, Lien S, Als TD, Hoyheim B, Skaala O. A comparison of SNP and STR loci for delineating population structure and performing individual genetic assignment. BMC Genetics 2010; 11: doi: 10.1186/1471-2156-11-2

[60] Hohenlohe PA, Bassham S, Etter PD, Stiffler N, Johnson EA, Cresko WA. Population genomics of parallel adaptation in threespine stickleback using Sequenced RAD Tags. PLOS Genetics 2010; 6: doi: 10.1371/journal.pgen.1000862

[61] Emerson KJ, Merz CR, Catchen JM, Hohenlohe PA, Cresko WA, Bradshaw WE, Holzapfel CM. Resolving postglacial phylogeography using high-throughput sequencing. Proceedings of the National Academy of Sciences 2010; 107: 16196–16200.

[62] Garrick RC, Caccone A, Sunnucks P. Inference of population history by coupling exploratory and model-driven phylogeographic analyses. International Journal of Molecular Science 2010; 11: 1190-1127.

[63] Hickerson MJ, Carstens BC, Cavender-Bras J, Crandall KA, Graham CH, Johnson JB, Rissler L, Victoriano PF, Yoder AD. Phylogeography's past, present, and future: 10 years after Avise, 2000. Molecular Phylogenetics and Evolution 2010; 54: 291-301.

[64] Knowles LL. The burgeoning field of statistical phylogeography. Journal of Evolutionary Biology 2004; 17: 1-10.

[65] Avise JC, Arnold J, Ball RM, Bermingham E, Lamb T, Neigel JE, Reeb CA, Saunders NC. Intraspecific phylogeography: the mitochondrial DNA bridge between population genetics and systematics. Annual Review of Ecology Evolution and Systematics 1987; 18: 489–522.

[66] Nei M. Estimation of average heterozygosity and genetic distance from a small number of individuals. Genetics 1978; 89: 583- 590.

[67] Heaney LR, Rickart EA. 1990 Correlations of clades and clines: geographic, elevational and phylogenetic distribution patterns among Philippine mammals. In Peters G, Hutterer R (eds.) Vertebrates in the Tropics. Bonn: Museum Alexander Koenig; 1990. p321-332.

Chapter 5

The Biogeography of the Butterfly Fauna of Vietnam With a Focus on the Endemic Species (Lepidoptera)

A.L. Monastyrskii and J.D. Holloway

Additional information is available at the end of the chapter

http://dx.doi.org/10.5772/55490

1. Introduction

Long term studies of Vietnamese Rhopalocera suggest that by using a taxonomic composition analysis of the modern fauna, with ecological and biogeographical characteristics and comparative data with butterfly faunas of adjacent regions, it is possible to offer a plausible account of the history and derivation of the Vietnamese fauna. In former works on the butterfly fauna of Vietnam and of the Oriental tropics generally, we completed the first steps in understanding possible derivation mechanisms for the group. In particular, all Vietnamese butterfly species have been classified according to their global geographical ranges (Holloway, 1973; 1974; Spitzer *et al.*, 1993; Monastyrskii, 2006; 2007), from the most restricted to the most widespread (Methods). A similar approach for notodontid moths in Thailand has been adopted by Schintlmeister & Pinratana (2007). Moreover, depending on the representation of various species distribution range categories, a scheme of biogeographical zonation has been suggested (Monastyrskii, 2006; 2007).

In continuing studies on the specificity and derivation of the modern Vietnam butterfly fauna, aspects of species range configuration and other parameters of butterfly distributions are considered in the current work. For example, it is possible to assign genera to groups according to both their overall range and variation of their species-richness across that range (Holloway, 1969, 1974) or according to representation of particular species range types within the genera (Holloway, 1998). Application of the first approach led to recognition of several generic distribution types within the Oriental Region that provide a foundation for the discussion of species ranges presented in this paper, such as: genera with a species-richness generally distributed from Assam to Sundaland (Indo-Burmese in this paper); genera with their greatest richness in Sundaland (Sundanian in this paper); and genera with a strong centre of richness in western China and the eastern Himalaya (Sino-

Himalayan in this paper). Representation of genera in the third category was low in the analysis by Holloway (1969) because of the inadequacy of data available at that time and also because of the weakness of many generic concepts, but the category is epitomized by the *Zephyrus* group of genera covered by Koiwaya (2007). Though some of the taxonomic concepts in Koiwaya's work need further investigation for the Indochinese fau na, the gross figures indicate that over 30 species in this diverse generic complex occur in northern Vietnam and Laos, but very few penetrate further south than this. This will be seen to hold for the butterfly fauna in this generic category generally except for a small outpost in the Da Lat Mountains. Recent important studies on the biogeographical features of Vietnam, including relatively new geological and palaeontological information, are also considered (Takhtajan, 1986; Holloway & Hall, 1998; Tougard, 2001; Averyanov *et al.*, 2003).

Consequences of tectonic collisions of the Indian Plate with the Eurasian Plate will have inevitably facilitated the mixing of previously isolated groups of plants and animals (Hall, 1998). This mixing will have promoted competition between taxa and resulted in the relative success of some taxonomic groups and the extinction of others. Further geological events included the rapid growth of the Himalayan mountain range whose development has split the formerly adjoined Asiatic and Southeast Asiatic faunas and floras (Hall, 1998; Sterling *et al.*, 2006). As well as these processes, global cooling and glacial events have also had an impact on the topographic and climatic history of this region and have greatly transformed compositions of many faunas (Tougard, 2001; Outlaw & Voelker, 2007) including butterflies (Holloway, 1969; 1974). With the appearance of the Arctic ice sheet at the beginning of Pleistocene, large-scale global glaciations began. During this epoch a series of alternating processes of global warming and cooling have resulted in the cyclic reduction and extension of mainland and island areas, and the disappearance and appearance of connecting land bridges (Hanebuth *et al.*, 2000; Voris, 2000). Palynological data for the Late Quaternary in the Indochinese Peninsula are sparse, but suggest that conditions in the Late Glacial Maximum in the Peninsula and in southern China were cooler and drier than at present, with a change to warmer and wetter conditions at about 9000 years B.P. (Maxwell & Liu, 2002). These authors review data from lake sediments in the lowlands of the north-east of both Thailand and Cambodia that indicate development of dense forest with reduced fire activity in the warmer period, with evergreen 'islands' embedded in dry deciduous forest, the latter now strongly influenced by anthropogenic burning.

In accepting the landscape reconstructions of these epochs, as suggested by the Russian geologist Synitsin (1962, 1965) and later confirmed by many authors (e.g. Hall, 1998; 2002), from the beginning of Palaeocene, and perhaps even earlier, a geographically stable area of land has developed in Southeast Asia to form the Indochinese Peninsula. Configuration of this part of the mainland has changed insignificantly since the Mesozoic era. With such relative stability of the mainland, landscapes and climate weakly supported the forming and transforming of floristic and faunistic zonation. As a result the fauna and flora of this area demonstrate small changes even during major global climatic fluctuations. However, of particular relevance to Vietnam and the Indochinese Peninsula generally is the uplift of a series of mountain ranges on the eastern margin of the Peninsula. This uplift occurred in various eras and epochs, but it has been more intensive during the Neogene. In this period several Asiatic and, in particular, Indochinese mountain systems have reached the elevations seen today (Averyanov *et al.*, 2003; Rundel, 1999). Such factors have impacted on the Vietnamese butterfly fauna, the modern composition and biogeographical structure of which are described below.

2. Methods

2.1. Study area and the collecting of material

The current studies are based on the materials collected in more than 60 sites of Vietnam, including 20 sites in 13 administrative provinces of northern of Vietnam; 30 sites (13 provinces) in central Vietnam and 10 sites (8 provinces) in southern part of the country. Site descriptions are represented in detail in Monastyrskii (2005, 2007). The collecting programme has been carried out from 1994 to 2008, managed by different Vietnamese research organizations and conservation NGO's based in Vietnam. A significant part of the research material has been provided by the collections of the Natural History Museum in London (BMNH) and the National Museum of Natural History in Paris (MNHN). Individuals were collected with different kinds of net allowing catching specimens from different strata within natural forests from the ground to canopies that can be as high as 8 metres. Standard butterfly traps were also operated during field works for collecting fruit-feeding butterfly species (DeVries, 1988; Austin & Riley, 1995; Tangah *et al.*, 2004; Monastyrskii, 2011).

2.2. Taxonomic foundation

Identification work has been carried out using modern taxonomic literature concerning the butterfly fauna of Vietnam (Monastyrskii, 2005; 2007, 2011) and adjacent areas (Corbet, Pendlebury & Eliot, 1992; Ek-Amnuay, 2006 *etc.*). Moreover an important part of the identification process has been based on original comparative work due to demonstrate distinctive characteristics of the local taxa. During this work over one hundred new species and subspecies representing all butterfly families have been described from 1995 up to date.

Biogeographical data can be classified according to (1) gross range types and (2) more topographical and habitat-based data from within Vietnam.

1. Global geographical ranges of Vietnamese butterflies suggested in our previous publications (Monastyrskii, 2006; 2007; 2010b) include nine categories: 1. Endemics of Indochina; 2. Sino-Himalayan species; 3. Indo-Burmese species; 4. Species with an Oriental (particularly Sundanian) distribution; 5. Species with an Indo-Australian distribution; 6. Species with a Palaearctic distribution extending into the Oriental region; 7. Old-World tropical species; 8. Holarctic species extending into the Oriental region; and 9. Cosmopolitan species (Fig. 1)

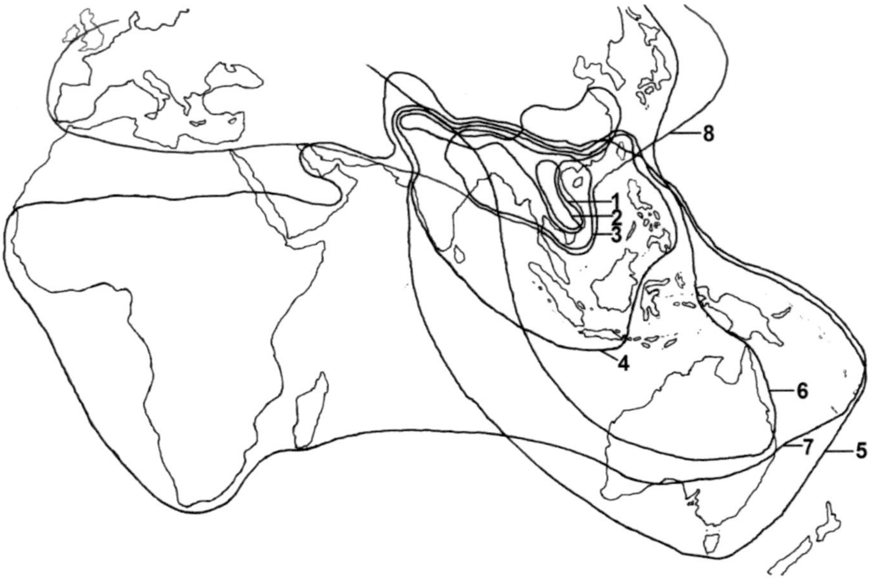

Figure 1. Boundaries of the Vietnamese butterfly biogeographical ranges: (1) Indochinese endemics, (2) Sino- Himalayan species, (3) Indo-Burmese species; (4) Indo-Malayan species, (5) Indo-Australian species, (6) Australo-Oriento-Palaearctic species; (7) Palaeotropical species and (8) Holarctic species. The boundary of the sole cosmopolitan species (9) *Vanessa cardui* (Nymphalinae) is not shown.

2. Configurations of butterfly ranges in Vietnam, and in Indochina discussed in the current work, include the following types: **a.** isolated endemic ranges (Fig. 2A): 1. – *Lethe philemon* (Nymphalidae, Satyrinae); 2. – *Heliophorus smaragdinus* (Lycaenidae); 3. – *Euthalia hoa* (Nymphalidae, Limenitidinae) **b.** continuous and mosaic ranges (Fig. 2B): *Ypthima baldus* (Nymphalidae, Satyrinae); **c.** disjunct ranges (Fig. 2C): *Mycalesis unica* (Nymphalidae, Satyrinae); and **d.** vicarious ranges (Fig. 2D): six representatives of *Ypthima sakra* group (Nymphalidae, Satyrinae).

The great diversity of isolation factors can be demonstrated by the schematic landscape profiles drawn in the north-south direction across the entire Vietnam territory (Fig. 4); they reveal considerable variation in the altitudes. One profile (I) runs along the principal mountain ranges (above 2000 m) of Hoang Lien Son in the north and Truong Son in the central part of Vietnam (including Kon Tum and Da Lat Plateaux). The other profile (II) runs across the plains and low mountains (0–500 m) along the coastline. According to this diagram, there are two types of isolating barriers in Vietnam. Firstly, there are significant fluctuations in altitude in the north-south mountain ranges, isolating mountain faunas of the Truong Son Range (Da Lat and Kon Tum Plateaux, the northern Truong Son) and the Hoang Lien Son Range (the southern part of Yunnan Mountains). The relative position of altitude belts and the previously proposed subdivision of biogeographical provinces associated with them are shown in Fig. 1. Secondly, these mountain ranges themselves separate the coastal zone, itself also hilly, from other lowlands of the Indochinese Peninsula, which are found west of Profile I in the diagram.

http://dx.doi.org/10.5772/55490

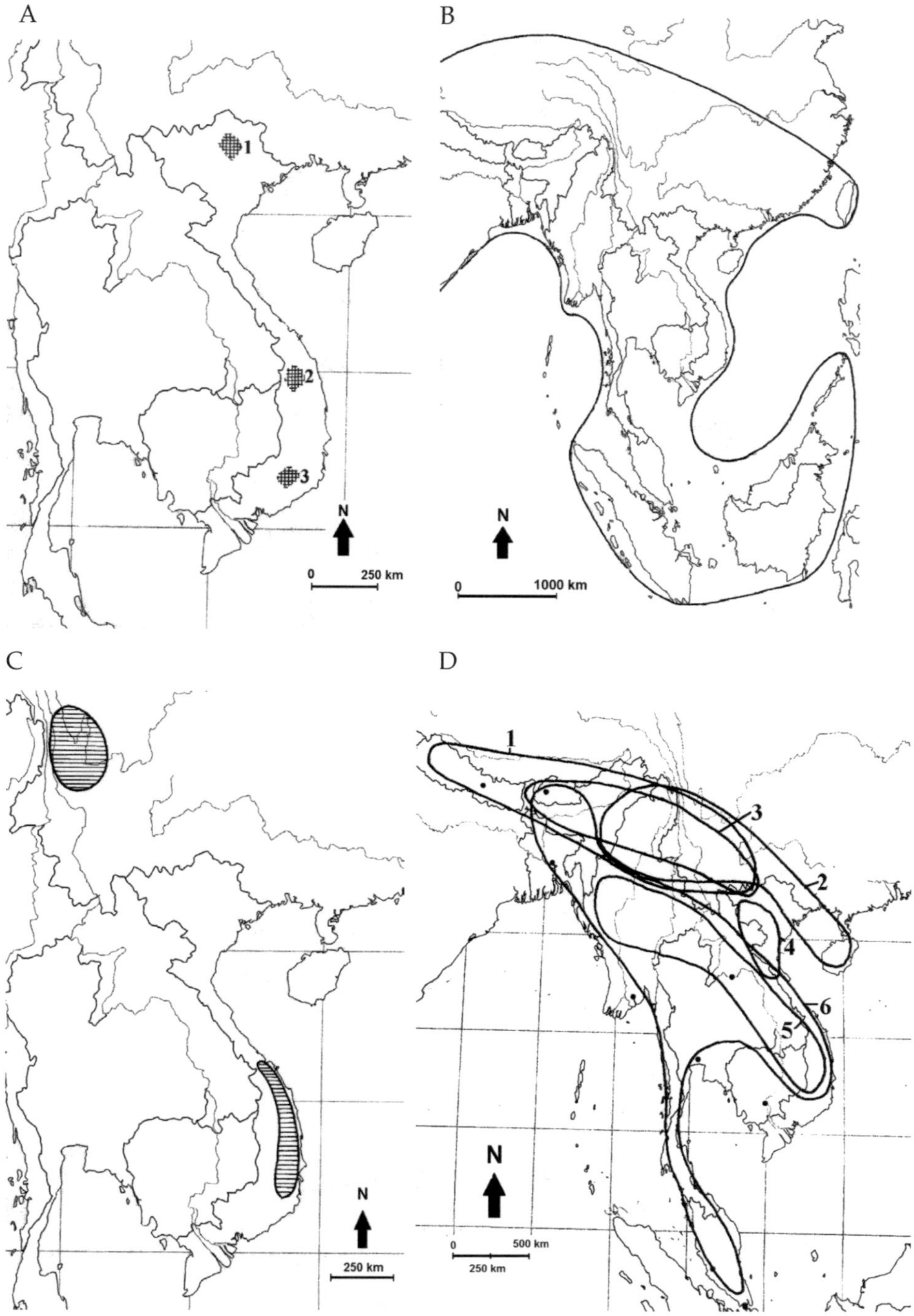

Figure 2. The main types of configurations of the butterfly ranges in Vietnam: A – Isolated (1 – *Lethe philemon*; 2 – *Heliophorus smaragdinus*; 3 – *Euthalia hoa*); B – Continuous (*Ypthima baldus*); C – Disjunct (*Mycalesis unica*); D - Vicarious (*Ypthima sakra* group): 1 – *Y. sakra*; 2 – *Y. atra*; 3 – *Y. persimilis*, 4 – *Y. pseudosavara*; 5 – *Y. evansi*; 6 – *Y. dohertyi*

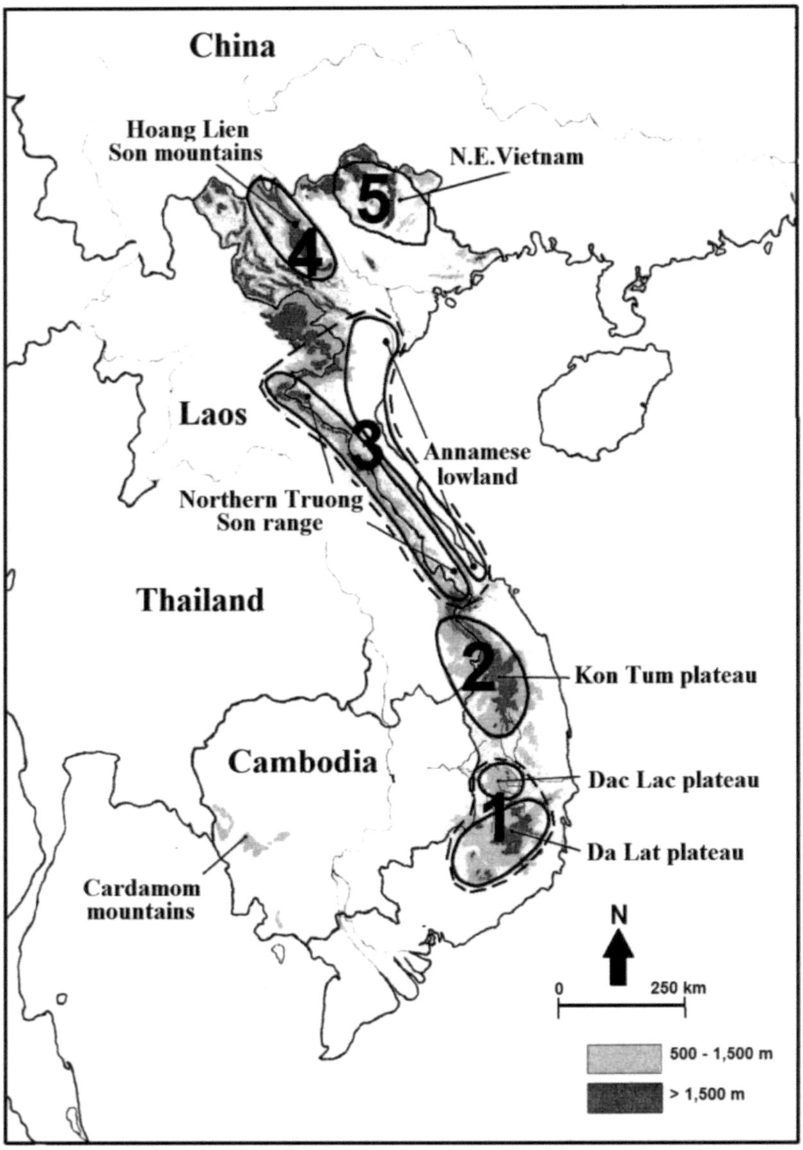

Figure 3. Butterfly endemism centres in Vietnam

3. Ranges of endemic Vietnamese butterflies

There are over 1100 butterfly species currently known from Vietnam. Approximately seven percent of all species are considered as endemic to the Indochinese Peninsula (Vietnam, Laos, Cambodia and eastern Thailand) (Monastyrskii, 2010a). These distinctive species, listed in the Appendix, are restricted to within the Peninsula border and have not yet been found in adjacent areas (Figs. 5-7).

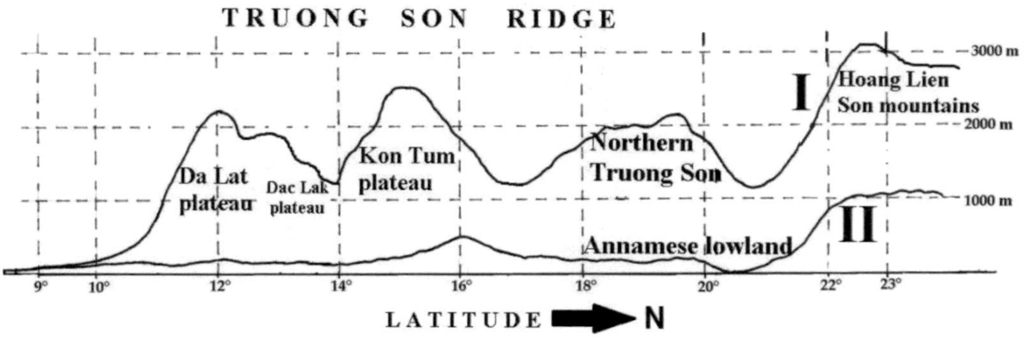

Figure 4. North-south Profiles of the Vietnamese landscapes through the main areas of endemism (indicated): I - Main ridges above 2000m; II - Lowland landscapes (0-500m) along the shoreline

The majority of endemic butterfly species range over isolated mountain massifs of the central Vietnamese Highlands and some areas in the northern part of the country (Fig. 3). Most of the smaller number of endemics that occur in the most southerly of these isolated montane areas, such as the Kon Tum and Da Lat (including small Dac Lac plateau) plateaus, are unknown in other parts of the Peninsula although there is a relatively small and lower altitude massif of mountains in western Cambodia called the Cardamom Mountains. However, according to preliminary studies, this area supports a much lower number of endemic butterfly taxa.

In Vietnam, endemic butterfly taxa consist mainly of geographically isolated populations. These species and subspecies are usually separated for hundreds or even thousands of kilometres from their nearest relatives. However, in Vietnam there are often very short distances (up to a few tens of kilometres) between isolated species populations and other parts of the range of a taxon. Such cases demonstrate that even small gaps, characterised by specificity of landscapes and habitats, are enough to break the process of genetic interchange and to promote development of separate taxa.

The concentration of endemic butterfly species is much higher in: the Da Lat and Dac Lac plateaus (Lam Dong and Dac Lac provinces) **(1)**; Kon Tum plateau (Gia Lai and Kon Tum provinces) **(2)**; northern Truong Son range and Annamese lowlands (Nghe An, Ha Tinh, Quang Binh and Quang Tri provinces) **(3)**; Hoang Lien Son range **(4)**; and the eastern region of N. Vietnam (Bac Kan and Lang Son provinces) **(5)** (Fig. 3) (Monastyrskii, 2007). These Vietnamese endemic butterfly species exhibit links to relatives distributed in different biogeographical zones. A number of Vietnamese endemic species have closely related species among representatives of the Sino-Himalayan and Sundanian faunas (Figs. 5 and 6). Another group of endemic taxa belongs to the local autochthonous Indo-Burmese fauna (Holloway, 1973) (Fig. 7). Distribution of the endemic butterfly species in Vietnam and their range features is described below.

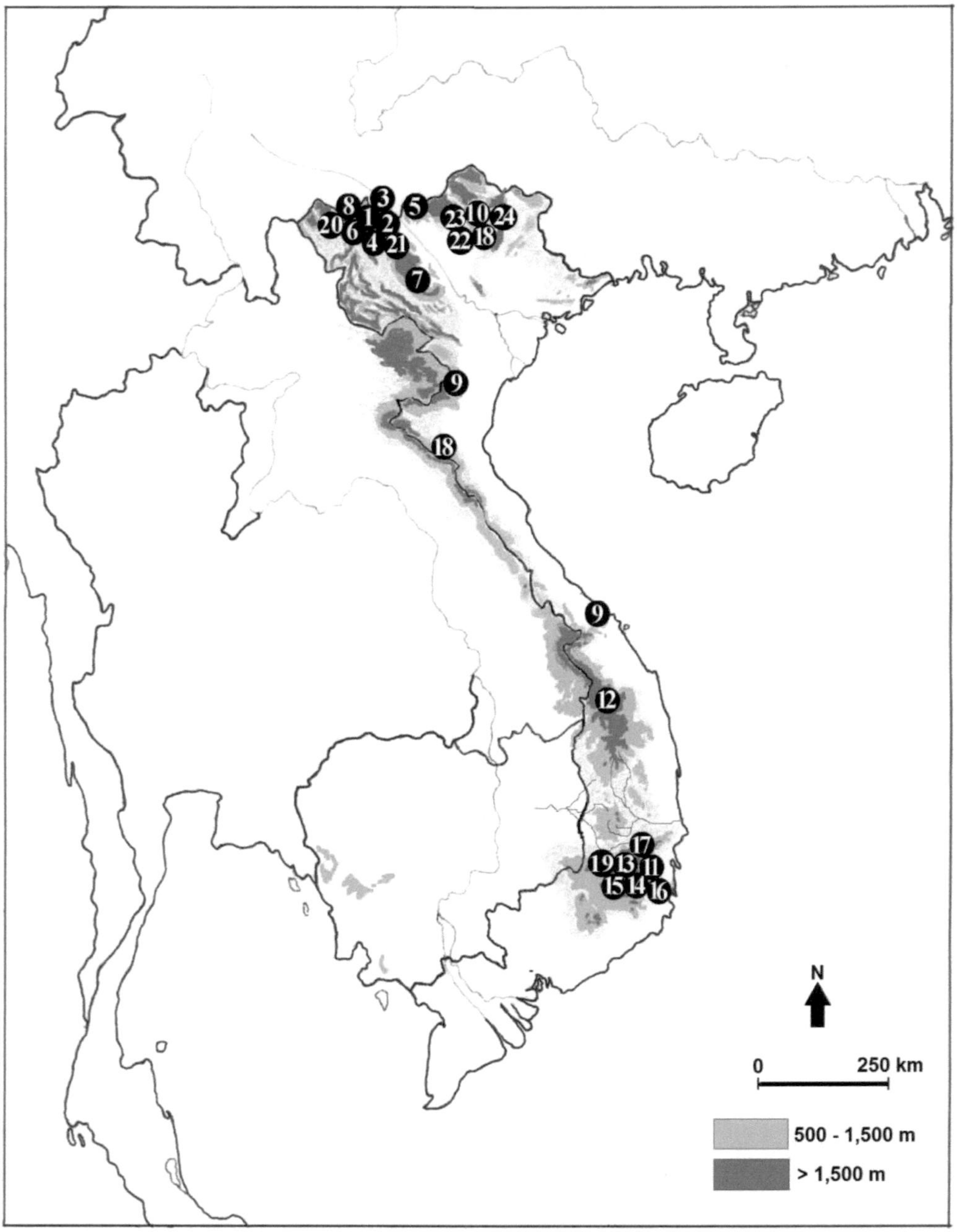

Figure 5. Endemic butterfly taxa of Indochina showing link with Sino-Himalayan fauna: 1- *Ypthima frontierii*; 2 – *Euthalia khambounei*; 3 – *Euaspa nishimurai*; 4 – *Shirozuozephyrus masatoshii*; 5 – *Proteuaspa akikoae*; 6 – *Chrysozephyrus vietnamicus*; 7 – *Lethe berdievi*; 8 – *Chrysozephyrus hatoyamai*; 9 – *Chrysozephyrus wakaharai*; 10 – *Calinaga funeralis*; 11 – *Euthalia hoa*; 12 – *Heliophorus smaragdinus*; 13 – *Euaspa minaei*; 14 – *Neptis transita*; 15 – *Chilasa imitata*; 16 - *Phaedyma armariola*; 17 - *Euthalia strephonida*; 18 - *Mycalesis inopia*; 19 – *Shirozuozephyrus alienus*; 20 – *Coladenia koiwaii*; 21 - *Praescobura chrysomaculata*; 22 – *Celaenorrhinus victor*; 23 - *Scobura eximia*; 24 – *Celaenorrhinus phuongi*

http://dx.doi.org/10.5772/55490

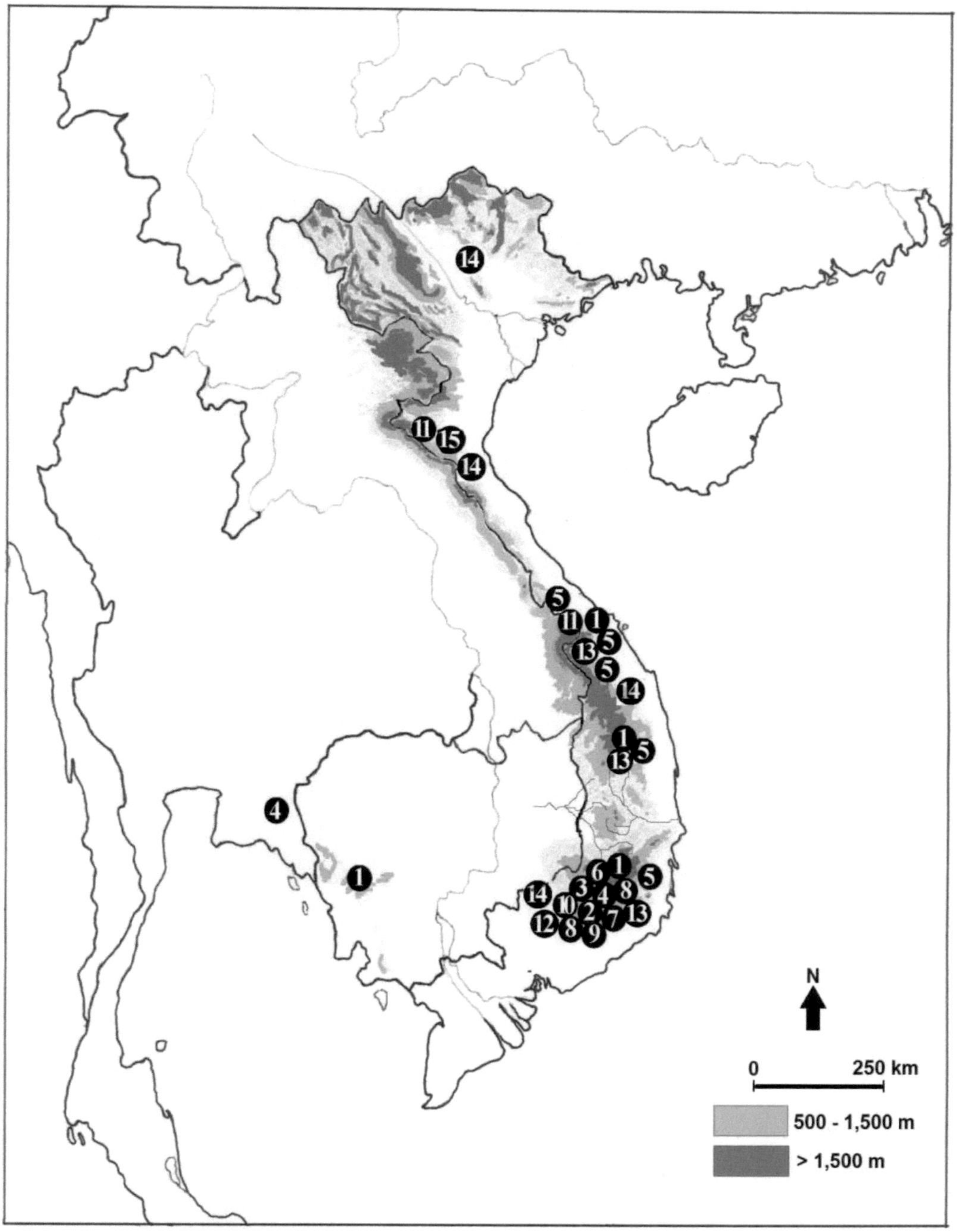

Figure 6. Endemic butterfly taxa of Indochina showing link with Sundanian fauna: 1- *Delias vietnamensis*; 2 – *Discophora aestheta*; 3 – *Cyllogenes milleri*; 4 – *Euploea orontobates*; 5 – *Zeuxidia sapphirus*; 6 – *Ypthima daclaca*; 7 – *Deramas cham*; 8 – *Tanaecia stellata*; 9 – *Tajuria sekii*; 10 – *Tajuria shigehoi*; 11 – *Elymnias saola*; 12 – *Eurema novapallida*; 13 – *Faunis bicoloratus*; 14 – *Suada albolineata*; 15 – *Neomyrina* sp.

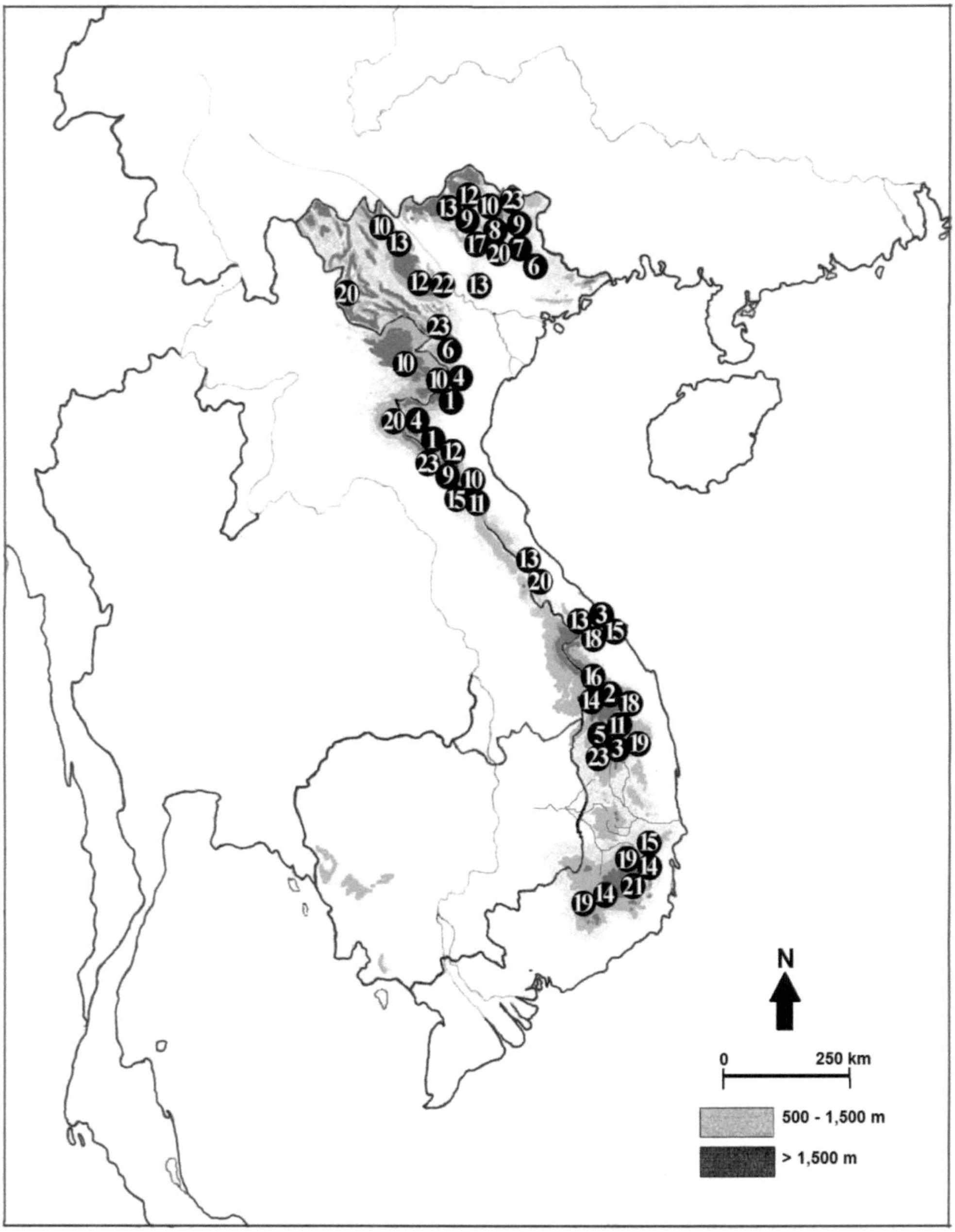

Figure 7. Endemic butterfly taxa of Indochina showing link with Indo-Burmese fauna: 1 – *Halpe paupera*; 2 – *Lethe melisana*; 3 – *Aemona simulatrix*; 4 – *Ypthima pseudosavara*; 5 – *Lethe konkakini*; 6 – *Lethe philesanoides*; 7 – *Lethe huongii*; 8 – *Lethe philemon*; 9 – *Lethe philesana*; 10 – *Graphium phidias*; 11 – *Dodona katerina*; 12 – *Aemona implicata*; 13 – *Aemona tonkinensis*; 14 – *Dodona speciosa*; 15 – *Pintara capiloides*; 16 – *Aemona kontumei*; 17 – *Penthema michallati*; 18 – *Stichophthalma eamesi*; 19 – *Stichophthalma uemurai*; 20 – *Stichophthalma mathilda*; 21 – *Aemona falcata*; 22 – *Aemona berdyevi*; 23 – *Taxila dora*

http://dx.doi.org/10.5772/55490

3.1. Endemics of the Da Lat plateau

There are twenty nine endemic butterfly species recorded within the border of Da Lat plateau. Twenty species have not been recorded outside of this mountain region so far. Additionally, several other species show distinct subspecific differences on the plateau (Monastyrskii, 2010a). The Da Lat endemics show a diversity of phylogenetic relationships with representatives of other biogeographic regions.

The endemic swallowtail *Chilasa imitata,* nymphalids *Euthalia hoa, E. strephonida, Phaedyma armariola, Neptis transita,* and lycaenids *Euaspa minaei* and *Shirozuozephyrus alienus* (Fig. 5) are related to species from Tibet, E. Himalayas, W. & C. China (Monastyrskii & Devyatkin 2003; Monastyrskii, 2005; Koiwaya & Monastyrskii, 2010). Some endemic species of the Da Lat plateau and their Sino-Himalayan relatives are separated by hundreds to thousands of kilometres (Appendix).

Ranges of some other relatives of endemic taxa are located in close proximity to the Da Lat plateau. For example, the closest relation to the recently described *Chilasa imitata* (Papilionidae) is *Ch. epycides,* which is widely distributed from Nepal, Tibet and W. China to Kon Tum plateau, and only occupies habitats above 1,000 – 1,500m. The continuous range of *Euthalia strephon* extends widely from Tibet to the Kon Tum plateau, while the closely-related endemic species *E. strephonida* is restricted to the Da Lat plateau.

Another group of endemic butterfly species of the Da Lat plateau includes taxa of Sundanian derivation. These are pierid *Delias vietnamensis,* nymphalids *Tanaecia stellata, Cyllogenes milleri, Faunis bicoloratus, Zeuxidia sapphirus, Discophora aestheta* and *Ypthima daclaca,* lycaenids *Tajuria sekii, T. shigehoi, Deramas cham* and hesperiids *Suada albolineata* (Fig. 6). These species occur far from their relatives living in the Malay Peninsula and Sunda Islands (Appendix).

Most (8 out of 12) of the endemics of Sundanian origin mentioned above have only been found in the Da Lat plateau. However, an exception is the pierid *Delias vietnamensis* which has also been found in other isolated mountain areas of Indochina (Fig. 5). The only species of Sundanian origin found in a locality other than Da Lat is the nymphalid *Elymnias saola* in the northern Truong Song Ridge.

Endemic butterfly taxa of the Da Lat plateau that demonstrate links with the faunas of Malaya and Sundaland (Fig. 6) are the most remarkable feature of the local fauna, with more than 60% of butterfly species found in the Da Lat plateau characterised by Sundaland derivation. The majority of these species still maintain this link with the archipelago through the Malay Peninsula. For this reason endemism of butterfly taxa in the Da Lat plateau should be noted as a rather unusual event. For example, the satyrid *Cyllogenes milleri,* recently discovered in Da Lat plateau of Vietnam, has a sole relative *C. woolletti* in northern Borneo. Both species are quite similar and suggest confirmation of the former land connection bridge between the mainland and the Greater Sunda Islands (Voris, 2000). It is notable that in comparison with endemic butterfly taxa of Sino-Himalayan origin, endemic butterfly taxa of the Sundanian fauna are mainly located at lower elevations, thus demonstrating the segregation on biogeographic lines of butterfly groups that have come into contact during climatic fluctuations in the last Ice Age.

The list of nationally endemic butterfly species found in the Da Lat plateau is extended by including taxa of Indo-Burmese origin (Fig. 7). Some of these species also occur on the Kon Tum plateau, for example *Stichophthalma uemurai* and *Dodona speciosa*.

3.2. Endemics of the Kon Tum plateau

There are sixteen endemic butterfly species belonging to families Pieridae (1), Nymphalidae (10), Riodinidae (3), Lycaenidae (1) and Hesperiidae (1) (Appendix). Generally, the biogeographical pattern of endemics of the Kon Tum plateau is similar to that of the Da Lat plateau (Figs. 5-7). In comparison with the Da Lat plateau, at higher elevations of the Kon Tum Mountains (above 1,500m) there are only two endemic butterfly species showing relationship with the Sino-Himalayan fauna, for example two lycaenids *Heliophorus smaragdinus* and *Chrysozephyrus wakaharai*, even though the total number of Sino-Himalayan species is rather high (over 16%). Strong morphological differences are becoming apparent in local populations of Sino-Himalayan species; these populations may well be described as new subspecies when additional material has been obtained.

The number of endemic butterfly species demonstrating a Sundanian origin is also less than on the Da Lat plateau. As in Da Lat, these endemics are distributed mainly at middle elevations (900-1,400m), for example *Delias vietnamensis, Elymnias saola, Zeuxidia sapphirus*. Endemic butterfly species of Indo-Burmese origin on the Kon Tum plateau are noticeably predominant (Fig. 7). Many of them are geographically unique and to date have only been found in this area and in the neighbouring Da Lat plateau and the northern Truong Son range: nymphalids *Lethe melisana, L. konkakini; Aemona kontumei, A. simulatrix, Stichophthalma uemurai, S. eamesi*; riodinids: *Dodona speciosa, D. katerina*; and hesperiid: *Pintara capiloides*.

3.3. Endemics of the northern Truong Son ridge

To the north of the Kon Tum plateau (northern Truong Son ridge and Annamese lowland **(3)**) the number of endemic butterfly species (26 species) is similar but with a different biogeographical pattern of endemism (Fig. 5-7). For example, the number of endemics (3 species) revealing a link with the Sundanian fauna is significantly reduced (*Elymnias saola, Zeuxidia sapphirus, Neomyrina* sp.) (Fig. 6) and the number of endemic species of Sino-Himalayan origin is also not high (*Papilio doddsi, Mycalesis inopia, Chrysozephyrus wakaharai*) (Fig.5). The majority of endemic species belong to the local Indo-Burmese fauna (73% of all endemics) (Fig. 7). Six endemics are unique to this territory.

3.4. Endemics of Hoang Lien Son range

The fauna of Hoang Lien Son range (the Fansipan massif) is considered as a part of the Southern Chinese mountain fauna (Monastyrskii, 2007). The massif includes southern ridges of the Yunnan Mountains with peaks reaching 3,000 m and above. The butterfly species composition of the Hoang Lien Son massif and the butterfly range structure in this area are distinctive and significantly differ from the populations of the other regions of the Indochinese Peninsula (Monastyrskii, 2007, 2010a). The species characterized by Sino-Himalayan ranges (44.3%) are

http://dx.doi.org/10.5772/55490

predominant, extending to the Chinese provinces of Yunnan and Sichuan. At the same time the butterfly species endemism in this area is rather low. There are fourteen endemic species (3.6%) ranges of which are restricted by the massif. Nine species are relatives of representatives with the Sino-Himalayan ranges, for example, nymphalid *Euthalia khambounei*, lycaenids *Euaspa nishimurai, Chrysozephyrus vietnamicus, C. hatoyamai, Shirozuozephyrus masatoshii*, and hesperiid *Praescobura chrysomaculata*; five endemic species demonstrate a link with Indo-Burmese fauna: *Graphium phidias; Aemona tonkinensis, A. berdyevi, A. implicata* and *Taxila dora,*

3.5. Endemics of N.E. Vietnam

A total 26 species, inhabiting eastern areas of N. Vietnam (east of the Red River), are endemic to the Indochinese Peninsula. Fifteen species extend south to the territories of northern Truong Son ridge and Annamese lowland (Appendix), and four of these endemics are found to west of the Red River. The ranges of eleven endemic species are bounded only by the eastern areas of North Vietnam.

3.6. Summary

It is evident from the data in Appendix that all except one of the Sundanian species is in Da Lat plateau, with little extension to the north. The Indo-Burmese species are dispersed more or less evenly from the north to south with definite localization. The Sino-Himalayan endemic species are concentrated in the two most northerly areas of endemism with disjunction also in Da Lat (Table 1); all seven of the Sino-Himalayan endemics in Da Lat are also exclusive to that area.

Centres of endemism in Vietnam	Biogeographical provinces (Monastyrskii, 2007)	Average latitude of area studied	Total no. Vietnam endemic species	Biogeographical elements		
				Sino-Himalayan (total of 26 endemic to Vietnam)	Indo-Burmese (total of 35 endemic to Vietnam)	Sundanian (total of 15 endemic to Vietnam)
Hoang Lien Son	Sikang-Yunnan	22°	14	9	5	0
N. & N.E. Vietnam	South Chinese	21°	26	7	18	1
Nothern Truong Son	North Annamese	18°	26	4	19	3
Kon Tum plateau	Central Annamese	14,5°	16	2	9	5
Da Lat plateau	Da Lat	11,5°	28	7	9	12

Table 1. Dispersion of the biogeographical elements of the butterfly species endemics in Vietnam

Each of the five centres of butterfly endemism in Vietnam contains species unique to it (Table 2).

Centres of endemism in Vietnam	Biogeographical provinces (Monastyrskii, 2007)	Average latitude of area studied	Total no. of unique endemic species	Biogeographical elements		
				Sino-Himalayan (total of 26 endemic to Vietnam)	Indo-Burmese (total of 35 endemic to Vietnam)	Sundanian (total of 15 endemic to Vietnam)
Hoang Lien Son	Sikang-Yunnan	22°	10	9	1	0
N. & N.E. Vietnam	South Chinese	21°	11	5	6	1
Nothern Truong Son	North Annamese	18°	6	1	4	1
Kon Tum plateau	Central Annamese	14,5°	6	2	4	0
Da Lat plateau	Da Lat	11,5°	19	7	4	8
Total			**52**	**24**	**19**	**10**

Table 2. Uniqueness of the butterfly species endemics in the Centres of endemism in Vietnam

This unique component is highest in the Hoang Lien Son massif (71%) and almost has high in the Da Lat plateau (66%). Amongst the former, 90% is of Sino-Himalayan affinity, whereas, in contrast, 42% of the latter is of Sundanian affinity.

It is also clear that there is a diversity of faunistic complexes that differ in origin, age and relationships, with the north-south grain of the landscape structure (Fig. 3) being a important factor in the development of this diversity, the topography providing both barriers to, and corridors for, butterfly dispersal.

The percentage of Indochinese endemic butterfly species noticeably decreases from the north of Vietnam to the south. There is a strong positive correlation between the latitude (X) and the percentage of species represented (Y): r =.532, $P < 0.05$ (Fig. 8) (Monastyrskii, 2010b).

4. Continuous and mosaic ranges of Vietnamese butterflies

Continuous ranges are typical of a number of Vietnamese butterflies, particularly eurybiont (or opportunistic) species. Many of these species are distributed throughout the country and also extend beyond its borders. High migratory activity, diffuse population boundaries and a high intensity of genetic flow are all contributing factors to increased similarity between populations of different species. Examples of such similarity may be seen among representatives of the families Papilionidae (genera *Papilio* and *Graphium*); Pieridae (genera *Appias, Prioneris* and *Catopsilia*); Danainae, and some groups of widely distributed Nymphalinae

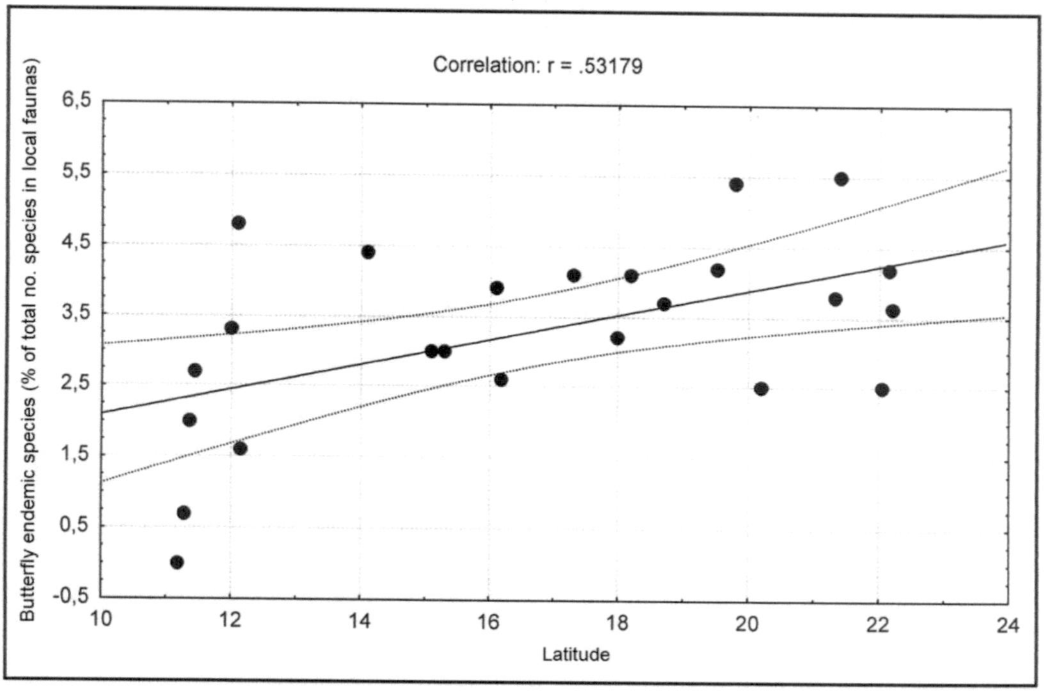

Figure 8. Correlation between the latitude (x-axis) and percentage endemism (y-axis) in localised inventories of Vietnamese butterflies (Monastyrskii, 2010b)

(genera *Kaniska, Junonia* and *Vanessa*) and also some other taxa that are characterised by long distance migrations. Conversely, the continuous ranges of stenotopic species have specific configurations corresponding with the geography of habitats and often demonstrate a mosaic character. These species often demonstrate a clinal variability of morphological characters; this is seen particularly in some other Papilionidae (*Byasa, Chilasa, Teinopalpus* and *Meandrusa*), Pieridae (*Delias*), and the majority of Satyrinae, Amathusiinae, Nymphalinae and Lycaenidae.

Clinal variability is exemplified by the widespread satyrine *Ypthima baldus* (Fig. 9). In populations of male *Ypthima baldus* the length of the forewing fluctuates insignificantly in central and southern parts of Vietnam while in the north this character depends greatly on habitats and landscapes. Populations occupying the northern mountainous regions (from Hoang Lien Son to the northern part of the Truong Son ridge) have a shorter forewing length though in Vu Quang (northern Truong Son ridge) this character varies widely. In terms of pattern of Vietnamese landscapes (Figs. 2, 3), the northern mountainous region maintains a continuous belt-like zone of intergradation between mountain and lowland habitats.

Mosaic ranges are exemplified by the very local, montane, seasonal amathusiine species *Faunis aerope* (Fig. 10) which is distributed in habitats above 1,500m, and where geographical population gaps can be large or small. Habitat isolation and high stenotopic behaviour have influenced morphology of the species' male genitalia. The pattern of the clasp apex from different sites of N. and C. Vietnam is illustrated in figure 10. Males from the central part of the country have a rather broad clasp, the apex of which is covered by several rows of much larger spines. Even populations of males from different localities of N. Vietnam are characterised by constant differences in the apical structure of the clasp (Monastyrskii, 2004).

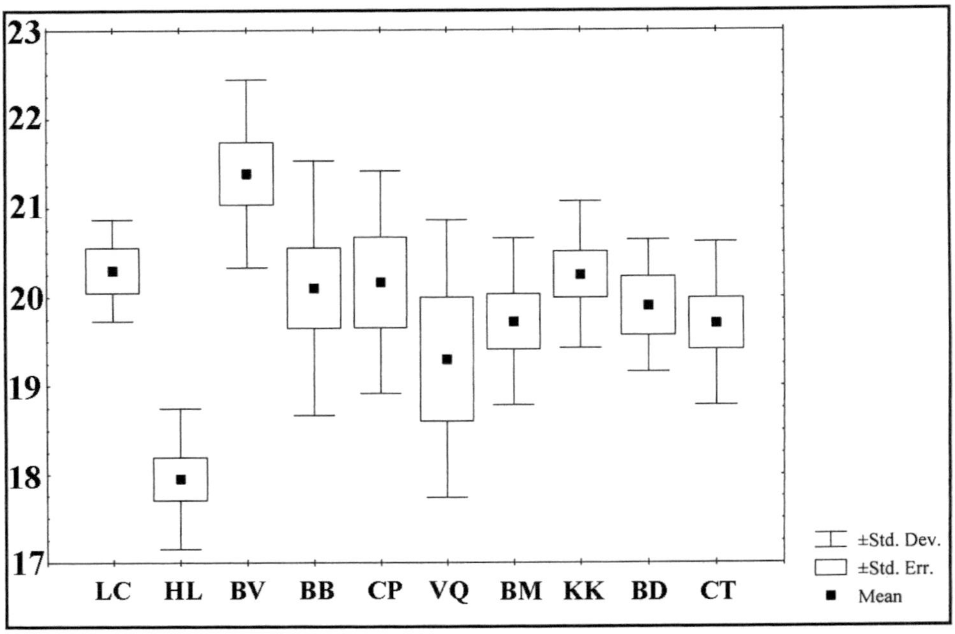

Figure 9. Cline variability of the forewing length in *Ypthima baldus* (Nymphalidae, Satyrinae); x – areas studied from north to south (from left to right) and latitude: LC – Lai Chau (22,3°N); HL – Hoang Lien (22,1°N); BV – Ba Vi (21,05°N); BB – Ba Be (22,2°N); CP – Cuc Phuong (20,1°N); VQ – Vu Quang (18,2°N); BM – Bach Ma (16,05°N); KK – Kon Ka Kinh (14,3°N); BD – Bi Doup (12,0°N); CT – Cat Tien (11,3°N); y – length of the forewing (in mm.) Std. Dev. – the standard deviation; Std. Err. – the standard error; mean – average

It is well known that continuous variability occurs in a latitudinal manner (Mayr, 1969; 1970). In Vietnam there are many butterfly species with geographically separate populations which vary in distinct characteristics such as colour and wing patterns, size and the development of some organs. Species are sometimes distributed very widely and occur in different kinds of landscapes and habitats. In such cases it is difficult to make conclusions regarding contact zones between subspecies. In other cases distinctive butterfly populations are divided by insuperable natural barriers. This latter variability is rather typical of populations of many Vietnamese butterflies.

http://dx.doi.org/10.5772/55490

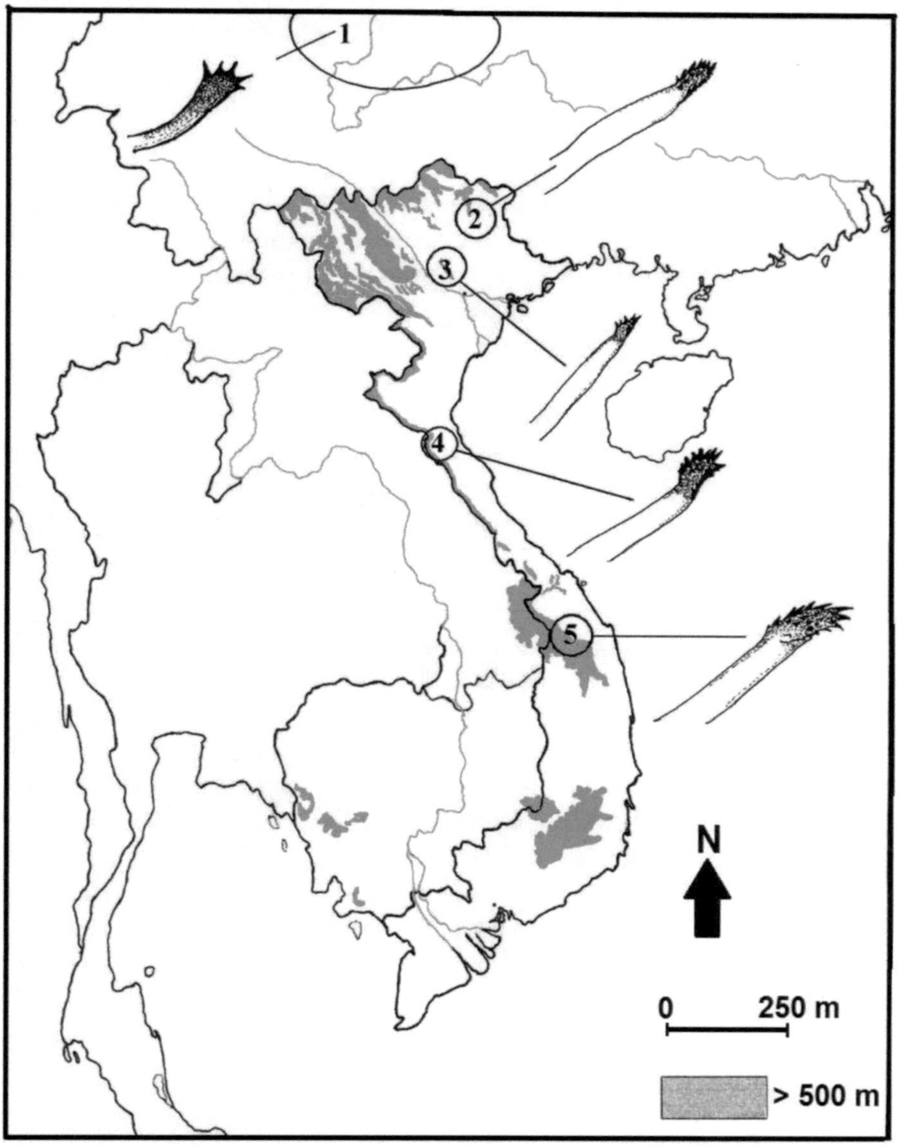

Figure 10. The pattern of the clasp apex in the males of *Faunis aerope* (Nymphalidae, Amathusiinae) from different sites of N. and C. Vietnam: 1 – ssp. *aerope* (C. & S. China); 2, 3 – ssp. *excelsa* (N. Vietnam); 4 – ssp. *excelsa* (northern Truong Son); 5 – ssp. *centrala* (the Kon Tum plateau).

5. Disjunct ranges of Vietnamese butterflies

Geographical gaps between populations of species caused by natural factors are not rare occurrences in the butterfly faunas of Indochina and Southeast Asia. Disjunctions observed differ in their distance and direction.

5.1. Distances of disjunctions

In some cases disjunctions between populations may only be a few tens of kilometers, but strong factors such as climate, river basins and montane ridges become geographical barriers which may cause and maintain divergence. For example, populations of many montane species are separated between the Da Lat and Kon Tum plateaus and also between the Kon Tum plateau and the northern Truong Son ridge and S. Yunnan mountain system. The Indo-Burmese swallowtail *Meandrusa lachinus* is distributed from Nepal to Indochina and consists of a number of subspecies, three of which are found in Vietnam. The subspecies *M. l. sukkity* is distributed from N.E. Thailand to C. Laos and the central Vietnamese Kon Tum plateau. This taxon does not cross the lower Dac Lac plateau and water barriers such as the Song Ba and Song Da Rang rivers; nor does it overlap populations of the distinctive subspecies *M. l. helenusoides* which is restricted to Da Lat plateau. There are many other examples similar to that of *M. l. sukkity* that are known.

In the majority of cases the natural disjunctions between Vietnamese populations of butterflies can occur over several hundreds or thousands of kilometres. Reasons for disjunctions between butterfly populations may also include human activity such as burning. For example, lowland forest habitats in coastal areas of Vietnam have been cleared leading to fragmented butterfly populations clinging to isolated habitats. It is now almost impossible to gather data on the nature of the original forests, though some information from palynology is becoming available (Maxwell & Liu, 2002). It is therefore difficult to reconstruct the possible composition of the original butterfly fauna. Altered coastal climate and remaining fragments of coastal forests with their plant communities point to the high diversity of mosaic habitats in recent time. It is also possible, however, that disjunctions were a natural characteristic of the local species ranges in these previously coastal forests. Nevertheless, logging of timber and other kinds of human activity may have intensified these gaps and exacerbated difficulties in explaining these geographical differences in the modern context.

5.2. Directions of disjunctions

These examples may be extended by disjunctions occurring over a few thousands of kilometres. Likewise the butterfly taxa of Indochina demonstrate links with butterfly faunas distributed in different directions from Vietnam (similar elements in the notodontid moth fauna of Thailand were indicated by Schintlmeister & Pinratana (2007): Yunnan; Pacific; Himalayan; Sundanian), with range disjunctions also along the same geographical orientation:

1. W. and C. China:

http://dx.doi.org/10.5772/55490

The majority of disjunctions in the Sino-Himalayan ranges is observed between populations of northern Vietnam (e.g. Hoang Lien Son mountains) and northern part of central Vietnam (northern Truong Son ridge) and populations of W. China and E. Himalaya: Nymphalidae: *Euthalia confucius, E. strephon, Mycalesis unica, Lethe ocellata, L. umedai*: Lycaenidae: *Euaspa milionia, Euaspa hishikawai, Howarthia kimurai, Teratozephyrus kimurai, Chrysozephyrus tytleri, Chrysozephyrus intermedius, Kawazoezephyrus jiroi, Yamomotozephyrus kwangtungensis etc.*

2. S.E. China, Taiwan and Hainan:

Examples of these taxa include swallowtail *Teinopalpus aureus*, nymphalid *Athyma minensis*, groups such as the Lycaenidae Hairstreaks *Zephyrus*, including *Ravenna nivea, Yamomotozephyrus kwangtungensis*, representatives of the genera *Chrysozephyrus* and *Euaspa*, and also some unique Hesperiidae that have long been regarded as endemics of S.E. China.

3. Burma and N.E. India:

Euthalia iva; Cyllogenes janetae, Penthema michallati.

4. Malay Peninsula and Sunda Islands:

Delias malayana, Elymnias panthera, Zeuxidia masoni, Papilio prexaspes and Kallima albofasciata.

Natural causes of disjunctions between butterfly populations are important in understanding the evolutionary processes that have resulted in the taxonomic composition of the modern fauna, and also for the prediction of its future transformations. In Vietnam populations of many butterfly species have lost links with the main part of their ranges, and have adapted to new natural conditions. This adaptation has been accompanied by the appearance of new taxonomic units (new species and subspecies). Fig. 11 shows range disjunctions for some species belonging to the genus *Ypthima*, for example *Y. norma* (1); *Y. watsoni* (2) and *Y. sarcaposa* (3), which are all distributed in the Indochinese subregion.

Some butterfly species in Vietnam are distributed mainly according to climatic factors. Changes in local climate appear to influence strongly the distribution of those butterfly species that are restricted to Vietnam's mountain areas. Survey reports suggest that some N. Vietnam/ S. Yunnan montane butterfly species (e.g. *Neorina neosinica* and *Teinopalpus imperialis*) also occur in the highlands of the Kon Tum plateau – montane habitats that are separated by hundreds of kilometres. This pattern might reflect the fragmentation of a once broader range that these butterflies occupied when montane habitats extended to lower elevations during cooler glacial periods. During the warmer eras, the species may have become isolated when these habitats receded to higher altitudes. Such cycles of habitat change may also have led to varying degrees of divergence in some groups of butterflies. Today this scenario presents a suitable explanation for range disjunctions for many separate montane butterfly taxa in Vietnam.

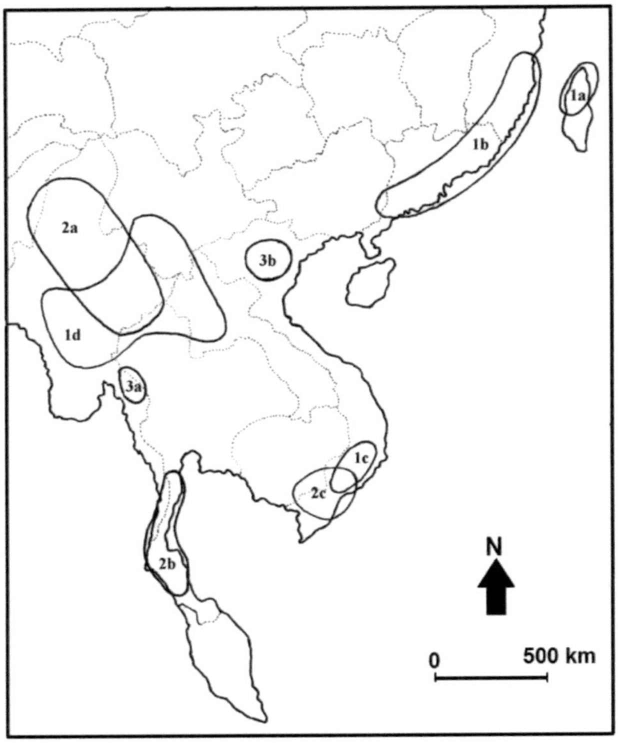

Figure 11. Disjunct ranges of some *Ypthima* species (Nymphalidae, Satyrinae): *Y. norma* (1); *Y. watsoni* (2) and *Y. sarcaposa* (3)

6. Vicarious ranges of Vietnamese butterflies

Examples of geographically vicarious butterfly species found in Vietnam are provided by stenotopic taxa representatives. Notable chains of vicariants include species belonging to the genera *Aemona* and *Stichophthalma* (Nymphalidae, Amathusiinae) (Figs. 12, 13). The range of *A. berdyevi* (1) in the north of the country (Hoang Lien Son mountains) is the vicariant of *A. oberthueri* ranging through the mountain areas of W. China (Sichuan and N. Yunnan) (Fig. 12). N. Vietnam and northern part of C. Vietnam is ranged by the sympatric taxa *A. tonkinensis* (2) and *A. implicata* (3) which are similar in size and wing colour pattern but have very distinctive genitalia. Ranges of these species reach the central highlands where they cede similar habitats to *A. kontumei* (4) and *A. simulatrix* (5). The southern Da Lat plateau is occupied by *A. falcata* (6) which has a distinctive wing pattern and genitalia (Fig. 12).

Ranges of *Stichophthalma* species in Vietnam follow a similar pattern (Fig. 13). During a recent new revision of Vietnamese *Stichophthalma*, the taxonomic status of some taxa has been changed (Monastyrskii & Devyatkin, 2008). The range of the Yunnan species *S. howqua iapetus* has borders with that of *S. mathilda* (4), *S. suffusa tonkiniana* (2) and *S. fruhstorferi* (3). The montane taxon *S. mathilda* reaches the central Vietnamese highlands (Gia Lai province); both other taxa, *S. s. tonkiniana* and *S. fruhstorferi*, are distributed through the lowlands of N. Vietnam

http://dx.doi.org/10.5772/55490

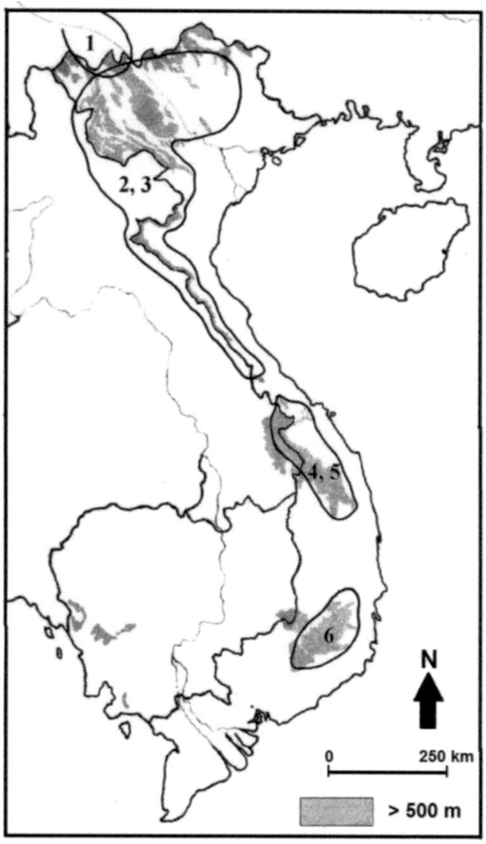

Figure 12. Vicarious ranges of the *Aemona* spp. (Nymphalidae, Amathusiinae): 1. *A. berdievi*; 2. *A. tonkinensis*; 3. *A. implicata*; 4. *A. simulatrix*; 5. *A. kontumei*; 6. *A. falcata*.

and northern part of C. Vietnam. The greater part of the Kon Tum plateau is populated by *S. eamesi* (5) where it overlaps with the range of *S. uemurai* (6), a species that covers the entire Da Lat plateau. The next vicariant species is *S. cambodia* (7) which ranges through the mountains of W. Cambodia and E. Thailand.

The ranges of these six species of *Aemona* and seven species of *Stichophthalma* found in Vietnam and adjacent countries coincide with floristic provinces proposed by Takhtajan (1986). These provinces belong to the Indomalesian subkingdom characterised by remarkably high levels of endemism including 16 endemic families of vascular plants and a great number of endemic genera and species.

Sometimes the pattern of vicarious ranges appears to have been modified by subsequent dispersals, leading to overlap of what were probably previously allopatric species. An example is mapped in Fig. 2d: the *Ypthima sakra* group of species. In a northern centre of diversity, three species (*Y. sakra, Y. atra, Y. persimilis*) partially overlap in the eastern Himalayas, and this overlap zone extends to N. Vietnam. To the south, these species are replaced by one very

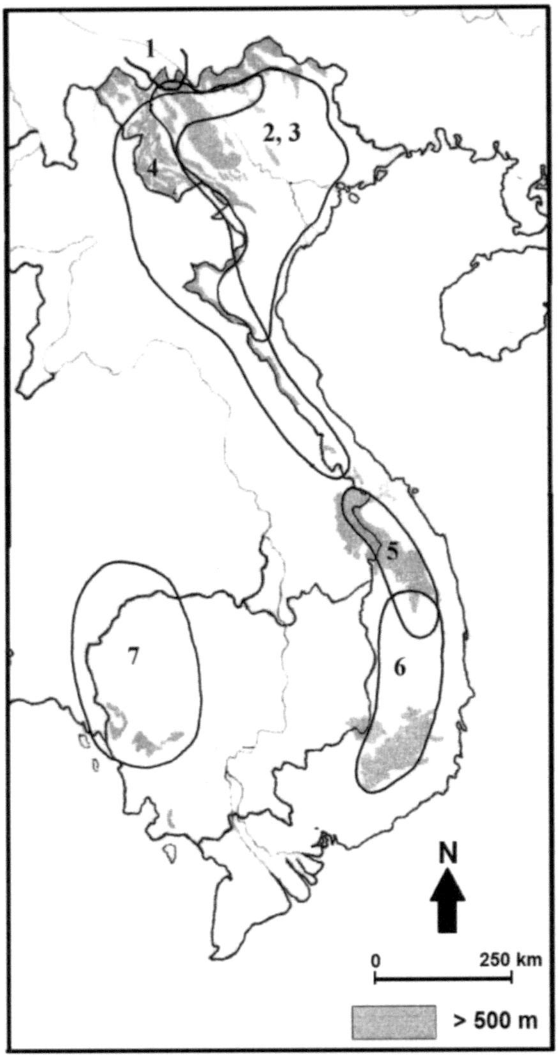

Figure 13. Vicarious ranges of the Stichophthalma spp. (Nymphalidae, Amathusiinae): 1. S. howqua iapetus; 2. S. suffusa tonkiniana; 3. S. fruhstorferi; 4. S. mathilda; 5. S. eamesi; 6. S. uemurai; 7. S. cambodia.

localised species, *Y. pseudosavara,* that is entirely allopatric, and a species pair, where one member, *Y. evansi,* has a range completely nested within that of the other, *Y. dohertyi.*

7. Conclusion

Analysis shows that Vietnamese butterflies are characterised by various range configurations, including endemic, continuous, mosaic, disjunct and vicarious. This diversity of pattern suggests that the Vietnamese butterfly fauna is in a continuous state of evolutionary develop-

http://dx.doi.org/10.5772/55490

ment in response to changes in topography and climate, possibly at least partially cyclic, younger patterns being progressively overlain on older ones, with various links to the adjacent Sino-Himalayan, Sundanian and Indo-Burmese faunas. Thus, it is plausible that the north-south ranges of mountains in the east of the Indochinese Peninsula, mostly in Vietnam, may have provided both a route whereby Sino-Himalayan elements were able to penetrate further south in cooler periods, and also a refuge in the very south, perhaps in more clement maritime conditions of the eastern margin of the much expanded area of Sundaland (Voris, 2000) where Sundanian humid forest elements were able to persist when the interior became much drier. The current altitudinal segregation of Sino-Himalayan versus Sundanian endemics in Da Lat is consistent with this hypothesis. Such a scenario might be assessed further by conducting rigorous phylogenetic studies of those butterfly groups with vicariant endemism within the Indochinese Peninsula, particularly *Aemona* and *Stichophthalma*, and also of those groups such as that of *Ypthima sakra*, where considerable overlap of species ranges occurs.

Appendix

Species	Family	Centres of endemism in Vietnam					Nearest relatives	
		Hoang Lien Son	N. and N.E. Vietnam	Northern Truong Son ridge	Kon Tum plateau	Da Lat and Dac Lac plateaus	Species	Distribution
1	2	3	4	5	6	7	8	9
Chilasa imitata	Papilionidae					+	*Ch. epycides*	Sino-Himalayan
Papilio doddsi	Papilionidae		+	+			*P. dialis*	Sino-Himalayan
Graphium phidias	Papilionidae	+	+	+			-	Indo-Burmese
Delias vietnamensis	Pieridae				+	+	*D. georgina*	Sundanian
Eurema novapallida	Pieridae					+	*E. lacteola*	Sundanian
Euploea orontobates	Nymphalidae					+	-	Sundanian
Cyllogenes milleri	Nymphalidae					+	*C. woolletti*	Sundanian
Elymnias saola	Nymphalidae			+	+		*E. casiphone*	Sundanian
Penthema michallati	Nymphalidae		+				*P. lysarda*	Indo-Burmese
Lethe berdievi	Nymphalidae	+					*L. christophi*	Sino-Himalayan
L. melisana	Nymphalidae				+		-	Indo-Burmese
L. konkakini	Nymphalidae				+		*L. latiaris*	Sino-Himalayan
L. philemon	Nymphalidae		+				-	Indo-Burmese

Species	**Family**	**Centres of endemism in Vietnam**					**Nearest relatives**	
		Hoang Lien Son	**N. and N.E. Vietnam**	**Northern Truong Son ridge**	**Kon Tum plateau**	**Da Lat and Dac Lac plateaus**	**Species**	**Distribution**
1	**2**	**3**	**4**	**5**	**6**	**7**	**8**	**9**
L. philesana	Nymphalidae		+	+			-	Indo-Burmese
L. philesanoides	Nymphalidae		+	+			-	Indo-Burmese
L. huongii	Nymphalidae		+				-	Indo-Burmese
Ragadia critias	Nymphalidae			+	+	+	-	Indo-Burmese
Mycalesis inopia	Nymphalidae		+	+			-	Sino-Himalayan
Ypthima frontierii	Nymphalidae	+					*Y. megalomma*	Sino-Himalayan
Y. pseudosavara	Nymphalidae		+	+			*Y. savara*	Indo-Burmese
Y. daclaca	Nymphalidae					+	*Y. pandocus*	Sundanian
Faunis bicoloratus	Nymphalidae				+	+	*F. canens*	Sundanian
Aemona tonkinensis	Nymphalidae	+	+	+			-	Indo-Burmese
A. kontumei	Nymphalidae				+		-	Indo-Burmese
A. simulatrix	Nymphalidae				+		-	Indo-Burmese
A. implicata	Nymphalidae	+	+	+			-	Indo-Burmese
A. falcata	Nymphalidae					+	-	Indo-Burmese
A. berdyevi	Nymphalidae	+					*A. oberthuri*	Indo-Burmese
Stichophthalma fruhstorferi	Nymphalidae		+	+			*S. cambodia*	Indo-Burmese
S. uemurai	Nymphalidae				+	+	*S. cambodia*	Indo-Burmese
S. mathilda	Nymphalidae		+	+			*S. louisa*	Indo-Burmese
S. eamesi	Nymphalidae				+		*S. louisa*	Indo-Burmese
Zeuxidia sapphirus	Nymphalidae			+	+	+	*Zeuxidia spp.*	Sundanian
Discophora aestheta	Nymphalidae					+	*Discophora spp.*	Sundanian
Neptis transita	Nymphalidae					+	*N. noyala*	Sino-Himalayan
Phaedyma armariola	Nymphalidae					+	*P. aspasia*	Sino-Himalayan
Tanaecia stellata	Nymphalidae					+	*T. godartii*	Sundanian
Euthalia hoa	Nymphalidae					+	*T. thibetana*	Sino-Himalayan

Species	Family	Centres of endemism in Vietnam					Nearest relatives	
		Hoang Lien Son	N. and N.E. Vietnam	Northern Truong Son ridge	Kon Tum plateau	Da Lat and Dac Lac plateaus	Species	Distribution
1	2	3	4	5	6	7	8	9
E. khambounei	Nymphalidae	+						Sino-Himalayan
E. strephonida	Nymphalidae					+	*E. strephon*	Sino-Himalayan
Calinaga funeralis	Nymphalidae		+				*Calinaga spp.*	Sino-Himalayan
Dodona katerina	Riodinidae			+	+		*D. dipoea*	Indo-Burmese
D. speciosa	Riodinidae				+	+	-	Indo-Burmese
Taxila dora	Riodinidae	+	+	+	+		-	Indo-Burmese
Deramas cham	Lycaenidae					+	*D. jasoda*	Sundanian
Heliophorus smaragdinus	Lycaenidae				+		*H. tamu*	Sino-Himalayan
Euaspa minaei	Lycaenidae					+	*E. hishikawai*	Sino-Himalayan
E. nishimurai	Lycaenidae	+						Sino-Himalayan
Proteuaspa akikoae	Lycaenidae		+					Sino-Himalayan
Chrysozephyrus wakaharai	Lycaenidae			+				Sino-Himalayan
Ch. vietnamicus	Lycaenidae	+						Sino-Himalayan
Ch. hatoyamai	Lycaenidae	+						Sino-Himalayan
Shirozuozephyrus alienus	Lycaenidae					+	S. hayashi	Sino-Himalayan
Sh. masatoshii	Lycaenidae	+						Sino-Himalayan
Neomyrina sp.	Lycaenidae			+			-	Sundanian
Tajuria sekii	Lycaenidae					+		Sundanian
Tajuria shigehoi	Lycaenidae					+	*T. luculenta*	Sundanian
Rapala persephone	Lycaenidae					+	*R. hades*	Indo-Burmese
Celaenorrhinus inexpectus	Hesperiidae		+				*C. maculosa*	Indo-Burmese
C. victor	Hesperiidae		+				*C. dayaoensis*	Sino-Himalayan
C. incestus	Hesperiidae			+			*C. maculosa*	Indo-Burmese
C. kuznetsovi	Hesperiidae			+			*C. oscula*	Taiwan

Species	Family	Centres of endemism in Vietnam					Nearest relatives	
		Hoang Lien Son	N. and N.E. Vietnam	Northern Truong Son ridge	Kon Tum plateau	Da Lat and Dac Lac plateaus	Species	Distribution
1	2	3	4	5	6	7	8	9
C. phuongi	Hesperiidae		+				*maculosa* group	Sino-Himalayan
Darpa inopinata	Hesperiidae		+	+			*D. striata*	Indo-Burmese
Coladenia tanya	Hesperiidae		+	+				Indo-Burmese
C. koiwaii	Hesperiidae	+					-	Sino-Himalayan
Pintara capiloides	Hesperiidae			+		+	other *Pintara*	Indo-Burmese
Tagiades hybridus	Hesperiidae			+			*T. gana, T. parra*	Indo-Burmese
Thoressa similissima	Hesperiidae		+	+				Indo-Burmese
Aeromachus cognatus	Hesperiidae					+		Indo-Burmese
Halpe frontieri	Hesperiidae		+				*H. nephele*	Indo-Burmese
Halpe paupera	Hesperiidae			+				Indo-Burmese
Halpe annamensis	Hesperiidae					+	*H. zema*	Indo-Burmese
Scobura eximia	Hesperiidae		+					Sino-Himalayan
Suada albolineata	Hesperiidae		+	+	+	+	*S. swerga*	Sundanian
Quedara flavens	Hesperiidae		+				*Q. albifascia*	Indo-Burmese
Praescobura chrysomaculata	Hesperiidae	+					*Scobura*	Sino-Himalayan

(Species marked with bold are restricted by the territory of Vietnam)

Table 3. Indochinese butterfly endemics and their distribution and nearest relatives.

Author details

A.L. Monastyrskii[1] and J.D. Holloway[2]

1 Ecology Department of Vietnam-Russia Tropical Centre, Nguyen Van Huyen Rd., Nghia Do, Cau Giay, Hanoi, Vietnam

2 Department of Life Sciences, The Natural History Museum, London, UK

References

[1] Austin, G. T. & Riley, T.J. (1995) Portable bait traps for the study of butterflies. *Trop. Lepidoptera*, 6, 1: 5–9.

[2] Averyanov, L.V., Phan Ke Loc, Nguyen Tien Hiep & Harder, D.K. (2003) Phytogeographic review of Vietnam and adjacent areas of Eastern Indochina. *Komarovia*, 3, 1-83.

[3] Corbet, A.S. & Pendlebury, H.M. (1992) *The butterflies of the Malay Peninsula* [4th edn, revised by J.N. Eliot]: i-x, 1-595, 69 pls – Kuala Lumpur.

[4] DeVries P.J. (1988) Stratification of fruit-feeding nymphalid butterflies in a Costa Rican rainforest. *J. Res. Lepidoptera*, 26: 98–108.

[5] Ek-Amnuay, P. (2006) *Butterflies of Thailand. Fascinating insects. Vol. 2 (1st edn)*. – Bangkok: Amarin Printing and Publishing. 849 pp.

[6] Hall, R. (1998) The plate tectonics of Cenozoic SE Asia and the distribution of land and sea. *Biogeography and Geological Evolution of SE Asia* (eds. R. Hall and J.D. Holloway), pp. 99-124. Backhuys, Leiden.

[7] Hall, R. (2002) Cenozoic geological and plate tectonic evolution of SE Asia and the SW Pacific: computer-based reconstructions and animations. *Journal of Asian Earth Sciences*, 20, 353-434.

[8] Hanebuth, T., Stattegger, K. & Grootes, P.M. (2000) Rapid flooding of the Sunda shelf: a late-glacial sea-level record. *Science*, 288, 1033–1035.

[9] Holloway, J.D. (1969) A numerical investigation of the biogeography of the butterfly fauna of India, and its relation to continental drift. *Biological Journal of the Linnean Society*, 1, 373-385.

[10] Holloway, J. D. (1973) The affinities within four butterfly groups (Lepidoptera: Rhopalocera) in relation to genera patterns of butterfly distribution in the Indo-Australian area. *Transaction of the Royal Entomology Society of London*. 125, 126-176.

[11] Holloway, J.D. (1974) The biogeography of the Indian butterflies. *Ecology and Biogeography in India* (ed. M. Mani). *Monographiae biologicae*, 23, 473-499. W. Junk Publishers.

[12] Holloway, J.D. (1998) Geological signal and dispersal noise in two contrasting insect groups in the Indo-Australian tropics: R-mode analysis of pattern in Lepidoptera and cicadas. *Biogeography and Geological Evolution of SE Asia* (eds. R. Hall and J.D. Holloway), pp. 291-314. Backhuys, Leiden, 291-314.

[13] Holloway, J.D. & Hall, R. (1998) SE Asian geology and biogeography. *Biogeography and Geological Evolution of SE Asia* (eds. R. Hall and J.D. Holloway), pp. 1-23. Backhuys, Leiden.

[14] Koiwaya, S. (2007) *The Zephyrus Hairstreaks of the World* (ed. H. Fujita), Mushi-Sha's Iconographic Series of Insects 5. Mushi-Sha.

[15] Koiwaya S. & Monastyrskli A.L. (2011) New species of *Shirozuozephyrus* (Lepidoptera, Lycaenidae) from Da Lat plateau (C. Vietnam). *Butterflies*, 56, 4-8.

[16] Maxwell, A.L. & Liu, K-B. (2002) Late Quaternary pollen records from the monsoonal areas of continental S and SE Asia. *Bridging Wallace's Line: the environmental and cultural history and dynamics of the SE-Asian-Australian Region* (eds. P. Kershaw, B. David, N. Tapper, D. Penny and & J. Brown). *Advances in Geoecology*, 34, 189-228. Catena Verlag, Reiskirchen

[17] Mayr E. (1969). *Principles of systematic zoology*. Cambridge, MA: Harvard University Press

[18] Mayr, E. (1970) *Populations, Species and Evolution*. The Belknap Press of Harvard University Press Cambridge, Massachusetts.

[19] Monastyrskii A.L. (2004) Infraspecific variation in Faunis aerope (Leech, 1890) and the description of a new subspecies from Central Vietnam (Lepidoptera: Nymphalidae, Amathusiinae). *Atalanta*. 2004. — Bd. 35, № ½. — P. 37–44.

[20] Monastyrskii, A.L. (2005) New taxa and new records of butterflies from Vietnam (3) (Lepidoptera, Rhopalocera). *Atalanta*, 36, 141-160.

[21] Monastyrskii, A.L. (2006). Fauna, ecology and biogeography of butterflies in Vietnam. *Butterflies*, 44, 41-55.

[22] Monastyrskii, A.L. (2007) Ecological and biogeographical characteristics of the butterfly fauna (Lepidoptera Rhopalocera) of Vietnam. *Entomology Review*, 87, 43-65.

[23] Monastyrskii, A.L. (2010a) On the origin of the recent fauna of butterflies (Lepidoptera, Rhopalocera) of Vietnam. *Entomology Review*, 90 (1), 39-58.

[24] Monastyrskii, A.L. (2010b) Butterfly fauna of Vietnam: origin and modern diversity – Author's abstract of Dr. Sc. dissertation. Moscow, A.N. Severtsov Institute Ecology and Evolution of Russian Asian Academy of Sciences. 47 pp. (in Russian)

[25] Monastyrskii, A.L. (2011) Fruit-feeding butterflies recorded by traps. – *in* Proceedings of the 4th National Scientific Conference on Ecology and Biological Resources. – Hanoi, 21 October 2011. – 753-756.

[26] Monastyrskii, A.L. & Devyatkin A.L. (2003) New taxa and new records of butterflies from Vietnam (2) (Lepidoptera, Rhopalocera). *Atalanta* 34, 471-492.

[27] Monastyrskii, A.L. & Devyatkin, A.L. (2008) Revisional notes on the genus *Stichophthalma* C. & R. Felder, 1862 (Lepidoptera, Amathusiinae). *Atalanta* 39 (1/4): 281-286.

[28] Outlaw, D.C. & Voelker, G. (2007) Pliocene climatic change in insular Southeast Asia as an engine of diversification in Ficedula flycatchers. *Journal of Biogeography*, 34, 1–14.

[29] Rundel P. (1999) Conservation priorities in Indochina — WWF Desk Study. Forest habitats and flora in Lao PDR, Cambodia, and Vietnam. - Hanoi: WWF Indochina Programme Office. 194 pp.

[30] Schintlmeister, A. & Pinratana, A. (2007) *Moths of Thailand Vol. 5. Notodontidae.* Brothers of St. Gabriel in Thailand, Bangkok.

[31] Spitzer, K., Novotny, V., Tonner, M. & Leps, J. (1993) Habitat preferences, distribution and seasonality of the butterflies (Lepidoptera, Papilionoidea) in a montane tropical rainforest, Vietnam. *Journal of Biogeography*, 20, 109-21.

[32] Sterling, E. J., Hurley, M. M. & Le Duc Minh. (2006) *Vietnam: a Natural History.* Yale Univiversity Press, New Haven, London.

[33] Synitsin, V.M. (1962) *Palaeogeography of Asia.* Academy of Sciences of USSR, Moscow-Leningrad. (*in Russian*).

[34] Synitsin, V.M. (1965) *Ancient Climates of Eurasia, Part I.* Leningrad State University, Leningrad (*in Russian*).

[35] Takhtajan, A.L. (1986) *Floristic regions of the World.* University California Press, Berkeley, Los Angeles, London.

[36] Tangah J., Hill J.K., Hamer K.C., Dawood M.M. (2004). Vertical distribution of fruit-feeding butterflies in Sabah, Borneo. Sepilok Bulletin, 1: 17-27.

[37] Tougard, C. (2001) Biogeography and migration routs of large mammal faunas in South-East Asia during the Late Middle Pleistocene: focus on the fossil and extant faunas from Thailand. *Palaeogeography, Palaeoclimatology, Palaeoecology*, 168, 337-358.

[38] Voris, H.K. (2000) Maps of Pleistocene sea levels in Southeast Asia: shorelines, river systems and time durations. *Journal of Biogeography*, 27, 1153–1167.

Chapter 6

Parascript, Parasites and Historical Biogeography

Hugo H. Mejía-Madrid

Additional information is available at the end of the chapter

http://dx.doi.org/10.5772/55459

1. Introduction

Eventually there may be enough pieces to form a meaningful language which could be called parascript - the language of parasites which tells of themselves and their hosts both of today and yesteryear (Manter, 1966) [1].

Few biological interactions have deserved so much attention from biologists during the latter part of the 20th century than host-parasite interactions. Parasites seem to throw a special light on the problems of ecology and evolution. Host-parasite interactions should be considered fine-grained biological models through which major changes in ecosystems can be monitored, e.g., global climate change [2,3]. In the following pages I will review as briefly as possible the main pathways that research on the historical biogeography of parasites has traversed ever since the American parasitologist Harold W Manter coined the term that is the subject matter of this chapter, *parascript*.

The historical biogeography of parasites is the concern of this chapter mainly because this discipline has gathered a great deal of information during the last two decades on both ecological and evolutionary studies that could be of extended use for future generations in order to know what to do with this planet.

In the late 19th century host-parasite interactions were under the scrutiny of evolutionary biologists ever since von Ihering [4,5,6] anticipated that the location of modern host and parasite biotas (he studied helminths and lice) could be evidence of past distributions. That was a time when Darwin's natural selection was under much debate, and host-parasite studies were used as proof of evolutionary change through channelled paths, called orthogenesis, an opposing view to natural selection. Nevertheless, thanks to von Ihering's anticipated insight continental drift and plate tectonics would become part of the core of recent parascript studies [6].

Klassen [6] and Brooks [7,8] concluded that the history of the impact of parasite studies in evolutionary biology had been significantly outstanding during the first half of the 20th century. During the critical years of debates on the mechanisms of evolution, e.g., selectionism vs. non-selectionist alternatives (end of 19th and first decades of the 20th century), parasites were at the core of such discussions. Yet, the demise of evolutionary studies on parasites occurred after the inception of the Modern Synthesis of Evolution [8], mainly because parasites fell into discredit as dead evolutionary ends, and as degenerate organisms living at the expense of their hosts. As Fahrenholz viewed it [6,8], parasite evolution just mirrored host evolution. So why bother study parasites under an evolutionary perspective?

American parasitologist Harold W Manter kept alive parasite evolutionary studies during the 1940's and through the rest of his life. These studies were mainly historical biogeographic, although he considered that the interplay between ecology and evolution is the language of parasitology. He viewed such studies as bilingual messages that parasites conveyed, one from the ecological realm and one from evolutionary biology. He named this type of studies, *parascript*. Today we can interpret parascript studies as global research programmes that study parasite ecology and evolutionary biology from the distinct standpoints of microevolution and macroevolution.

Parascript studies were initially explored by helminthologists [6,7,8,9] but unknowingly left out a great deal of information on insect ectoparasites as voiced by Ròzsa [10] (but see [11]). Parascript studies, therefore, should not be restricted to the type of parasite. Parascript studies should encompass all different types of parasites, whether ecto or endoparasitic. Yet, the differences between them help monitor distinct levels of ecosystem structuring. It is probable that helminth parasites have been surveyed more in relation to historical biogeographical research than ectoparasites in general mainly because Professor Manter was a helminthologist. Currently, parascript is the study of parasites that connect the phylogenetic, biogeographical, historical, and ecological realms, where parasites play an important role as 'thermometers' of environmental status and decidedly offer information on geomorphologic changes of the earth's crust, biogeography, and ecological status, where parasites as part of the interactor universe of their hosts can indicate the connections within trophic foodwebs, migrations, colonizations, and in situ speciation. They are an important if not one of the most important components of biomass in coastal ecosystems [12]. In the words of Hoberg and Klassen [9]: "parasites serve as keystones for understanding the history of biotas because of their critical value as phylogenetic, ecological and biogeographic indicators of their host groups."

2. Objectives

The aim of this chapter is to succinctly review past and present research on parasite historical biogeography and concludes what shape could take future research. Parasites have lent themselves to phylogenetic, ecological, and biogeographical analyses ever since von Ihering

http://dx.doi.org/10.5772/55459

maintained that parasites represent conservative lineages and evolve in isolation [4] (now called allopatric speciation). It was Metcalfe [6,8,13] who actually anticipated the necessity of having phylogenies of both hosts and parasites.

Phylogenetic systematics in particular has played a strong guiding role in parasite historical biogeography during the 20th century and well within the present one [8,14,15]. Parasite ecology has generally followed a distinct path (but see [16,17,8]) that is the consequence of the divorce between ecology and historical biogeography (16,17,18,19] but as rich in conclusions as the evolutionary part. The integration of both disciplines has been named 'parascript' and to a considerable extent, is part of historical ecology studies [1]. Parascript studies have generally dealt with the reconstruction of ancient distributions and geological events, so generally parascript studies have been equated with historical biogeography. Today, different 'branches' of historical biogeographical research have expanded into two seemingly different research programmes: event-based historical biogeography and discovery-based historical biogeography ('pattern based' of Ronquist and Sanmartin [20]). Parasite historical biogeography has benefited from both approaches, but mainly from the latter [21].

Historical background notwithstanding, the present review is centered on metadata based on the relative number of studies published on parasites and historical biogeography that generally utilize phylogenies as initial hypotheses of distribution and area delimitation. When taxon cycles are involved in the discussion, I assume both vicariance and dispersal, according to Halas et al. [22].

It is inevitable to ask why, despite the previous work done [8,15], hotly debated, on methods of historical biogeography, parasite biologists insist on reconstructing host-parasite phylogenies first and add as secondary and unchanging information, geographic distribution? The answer offered by historical biogeography cannot be more persuasive, as this chapter unfolds.

3. Definitions

Several definitions are necessary when discussing historical biogeography and parascript. Terms have been discussed in several renderings [7,8,15,16,23]. It is outside the scope of this chapter to enter such a discussion. Although the most debated terms in evolutionary biology of parasites have revolved around the words 'coevolution' and 'coadaptation' (and its derivatives), these definitions are nearly related to historical biogeographical concepts, especially when 'coevolution' is interpreted as homologous to 'vicariance'. Historical biogeography is the study of the phylogenetic relationships of different taxa and the areas where they currently live in and where they probably were previously distributed. For some authors [24] it is the study of the evolution of areas and their taxa inhabiting them. The point of departure of all these definitions is the fact that earth and biota evolve simultaneously, at least as a starting or null hypothesis. It is better to say that earth and biota can chronologically evolve in parallel because simultaneity could confound the timing of vicariant and dispersal phenomena.

Vicariance in temporal terms actually recovers only that part of the evolution of earth and biota that occur simultaneously if earth evolution is deemed as the separation of landmasses, major continental blocks, ocean and river basins, and mountain uplifting that leaves a permanent effect on species. These effects can be traced to speciation events and host-switching, or hybridization, among other phenomena. Dispersal under these terms is the movement, idiosyncratic or concerted (as in range expansions or geodispersal) of whole populations or communities of organisms over those earthly barriers already in existence, due to changes in climate or the breakdown of previous barriers.

4. Methods

Database information today is a primer for further research. It is desirable that databases are compiled and then published for the rest of colleagues interested in following some lines of research, especially those who are newcomers to a field of study.

Databases consulted for the present chapter included mainly Web of Science® (WS 1899-present) because other databases (Current Contents Connect® (1998-present), Biological Abstracts® (1993-present), Zoological Record® (1976-present), and Journal Citation Reports®), are integrated to the WS, have a smaller year-span search record, and the records found in them approximate but are not as complete as those of WS.

I followed in the lead of Poulin and Forbes [25] on the web-based research they employed on host-parasite interactions. The database was developed as a result of the current objective experience that is contained in the literature and research programmes that exploit to its full extent the parascript concept, as defined by Manter [1], and further developed by Brooks and McLennan [8], Hoberg and Klassen [9] and Hoberg et al. [26], among others and in posterior publications by themselves and other researchers. Results were then incorporated into the following categories.

4.1. Database entries

Entries were included accordingly as: general type of macroparasite, inferred historical biogeographical patterns, time dimension, terrestrial geomorphological features, taxon level analyzed, methods applied to historical biogeography analysis, and number of papers. Entries included word combinations as 'metadata* parasites* historical biogeography', 'parascript* parasites', 'parasites* biogeography', 'parasites* historical biogeography', 'parascript' as a stand-alone, 'parasite* biogeography' and finally 'parasite* historical biogeography'.

4.1.1. General type of macroparasite

Helminths, arthropods –three distinct entries were developed, one that included simultaneously ecto and endohelminths, a second that only included ectoparasites such as mites, ticks and lice, and a third one that included other types of arthropod parasites, e.g., Coleoptera, Lepidoptera, Hymenoptera, Crustacea (Copepoda), and so forth. Pests are not included, although agricultural studies represent an area where several discoveries on parasite-host interactions have had their point of departure [27].

4.1.2. *Inferred historical biogeographical patterns*

General type of inferred speciation was used as explanation for perceived patterns of historical biogeography. I only grouped all inferred phenomena under two headings – vicariance and dispersal. In the former I considered several names by which vicariance has come down in the literature: coevolution (of parasites/areas), structure of trees not attributable to chance, host-shifts promote speciation ≈ vicariance, cospeciation. Dispersal could be recovered from the records as colonization, chance, non-vicariant processes, range expansion, and geodispersal. Whether all of these designations are equivalent or not exactly equivalent to vicariance or dispersal should not concern us here, as the major debates over historical biogeography clearly are between 'vicariancists' and 'dispersalists' with a variety of definitions according to patterns observed [23]. In the case of dispersion there is evidence that it is a phenomenon not due to chance solely but owes its resulting patterns to other simultaneous events in time, or nearly simultaneous events in time such as environmentally promoted range expansion [28]. When the pattern inferred includes both vicariance and dispersal, I included a third entry.

4.1.3. *The time dimension*

Time is another entry that should be considered [29,20]. Needless to say, time is of central importance in historical biogeographical studies [8]. Yet only in later papers time has become more explicit a variable, and not just a framework, as molecular clocks have entered the arena of historical biogeography through phylogeography [26,30-35].

I recorded entries according to the The Beringian Coevolution Project (BCP, [26]) publications that have a clear use of the terms "deep-time" and "shallow-time". Therefore, I recorded deep time as $>1x10^6$ years and shallow time as $<1x10^6$ years. As many authors seem to combine in their researches explanations that include both age groupings, -in recent papers there seems to be an increase in the use of molecular clock data and phylogeography- I added the category deep/shallow time.

4.1.4. *Terrestrial geomorphological features*

The terrestrial geomorphological features by scale were included in the analysis according to the hierarchical classification of Baker [36]. Authors hardly mention any of these features. The data were entered according to Table 1 but deliberately left out most of those areas that are not mentioned. Area delimitation is still a problem in historical biogeography. No two authors could really agree as to what an area is actually in historical biogeographical studies. 'General areas' is a term often found in the earlier literature on historical biogeography. The first attempts in parasite historical biogeography (summarized in [8]) clearly used drifting continental masses through time, which represents apparently unequivocal designation to discrete areas. Yet, when other geomorphological features are analyzed, authors have resorted to ocean basins, river basins, intermontane geological features, subcontinental regions or vague geographical references, like 'eastern' or 'western' areas. There should be an explicit hierarchical usage of these areas for historical biogeographical phenomena operate at different geographical and time scales. Other authors prefer to substitute areas with events [37].

Order	Approximate Spatial Scale (km^2)	Characteristic Units (with examples)	Approximate Time Scale of Persistence (years)
1	10^7	Continents, ocean basins	$10^8 - 10^9$
2	$10^5 - 10^6$	Physiographic provinces, shields, depositional plains, continental-scale river drainage basins (e.g., Amazon, Mississippi Rivers, Danube, Rio Grande)	10^8
3	10^4	Medium-scale tectonic units (sedimentary basins, mountain massifs, domal uplifts	$10^7 - 10^8$
4	10^2	Smaller tectonic units (fault blocks, volcanoes, troughs, sedimentary sub-basins, individual mountain zones)	10^7
5	$10 - 10^2$	Large-scale erosional/depositional units (deltas, major valleys, piedmonts)	10^6
6	$10^{-1} - 10$	Medium-scale erosional/depositional units or landforms (floodplains, alluvial fans, moraines, smaller valleys and canyons)	$10^5 - 10^6$
7	10^{-2}	Small-scale erosional/depositional units or landforms (ridges, terraces, and dunes)	$10^4 - 10^5$
8	10^{-4}	Larger geomorphic process units (hillslopes, sections of stream channels)	10^3
9	10^{-5}	Medium-scale geomorphic process units (pools and riffles, river bars, solution pits)	10^2
10	10^{-8}	Microscale geomorphic process units (fluvial and eolian ripples, glacial striations)	$10^{-1} - 10^4$

Table 1. Classification of Terrestrial Geomorphological Features by Scale. Modified from Baker [36] (http://disc.sci.gsfc.nasa.gov/geomorphology/GEO_1/GEO_CHAPTER_1.shtml).

4.1.5. Taxon level analyzed

Parasites and hosts have decoupled evolutionary histories [8,23,38] when colonization, host-switching or failure to speciate concurrently with hosts has occurred. Analyzes involving distinct taxon levels have made it clear that parasites seem to speciate in correlation with a change in their physical conditions [39]. The level at which parasites seem to speciate more frequently is at the family level of hosts, correlated with dispersal [38-40]. A distinction between host and parasite levels involved in historical biogeography is at times explicit in such studies. Parasite taxon and host level were recorded as: 1=species (or isolate)/genus, 2=genera (or tribes)/family or subfamily, 3=family/order, 4=order/class, and 5=multiparasite assemblages. When families belonged to the same order, order level was entered; when families corresponded to different orders, multiparasite assemblage was entered instead. I recorded intermediate hierarchical taxon levels as the immediate level above.

4.1.6. Methods applied to historical biogeography analysis

Not all methods were incorporated in the analysis, but only those that have been most widely used [20,41].

Panbiogeography is not considered here a historical biogeographic method for it does not consider the time dimension. Interesting research on panbiogeographic tracks of helminth parasites have been published, especially for central Mexico [42,43]. Nevertheless, it is considered here that historical biogeography should begin with phylogenetic reconstructions, where the time dimension is implicitly or explicitly incorporated into such explanations. Parsimony analysis of endemisms (PAE) papers were not considered as well, as PAE is a non-historical method. PAE relies on current distribution information of organisms, as it analyzes areas of endemism rather than phylogenetic frameworks of the groups studied rendering it unsuitable as a method of historical biogeography [44].

Separate entries for method employed in historical biogeographical inference were incorparated into the analysis. The combinations of words for generating these data were: Topic=(PARASITES* TREEMAP); (PARASITES* BROOKS PARSIMONY ANALYSIS* HISTORICAL BIOGEOGRAPHY), (PARASITES* PARSIMONY* ANALYSIS* FOR COMPARING TREES* PACT* HISTORICAL BIOGEOGRAPHY) (PARASITES* DISPERSAL* VICARIANCE* ANALYSIS* HISTORICAL BIOGEOGRAPHY).

When explanation for a pattern is referred to a previous work by the same author it is considered as extending her/his hypotheses to works examined.

4.1.7. Number of papers

The number of papers based on the indicated word combinations was recovered as well as the number of citations per year. I justify this part because it is interesting how the number of publications on historical biogeography of parasites, especially eukaryotes, has fluctuated since the early 1980's. The number of citations was taken into account as a measure of how many times published works have been used among researchers of historical biogeography of parasites.

5. Results

The analysis of the database herein presented comprises mainly metazoan parasites of vertebrates, because most of the work on historical biogeography of parasites comes from these phyla. To my knowledge, no one has attempted a complete metanalysis of the works published on the historical biogeography of parasites from its beginnings to this time. The following pretends to be a brief account of the data base search undertaken.

No entries for 'metadata* parasites* historical biogeography' were found. This means that there are no metadata analyses of the historical biogeography of parasites. When the words 'parascript* parasites' was entered only 2 entries were recovered in all databases mentioned above, i.e., Brooks and McLennan's [8] book on parascript and Nadler's [45] review in *Science*. Nevertheless, what is probably the only attempt of reviewing the data on marine parasites from a historical biogeographical standpoint was published nearly 10 years ago [9]. Therefore, more than 20 searches were made by combining 'parasites* biogeography', 'parasites* historical biogeography', 'parascript', among others. The entries 'parasite* biogeography' gave 2677 records, while narrowing to 'parasite* historical biogeography' gave 209 records in an early search (136 in a later one, the origin of that difference could not be assessed). Most of the latter records were contained in the former and because the former did not contain additional information on historical biogeography, I chose the latter 209 records for a metadata analysis.

From the initial 209 entries recovered from the WS, 205 qualified initially for historical biogeography and parasites. When research was narrowed to those papers that concluded with historical biogeography + parasites results, only 75 papers that explicitly report results on the historical biogeography of parasites could be detected. Among these papers blood parasites [46,47,48], plant parasites, mistletoes in South America [49], and fungi [50] are included because it seems that there is a growing interest in historical biogeographical research in non-metazoan eukaryotes that have been used as tags for migratory vertebrates.

Despite the importance of parasites and the consequences of parasitism in modern times, as exemplified by the appearance of emerging infectious diseases [51], the evidence of the interplay between taxon pulses and ecological fitting [28] in the structuring of host-parasite communities in the Holarctic region (and purportedly in other regions of the globe) and its restructuring derived from climatic cycling and current climatic change [26], it is surprising that only circa 200 entries with the words 'parasite historical biogeography' could be recovered. It is evident that a certain number of published works that do not include, happen to mention, or were careful not to mention these words have been excluded from the aforementioned database. For example, Brooks and McLennan's [8,15,16] and references therein] works are not included, when they actually contain the words 'historical biogeography' and 'parasites' repeatedly. Not a single paper of Nieberding and Morand [30-34] is ever mentioned, or the recent book edited by Morand and Krasnov [35] on the biogeography of parasites.

5.1. General type of macroparasite

Metadata analysis of historical biogeographical studies of host/parasite/area (Figure 1) indicates that helminth phyla have been the most studied group and within these helminths of freshwater and marine fish, mammals, and birds of the Holartic region [26,30-34], followed afar by bird and mammal ectoparasites (lice and ticks) from northern latitudes, as well [11,23]. A similar situation was recorded 10 years ago from marine parasite historical biogeography [9, Table 1] where 68 works are recorded, among those 51 dealt with helminths (those authors had made clear they centered their analysis on these phyla) and 8 with arthropods, plus 8 theoretical works (20 up to 2012). Researchers on arthropod ectoparasites such as lice and ticks seem to have preferred to study host-parasite coevolution rather than their historical biogeography [23,41] though paradoxically some of the first attempts at tracking historical biogeographical patterns used lice as tags for historical biogeography [13].

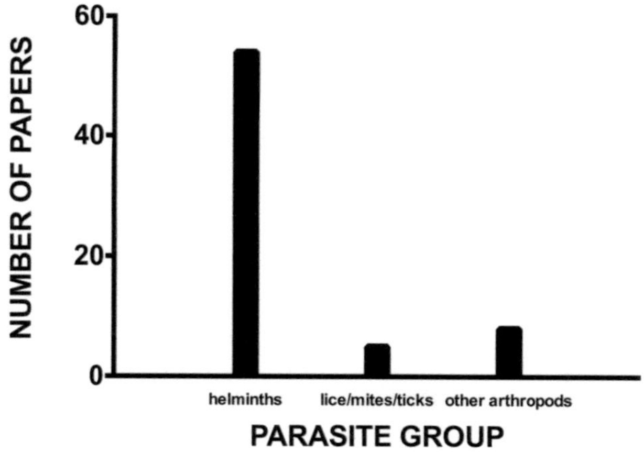

Figure 1. Metadata analysis of parasite historical biogeography. Parasites groups* and papers referring to their historical biogeography. Source of data: Web of Science® (1899-present). * virus, fungi or protozoans not included

5.2. General type of inferred pattern of historical biogeography

A significant conclusion of these analyses (Figure 2) is that 15% of the papers analyzed have recorded patterns of historical biogeography of parasites as vicariant phenomena that involve speciation (coevolution) whereas dispersal events, or host-switching events account for 45%. Papers that mention both vicariance and dispersal account for 40%, a figure near to that of papers that explain pattern with dispersal. If combined, 39% of papers favour vicariance as an explanation and 61% dispersal. Dispersion and related phenomena are favored in parasite historical biogeography as the explanation for modern and historical patterns of parasite distribution across and within continents. Differences in the relative occurrence of one or the other phenomenon rely on methods used. Generally, works that employ a priori considerations of parasite evolution and use vicariance as a constraint, recover vicariant patterns, as in the initial versions of TreeMap [23,52]. When no hypothetical considerations are entertained a priori, multiple instances of vicariance and dispersal are recovered [53] for multiple lineages of both parasites and hosts [54]. The consequences of this are manifold but at least a couple can be identified. Parasites tend to disperse from host taxon to host taxon without changing their morphology (but can modify their life cycles), i.e., they are resource trackers [55]. The other consequence relevant to historical biogeography is that a limited number of species of parasites will disperse into large areas invading new hosts and causing pandemics or even epidemics [51] and probably leave significant and discoverable tracks in geologic time due to coupled phenomena related to range expansion with little morphological change [55].

Brooks and McLennan [8,15] were the first to suggest that parasites exhibit stronger historical associations "with the areas in which they evolved and lived than with the particular species of hosts they inhabit" [13]. Such statement has been confirmed by the empirical data recovered by parascript studies. Metadata analysis herein included reinforces this view, where mention of a weak cophylogenetic signal is common in these papers. A similar conclusion had already been reached by Manter [56], under a different approach, when comparing helminth faunas of marine fish, although he added a second explanation, namely, that parasites lag behind their hosts in evolutionary time. The consequences of such a discovery has far-reaching implications in the management of large areas of the globe related to human health, livestock, agriculture, migrations, and climatic change.

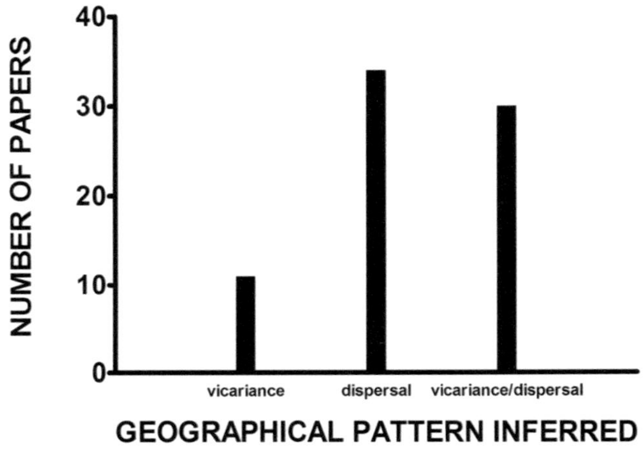

Figure 2. Geographical pattern. Source of data: Web of Science® (1899-present).

This has several implications for the present and future of parascript studies. First, it seems unreliable to ascertain that host/parasite relationships, in a historical perspective, correspond to what has been formerly called parasite specificity. It is now understood that parasites do not track host species, but tend to track host resources that can be represented across different taxa and therefore, are plesiomorphic. It is humans who define host taxa, not parasites [15]. A parasite-centered point of view would be that of "what hosts suits me is what host is my feeding site".

5.3. The time dimension

Previous analyses [9] and the one included in this chapter, reflect a deep concern of researchers of historical biogeography for deep time and deep time combined with shallow time (Figure 3). This is actually the case when an increase in works of phylogeography is recorded. Nevertheless, the WS database includes few of these. Major works on the phylgoeography and comparative phylogeography of parasites and hosts include explanations on recent (shallow) and ancient (deep) biogeographical phenomena [26, 30-34,57]. Now there is a whole new universe of research where there is growing room for inferring simultaneity of speciation of parasites, hosts, and historical divergence or dispersal into new areas. There have been serious statistical analyses involving simultaneity of divergence [58] in free living organisms, but still not enough on parasites. This is reflected in parascript studies in that most of the cladograms of parasites and areas published up to this day lack an explicit hypothesis of the timing of historical events [6,20,28]. In the case of parasites, a lack of fossil evidence seemingly hampers such a calculation, but the growth of research of molecular clocks for both parasites and hosts might be promising [28]. Speculation enters the arena here when we try to deduct the origin of a parasite clade derived from its probable most ancient host. Some attempts have been made earlier [59] with fossils of hosts as calibration points for parasite clades. Nevertheless, the lack of fossils for the parasite associate will always remain and heavy reliance on what host taxon was the original one adds up to this uncertainty. Despite this fact, hypotheses of the original hosts of several endoparasitic [9,60] and ectoparasitic taxa [54] have been utilized as departing points for assessing the origin of particular parasite clades. Parasite counts of modern clades and the use of appropriate net diversification intervals could give some insight as to the antiquity of some key clades [38].

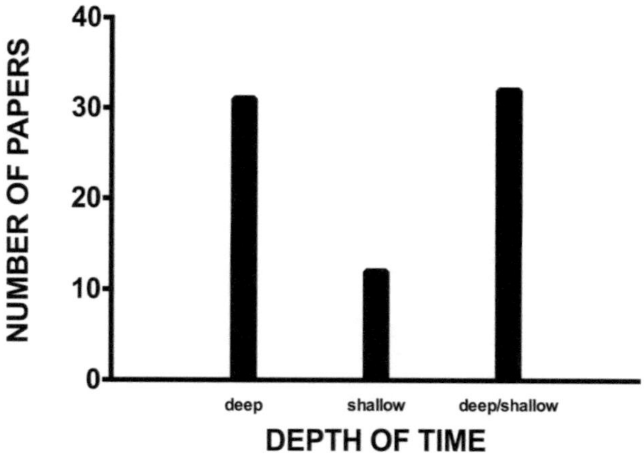

Figure 3. Metadata analysis of parasite historical biogeography. Depth of time. Web of Science® (1899-present).

5.4. Terrestrial geomorphological features

According to the classification of geomorphological features, historical biogeography parasitologists are deeply concerned with large continental areas in their analyses (Figure 4). As parasites speciate seemingly with geomorphological changes it is hardly surprising that the higher hierarchical levels of parasite/area were considered as the first targets of historical biogeography. The Holarctic regions has been the most intensively studied [26, 30-34,57]. Southern regions of the earth have been less explored; among these, South America and

Australia have been the most intensively studied, at the drainage level in the former (Amazon and Paraná drainages mainly) [61-64] and at the continental scale in the latter. It is important to note that areas as terminals in phylogenetic analyses are equal or less in numbers if compared to parasite terminals. Despite the quality of works done on the northern areas of this planet, there are still no independent estimates of the histories of areas [65], where geological studies need to be consulted by parasitologists. Nevertheless, during the modern era of parascript studies, there has been a concern for formulating independent area cladograms of e.g., the breakup of Pangea [8]. Despite the fact that molecular studies have increasingly become incroporated into the historical biogeography of parasites, the breakup of Pangea [66] has remained a very good starting point for historical biogeographical studies and a well supported hypothesis of tectonic plate movements. The latter studies will certainly incorporate more information to the point where it will probably be difficult to discover single independent area histories, especially if dispersal or range expansions are being identified as the engine of parasite speciation. Yet, it would be unvaluable information if independent geological information was explicitly incorporated into historical parascript studies [65].

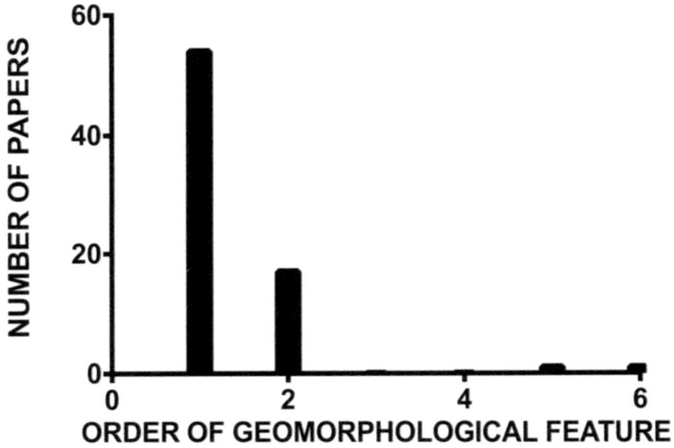

Figure 4. Metadata analysis of parasite historical biogeography. Geolomophological features. Source of data: Web of Science® (1899-present). See Table 1 for descriptions of orders.

5.5. Taxon level analyzed

Species level studies seem to be preferred over higher taxonomic levels or multi parasite assemblages (Figure 5). This might represent the difficulties in assessing parasite communities from host assemblages. Additionally, this could reflect that the study of parasite historical biogeography has centered on core species within parasite communities.

Quite a different result was recovered from hosts. A preference for multi host assemblages was recovered in the study of parasite historical biogeography (Figure 6). This could reflect the interest on different host taxa, the availability of different species of hosts or the presence of single parasite species in different hosts.

http://dx.doi.org/10.5772/55459

Despite the foregoing, a correlation appears between the distinct levels of parasite and host taxa involved in historical biogeographical studies (Figure 7). It is particularly interesting to note that a direct relationship exists between the host taxon level and parasite taxon level. This reflects that as the level of host taxon sampling increases there is an increase in the number of distinct parasite species sampled.

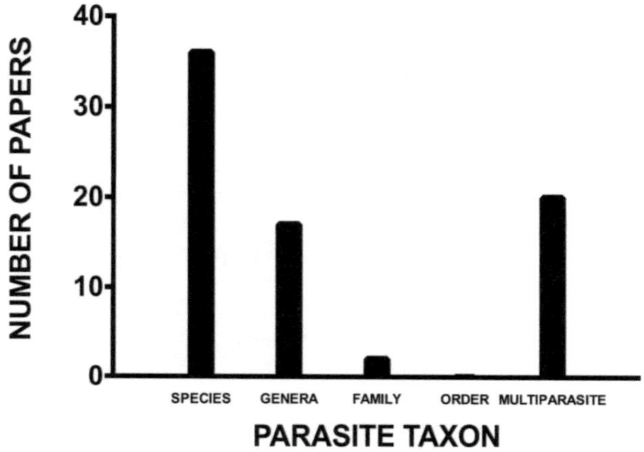

Figure 5. Parasite taxon levels analyzed in historical biogeographical studies.

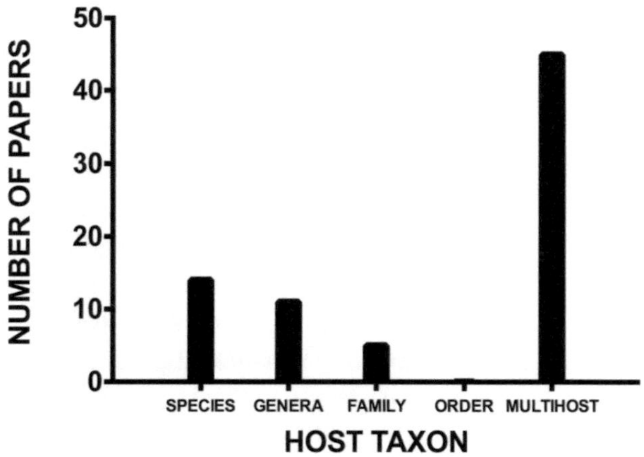

Figure 6. Metadata analysis of parasite historical biogeography. Host taxa levels analyzed in historical biogeographical studies. Source of data: Web of Science® (1899-present).

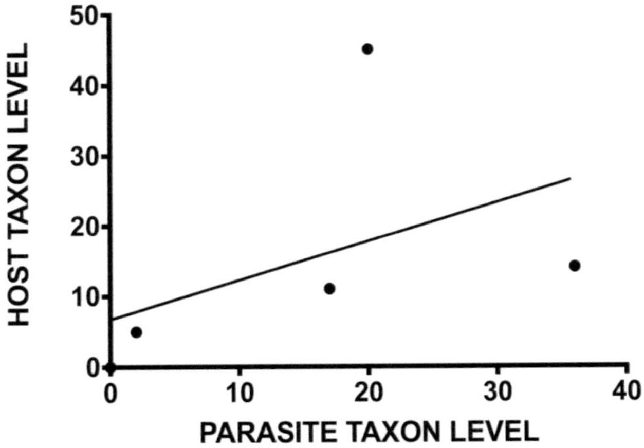

Figure 7. Correlation between host and parasite taxon level. (correlation coefficient = 0.46,t = 1,d.f. = 6, p>0.01).

5.6. Methods employed in historical biogeography of parasites

Parsimony analysis of host/parasite/area seems to be the dominant optimality criterion for proposing hypotheses of historical biogeography of helminth parasites (Figure 8) while other methods, i.e., component analysis, dispersal-vicariance, among others, have more often been implemented with helminth endoparasites and arthropod ectoparasites phylogenies. Nevertheless, other methods have recently gained acceptance and have been preferred over parsimony and component analyses for the study of historical biogeography [20] but have not been developed in relation to host/parasite/area biogeographic reconstruction. The number of citations amongst the different methods used during the development of parasite historical biogeography have been manifold, but all of them can be grouped mainly in two camps, although there is a growing tendency to use probabilistic methods, probably as a reflection of what is the general trend in phylogenetic reconstruction [20]. Among the parsimony methods and the non-parsimonious methods, I explored the number of citations for at least the four most recurrent used and cited methods: TreeMap [23 and references therein, 52], BPA [8, 15, 16, 67-69], PACT [70-72], and DIVA [73]. The most cited method is DIVA [73]. This could only mean that methods that include both dispersal and vicariance as their working hypothesis have been favored over those that favor maximum cospeciation. DIVA has been equated to secondary BPA [68]. Parsimony methods seemingly took a higher stand during the development of parasite historical biogeography. Nevertheless, statistical-based methods seem to be gaining ground [20] mainly because there is an actual increase in molecular phylogenies (and phylogeographical studies) as compared to recently published morphological phylogenies, although it must be kept in mind that statistical methods can be and have been applied to morphological phylogenies.

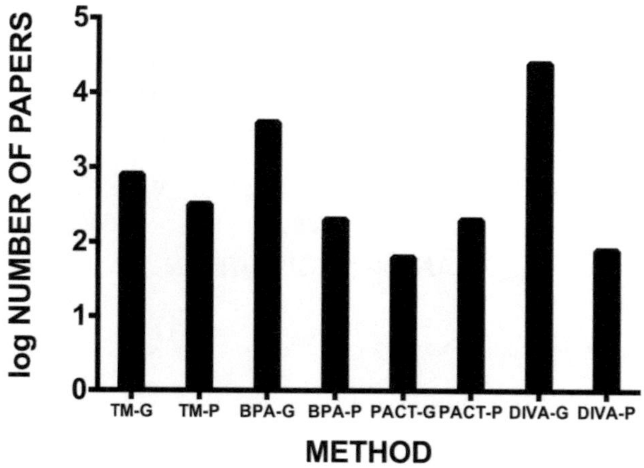

Figure 8. Number of citations per major method used for historical biogeography reconstruction of parasites. Source of data: Web of Science® (1899-present). G- methods used with other groups other than parasites; P- parasite groups.

Analytical methods of patterns and processes in historical biogeography have tended to favor other groups than parasites (Figure 8). DIVA, despite its widespread use, has been very limited in dealing with parasite groups. No wonder, BPA is the method that has been more commonly utilized by parasitologists.

5.7. Number of papers

Figures 9 and 10 bring together the number of papers written on the historical biogeography of parasites in general and the number of citations per paper. Number of papers is one and more generally two orders of magnitude below the number of citations per paper. The most cited paper is on the historical biogeography of *Drosophila* spp. in Africa [74]. The next most cited paper is a work by Rod Page that conflates genes, organisms, and areas without a distinction between hierarchical levels [75]. It is difficult to explain why the number of papers plot is bimodal whereas the citations plot is nearer to an exponential curve. It can be seen that the increase in the use of molecular biology in phylogenetic systematics and phylogeography has increased the number of publications. Interest on this research area has expanded to other regions of the world. As for citation increase, the only other conclusion that can be reached at this stage of research is that historical biogeography of parasites papers have had an enormous impact in areas beyond parasitologists traditional lines of research.

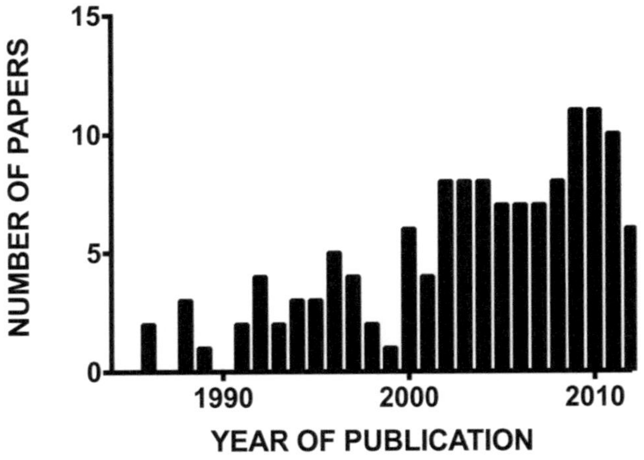

Figure 9. Number of publications on historical biogeography of parasites per year. Source of data: Web of Science® (1899-present).

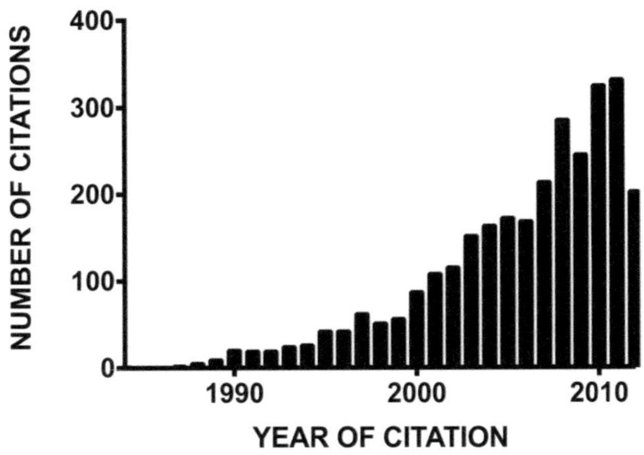

Figure 10. Number of citations on historical biogeography of parasites per year. Source of data: Web of Science® (1899-present).

6. Discussion

A metadata analysis of the historical biogeography of parasite studies had never been attempted before. The analyses practiced to the present data were kept as clear as possible. Several shortcomings stemmed from these type of analyses. The most immediate one is related to the combination of several taxa in one paper, e.g., helminths and arthropods. Nevertheless, I found only a single paper that included analysis both on parasitic copepods and endohelminths [76]. Several methods of analyses in a single paper are generally more common. Despite this fact, those papers recovered were substantially TreeMap-oriented or BPA-oriented. PACT is an analysis that has hardly been exploited. Probabilistic analyses are still in their beginnings, so we must see a substantial growth in usage of these methods in the present decade. An in-depth analysis of every single paper included in the present chapter would want from space and reading time. Let this brief account of the use of parascript studies, or studies related to the historical biogeographical part be a starting line for further accounts.

The most outstanding problem in modern historical biogeography a decade ago was related to the most approximate method(s) that recovered most of the information contained in parasite/hosts/area phylogenies in order to offer approximate historical biogeographical reconstructions. Nevertheless, numbers indicate there was more concern for reconstructing coevolutionary scenarios than for historical biogeography reconstructions. Under this heading methods have diversified, but today little attention is paid as to what method is used. Instead, the main concerns centers more and more as to the number of genes used to reconstruct phylogenies and then afterwards what the shape of the phylogeny tells us about the biogeography of the taxon or taxa studied. There are substantially excellent reviews on the state of the art in coevolution studies [20]. Yet, there is a need for an equivalent review on historical biogeographical methods that brings together the best ideas from each camp. New computer methods are being implemented, but the assumptions have remained the same. What is notable is that the null hypotheses for historical biogeographical studies depart each day more and more from the original 'coevolutionary' assumption. Parsimony methods have brought about this departure and have influenced all those methods that originally belonged to the 'maximum coevolution' camp. Parsimony methods have moved on and have incorporated cost analysis [41]. Yet some of the methods mentioned in Ronquist and Sanmartin [20] for free-living organisms have not been explored in host/parasite/area research programmes. Non-parsimony methods, such as ML and Bayesian, have not been incorporated yet into parascript studies but will certainly do in the near future.

7. Conclusions

There is little room for doubt that parascript studies, as envisioned by Harold Manter [1], are in the need to enter the application arena. The results obtained by major research programmes, namely the Beringian Coevolutionary Project (BCP), are moving into the direction of a more propositive agenda than ever. This does not mean that data collecting is going to be disregarded. On the contrary, there is today a growing need to increase the number of parasite specimens and hosts as never before.

From the foregoing analysis it seems that the state of the art in parascript studies will head towards a more comprehensive understanding of the biosphere [26]. Regardless of the method employed, it seems that careful and detailed phylogenetic reconstruction, both morphological and molecular, lies at the heart of a sound historical biogeographical reconstruction of events in the earth's past and present. The predictive nature of parascript studies is still being worked out, with significative advances stemming from the BCP. One lesson is that methods must lie deep within phylogenetic studies and especially should be fed by the backup and background supported by museum collections of parasites throughout the world [77]. Repositories of parasite specimens cannot be supplanted by any other means of information repository. The very nature of parascript studies depends on well documented specimens that must be deposited in recognized collections around the world. The very curatorial nature of parascript needs a complete overhaul around the most outstanding academic institutions of the world, where most of the information for the historical biogeography of parasites lies for future generations to study the biodiversity on this planet Earth.

Acknowledgements

This work was supported through a SNI grant 43282 from the CONACYT and Facultad de Ciencias, UNAM. Special thanks go to Dr. José G. Palacios-Vargas, head of the Laboratorio de Ecología y Sistemática de Microartrópodos, Facultad de Ciencias, and Dr. Rosaura Ruíz-Gutiérrez Director of Facultad de Ciencias, UNAM, for their unvaluable support during the writing of the present work.

Author details

Hugo H. Mejía-Madrid

Universidad Nacional Autónoma de México/Laboratorio de Ecología y Sistemática de Microartrópodos/Departamento de Ecología y Recursos Naturales, México

References

[1] Manter HW. The zoogeography of trematodes of marine fishes. Expermiental Parasitology 1966;4 62-86.

[2] Brooks DR, Pérez-Ponce de León G, León-Règagnón V. Enfoques contemporáneos para el estudio de la biodiversidad. México: IBUNAM y Fondo de Cultura Económica; 2001.

[3] Brooks DR, Hoberg EP. Triage for the biosphere: The need and rationale for taxonomic inventories and phylogenetic studies of parasites. Comparative Parasitology 2000;67 1-25.

[4] Von Ihering H. Die Helminthen als Hilfsmittel der zoogeographischen Forshung. Zoologischer Anzeiger 1902;2 42-51.

[5] Von Ihering H. On the Ancient Relations between New Zealand and South America. Transactions and Proceedings of the New Zealand Institute 1891;24 431-445.

[6] Klassen GJ. Coevolution: A history of the macroevolutionary approach to studying host-parasite associations. Journal of Parasitology 1992;78(4) 573-587.

[7] Brooks DR. Testing the context and extent of host-parasite coevolution. Systematic Zoology 1979;28, 299-307.

[8] Brooks DR, McLennan DA. Parascript. Parasites and the language of evolution. Washington and London: Smithsonian Institution Press; 1993.

[9] Hoberg EP, Klassen GJ. Revealing the faunal tapestry: co-evolution and historical biogeography of hosts and parasites in marine systems. Parasitology 2002;12 S3–S22.

[10] Ròzsa L. Speciation patterns of ectoparasites and "straggling" lice. International Journal for Parasitology 1993;23(7) 859-864.

[11] Hoberg EP, Brooks DR, Siegel-Causey D. Chapter 11. Host-parasite cospeciation: History, principles, and prospects. In: Clayton D H, Moore J. (eds.) Host-parasite evolution: General principles and avian models. U.K.: Oxford University Press, Oxford; 1997. p212-235.

[12] Kuris AM, Hechinger RF, Shaw JC. et al. Ecosystem energetic implications of parasite and free-living biomass in three estuaries. Nature 2008;454 515-518.

[13] Metcalf MM. Parasites and the aid they give in problems of taxonomy, geographical distribution, and paleogeography. Smithsonian Miscellaneous Collections 1929;81(8) 1-36.

[14] Henning W. Phylogenetic Systematics. USA: Chicago University Press; 1966.

[15] Brooks DR, McLennan DA.The Nature of Diversity: An Evolutionary Voyage of Discovery.USA: University of Chicago Press; 2002.

[16] Brooks DR, McLennan DA. Phylogeny, Ecology and Behavior. A research program in compararive biology. USA: University of Chicago Press; 1991.

[17] Brooks DR. Historical Ecology: A new approach to studying the evolution of ecological associations. Annals of the Missouri Botanical Garden 1985;72(4) 660-680.

[18] Poulin R. Evolutionary Ecology of Parasites. Second Edition. USA: Princeton University Press; 2006.

[19] Wiens JJ, Donoghue MJ. Historical biogeography, ecology and species richness. Trends in Ecology and Evolution 2004;19(12) 639-644.

[20] Ronquist F, Sanmartin I. Phylogenetic Methods in Biogeography. Annual Review of Ecology, Evolution, and Systematics 2011;42 441–64.

[21] Brooks DR, McLennan DA. A comparison of a discovery-based and an event-based method of historical biogeography. Journal of Biogeography 2001;28(6) 757–767.

[22] Halas D, Zamparo D, Brooks DR. 2005. A historical biogeographical protocol for studying biotic diversification by taxon pulses.Journal of Biogeography 2005;32(2) 249–260.

[23] Page RDM. (ed.) Tangled trees: phylogeny, and coevolution. USA: University of Chicago Press, Chicago; 2003.

[24] Platnick NI, Nelson G. A method of analysis for historical biogeography. Systematic Zoology 1978;27 1–16.

[25] Poulin R, Forbes MR. Meta-analysis and research on host-parasite interactions: past and future. Evolutionary Ecology 2012;26 1169-1185.

[26] Hoberg EP, Galbreath KE, Cook JA, Kutz SJ, Polley L. Chapter 1. Northern Host–Parasite Assemblages: History and Biogeography on the Borderlands of Episodic Climate and Environmental Transition. In: Rollinson D, Hay SI. Advances in Parasitology UK: Elsevier Limited; 79, 2012. p1-97.

[27] Price PW. Evolutionary Biology of Parasites. USA: Princeton University Press; 1980.

[28] Hoberg EP, Brooks DR.Chapter 1: Beyond vicariance: integrating taxon pulses, ecological fitting, and oscillation in evolution and historical biogeography In: Morand S, Krasnov BR (eds.) The Biogeography of Host-Parasite Interactions. U.K.: Oxford University Press, Oxford; 2010. p7–20.

[29] Donoghue MJ, Moore BR.Toward an integrative historical biogeography. Integrative Comparative Biology 2003;43 261–270.

[30] Nieberding C, Morand S, Libois R, Michaux J. A parasite reveals cryptic phylogeographical history of its host. Proceedings of the Royal Society London B 2004;271 2559–68.

[31] Nieberding C, Morand S, Douady CJ, Libois R, Michaux J. Phylogeography of a nematode (*Heligmosomoides polygyrus*) in the western Palearctic region: Persistence of northern cryptic populations during ice ages? Molecular Ecology 2005;14:765–779.

[32] Morand S, Krasnov BR, Poulin R (eds.) Micromammals and Macroparasites. From Evolutionary Ecology to Management. Tokyo Berlin Heidelberg New York: Springer-Verlag; 2006.

[33] Nieberding CM, Morand S. Chapter 15. Comparative phylogeography: The use of parasites for insights into host history. In: Morand S, Krasnov BR, Poulin R (eds.) Micromammals and Macroparasites. From Evolutionary Ecology to Management. Tokyo Berlin Heidelberg New York: Springer-Verlag; 2006. p277-293.

[34] Nieberding C, Morand S, Libois R, Michaux JR. Parasites and the island syndrome: the colonization of the western Mediterranean islands by *Heligmosomoides polygyrus* (Dujardin, 1845). Journal of Biogeography 2006;33(7) 1212–1222.

[35] Morand S, Krasnov BR (eds.) The Biogeography of Host-Parasite Interactions. UK: Oxford University Press; 2010.

[36] Baker VR. Introduction: Regional landforms analysis. In: Short, NM, Blair, RW, Jr. (eds.) Geomorphology from Space. A global overview of regional Landforms. USA: NASA; 1986. Available from http://disc.sci.gsfc.nasa.gov/geomorphology/GEO_1/GEO_CHAPTER_1.shtml (accessed 17 September 2012).

[37] Hovenkamp P. Vicariance events, not areas, should be used in biogeographical analysis. Cladistics 1997;13 67–79.

[38] Mejía-Madrid HH. Biogeographic Hierarchical Levels and Parasite Speciation. In: Stevens L. (ed.) Global Advances in Biogeography. Rijeka: InTech; 2012. p23-48. Available from: http://www.intechopen.com/books/global-advances-in-biogeography/biogeographic-hierarchical-levels-and-parasite-speciation (accessed 27 August 2012).

[39] Vrba, ES. Mass turnover and heterochrony events in response to physical change. Paleobiology 2005;31(2) 157-174.

[40] Pérez-Ponce de León G, Choudhury A. Biogeography of helminth parasites of freshwater fishes in Mexico: the search for patterns and processes. Journal of Biogeography 2005;32 645-659.

[41] Ronquist F. Parsimony analysis of coevolving species associations. In: Page RDM (ed.) Tangled trees. Phylogeny, cospeciation, and coevolution. USA: The University of Chicago Press; 2003. p22-64.

[42] Aguilar-Aguilar RR, Contreras-Medina R, Salgado-Maldonado G. Parsimony analysis of endemicity (PAE) of Mexican hydrological basins based on helminth parasites of freshwater fishes. Journal of Biogeography 2003;30 1861-1872.

[43] Aguilar-Aguilar RR, Contreras-Medina R, Martínez-Aquino, Salgado-Maldonado G, González-Zamora A. Aplicación del análisis de parsimonia de endemismos (PAE) en los sistemas hidrológicos de México: un ejemplo con helmintos parásitos de peces dulceacuículas. In: Llorente -Bousquets J y Morrone JJ (eds.) Regionalización biogeográfica en Iberoamérica y tópicos afines. México: Comisión Nacional para el Conocimiento y Uso de la Bidoviersidad y Universidad Nacional Autónoma de México; 2003 p227-239.

[44] Brooks DR, van Veller, MGP. Critique of parsimony analysis of endemicity as a method of historical biogeography. Journal of Biogeography 2003;30 819–825.

[45] Nadler SA. Non-Degenerates. Science New Series 1993;261(5123) 927-928.

[46] Hamilton PB, Cruickshank C, Stevens JR, Teixeira MMG, Mathews F. Parasites reveal movement of bats between the New and Old Worlds. Molecular Phylogenetics and Evolution 2012;6(2) 521-526.

[47] Jenkins T, Thomas GH, Hellgren O, Owens IPF. Migratory behavior of birds affects their coevolutionary relationship with blood parasites. Evolution 2012;66(3) 740-751.

[48] Silva-Iturriza A, Ketmaier V, Tiedemann R. Profound population structure in the Philippine Bulbul *Hypsipetes philippinus* (Pycnonotidae, Ayes) is not reflected in its *Haemoproteus* haemosporidian parasites. Infection Genetics and Evolution 2012;12(1) 127- 136.

[49] Amico GC, Nickrent DL. Population structure and phylogeography of the mistletoes *Tristerix corymbosus* and *T. aphyllus* (Loranthaceae) using chloroplast DNA sequence variation. American Journal of Botany 2009;96(8) 1571-1580.

[50] Peterson KR, Pfister DH, Bell CD. Cophylogeny and biogeography of the fungal parasite *Cyttaria* and its host *Nothofagus*, southern beech. Mycologia 2010;102 (6) 1417-1425.

[51] Brooks DR, Ferrao AL. The historical biogeography of coevolution: emerging infectious diseases are evolutionary accidents waiting to happen. J. Biogeogr. 2005;32 1291–1299.

[52] Page RDM. Parallel phylogenies: reconstructing the history of host-parasite assemblages. Cladistics 1995;10 155-173.

[53] Van Veller MGP, Kornet DJ, Zandee M. A posteriori and a priori methodologies for testing hypotheses of causal processes in vicariance biogeography. Cladistics 2001;7, 248–259.

[54] Smith VS, Ford T, Johnson KP, Johnson PCD, Yoshizawa K, Light, JE. . Multiple lineages of lice pass through the K-Pg boundary. Biology Letters 2011;7(5) 782-785.

[55] Agosta SJ, Janz N, Brooks DR. How specialists can be generalists: resolving the "parasite paradox" and implications for emerging infectious disease. Zoologia 2010;27(2) 151-162.

[56] Manter HW. The zoogeographical affinities of trematodes of South American freshwater fishes. Systematic Zoology 1963;12(2) 45-70.

[57] Choudhury A, Dick TA. Sturgeons and their parasites: Patterns and processes in historical biogeography. Journal of Biogeography, 2001;28 1411-1439.

[58] Hickerson MJ, Stahl EA, Lessios HA. Bayesian Test for simultaneous divergence using approximate computation. Evolution. 2006;60(12) 2435-53.

[59] Verneau O, Du Preez LH, Laurent V, Raharivololoniaina L, Glaw F, Vences M. The double odyssey of Madagascan polystome flatworms leads to new insights on the

origins of their amphibian hosts. Proceedings of the Royal Society B 2009;276 1575-1583.

[60] Hoberg EP, Jones A, Bray RA. Phylogenetic analysis among the families of the Cyclophyllidea (Eucestoda) based on comparative morphology, with new hypotheses for co-evolution in vertebrates. Systematic Parasitology 1999;42 51–73.

[61] Brooks, DR. Origins, diversification, and historical structure of the helminth fauna inhabiting neotropical freshwater stingrays (Potamotrygonidae). Journal of Parasitology 1992;78(4) 588-595.

[62] Lovejoy NR. Stingrays, Parasites, and Neotropical Biogeography: A closer look at Brooks et al.'s hypotheses concerning the origins of Neotropical freshwater rays (Potamotrygonidae). Systematic Biology 1997;46(1) 218-230.

[63] Boeger WA, Kritsky DC, Pie MR. Context of diversification of the viviparous Gyrodactylidae (Platyhelminthes, Monogenoidea). Zoologica Scripta 2003;32(5) 437–448.

[64] Bandoni SM, Brooks DR. Revision and phylogenetic analysis of the Amphilinidea Poche, 1922 (Platyhelminthes: Cercomeria: Cercomeromorpha). Canadian Journal of Zoology 1987;65, 1110–1128.

[65] Siddall ME, Perkins SL. Brooks Parsimony Analysis: a valiant failure. Cladistics 2003;19 554–564.

[66] Badets M, Whittington I, Lalubin F, Allienne J-F, MaspimbyJ-L, Bentz S, Du Preez LH, Barton D, Hasegawa H, Tandon V, Imkongwapang R, Ohler A, Combes C, Verneau O. Correlating early evolution of parasitic platyhelminths to Gondwana breakup. Systematic Biology 2011;60(6) 762–781.

[67] Brooks DR, vanVeller MGP, McLennan DA. How to do BPA, really. Journal of Biogeography 2001;28 343–358.

[68] Dowling APG. A rigorous test of accuracy between Brooks Parsimony Analysis and TREEMAP, the two most commonly used methods for determining coevolutionary patterns. Cladistics 2002;18 416–435.

[69] Brooks DR, Dowling APG, van Veller MGP, Hoberg EP. Ending a decade of deception: a valiant failure, a not-sovaliant failure, and a success story. Cladistics 2004;20, 32–46.

[70] Wojcicki M, Brooks DR. Escaping the matrix: a new algorithm for phylogenetic comparative studies of co-evolution. Cladistics 2004;20 341–361.

[71] Wojcicki M, Brooks DR. PACT: an efficient and powerful algorithm for generating area cladograms. Journal of Biogeography 2005;32 755–774.

[72] Arias JS, Garzón Orduña IJ, López-Osorio F, Parada Vargas E, Miranda-Esquivel DR. What is PACT really? Cladistics 2008;24 1–12.

[73] Ronquist F. Dispersal-vicariance analysis: a new approach to the quantification of historical biogeography. Systematic Biology 1997;46 195–203

[74] Lachaise D, Cariou ML, David JR, Lemeunier F, Tsacas L, Ashburner, M. Historical biogeography of the Drosophila-melanogaster species subgroup. Evolutionary Biology 1988;22 159-225.

[75] Page, RDM. Maps between trees and cladistic-analysis of historical associations among genes, organisms, and areas. Systematic Biology 1994;43(1)58-77

[76] Avenant-Oldewage A, Oldewage WH. The occurrence of fish parasites in the Kwando River, Caprivi, Namibia. Madoqua 1993;18(2) 183-185.

[77] Hoberg EP, Pilitt PA, Galbreath KE. Why Museums Matter: A Tale of Pinworms (Oxyuroidea: Heteroxynematidae) Among Pikas (*Ochotona princeps* and *O. collaris*) in the American West. Journal of Parasitology 2009;95(2) 490–501.

Chapter 7

Spatial Variability of Vegetation in the Changing Climate of the Baikal Region

A. P. Sizykh and V. I. Voronin

Additional information is available at the end of the chapter

http://dx.doi.org/10.5772/55481

1. Introduction

The systems of environments contact sites are somewhat models reflecting practically all changes occurring in any hierarchic systems. Recently different approaches to the assessment of such processes as paragenesis manifestation in the environments are proposed. There are some suppositions on manifestation of polyzonality (binarity) of the environments, especially at the local level of their organization of the background of climate changes. Here, on the author's opinion, the geomorphology peculiarities and edaphic conditions in polyzonality formation at the regional level of the environment organization are manifested. The validity of use of concrete terms characterizing one or other environments is discussed. In particular, conclusions on the opportunity of use the term "zonal habitat" in the characterization of flat interfluve vegetation and soils are very curious. In this context, the use of polysystem modeling method and of ones of systematic mapping analysis of environments organization and dynamics will promote resolution of concrete tasks for indication and forecasting of environments contact systems. The vegetation structure of the Prebaikalia reveals a certain relation to the evolution history of the natural environment of the entire Baikal region. In the tertiary era the territory of the present-day Prebaikalia was occupied by broad-leaved forests where valleys and dry depressions between mountains were dominated by xerophyte grass communities (Grichuk, 1955; Dylis, Reshchikov, Malyshev, 1965). Tectonic movements and changes of climate were responsible for the disappearance of the heat-loving flora. The landscapes of the Baikal region have attained their modern character during the last 10-12 thousand years. The development of the vegetative cover in the Prebaikalia dates back to the Holocene (Belova, 1975, 1985; Savina, 1986; Bezrukova, 1996, 2002). Climate fluctuations over the course of the Holocene were responsible for the characteristic properties of spatial variability and dynamics of the interrelationship between the various types of vegetation in the region, in the character of changes in the species composition, of the predominant kinds of layers, and of change sin the areas occupied by different types of communities (forest and steppe communities) at different periods of the Holocene. The relative increase in the amount of yearly mean summertime precipitation and yearly mean winter temperatures (Gustokashina, 2003) qualitatively alter the conditions of the forming environment, the cause for the tendencies of the region's vegetation (and the natural environment as a whole) to develop. A highly instructive example with regards to identifying the dynamic properties of the communities that develop in the zone of contact of the types of vegetation, and the factors that are responsible for them, is provided by a publication (Thomas T. Veblen, Diana C. Lorenz, 1988) which treats the problem of vegetation changes in the "forest-steppe" ecotone zone in Northern Patagonia.

For spatial variability of vegetation in the changing climate there are quit new information for Ural mountain systems (Shyatov et al., 2005; Kapralov et al., 2006, and others).

Some new information about current structure and tendency of the vegetation formation around Lake Baikal we have get for last years, just for some of territories of the Baikal region.

The aim of our studies is determining of main peculiarities of structural and dynamical communities organization forming under the conditions of mutual development of extra zonal steppes and taiga with identification of nowadays tendencies of communities genesis under the conditions of changing climatic situation and of dynamics of anthropogenic impacts in the region. The areas investigation there are on the map (Fig.1.).

2. Methods

This study is based on using the method of large-scale mapping of the vegetation in conjunction with field aerospace photography interpretation of a different scale, by generating maps on a scale 1 : 25 000 - 1: 100 000. By laying transect-profiles and using geobotanical descriptions for different years, it was possible to identify areas reflecting the whole spectrum of the typological composition of the region's communities. These model areas are representative throughout the entire spatial structure of vegetation and were the objects of monitoring of the dynamics and genesis of communities that develop in different environmental conditions and reflecting different types of the region's vegetation. A many-year (15 years) monitoring in the model areas using aerospace photographs from different years (1972-2002) for the territory of the Prebaikalia was instrumental in revealing the typological composition of communities, with a certain set of plant species, diagnostic tools for communities of different conditions of development. The selection of a territory where profiling is to be performed requires always natural phenomenon analysis, its concrete characteristics or a particular structure and is always individual. The relief structure, taking into account differences in relative heights, the situation of a territory in a mountain system, if available, as well as driangle system analysis (river basin, lake coast, etc) determine the profile site and length. A geobotanic profile aimed to reveal the spatial variability of communities structure is established taking into account the peculiarities of vegetation on a territory depending on the range – topologic, regional, zonal, etc. One of the methods for revealing structure, spatial variability and interaction of phytocenoses in environments contact sites with edaphic conditions, on our opinion, can be combined

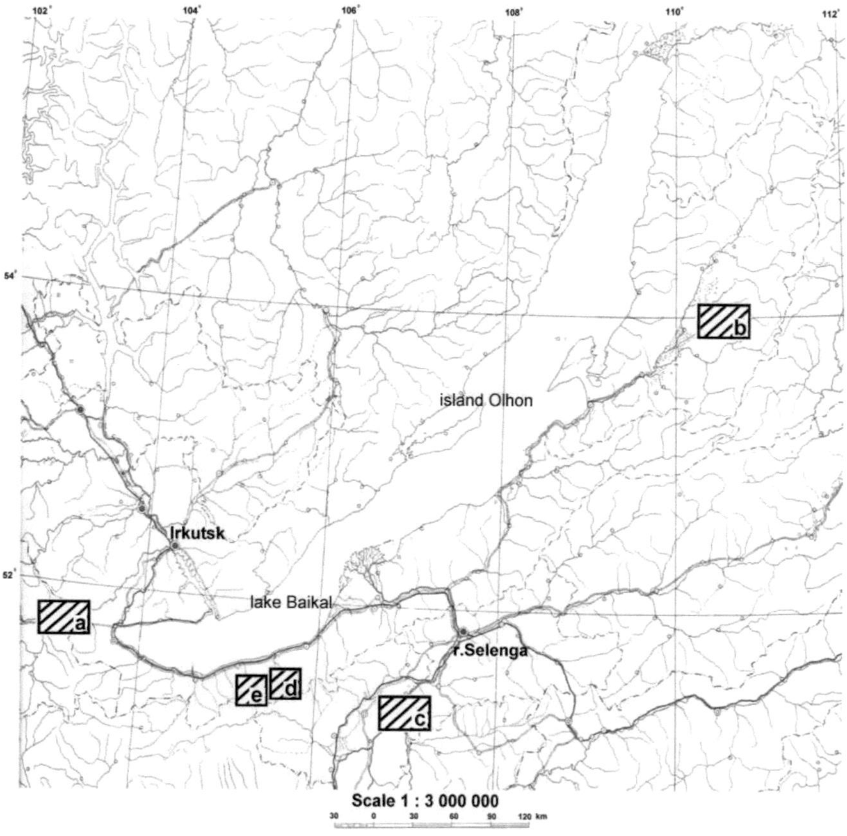

Figure 1. Areas of investigation, key territories: a - Tunka valley, b – Barguzin valley, c – Selenga river basin, e – around the Osinovka mountain, d – around the Lysaya mountain.

soil-geobotanic profiling. Due to the application with materials of perennial monitoring and geobotanic survey, soil-geobotanic profiling favored the resolution of such tasks as establishing of the structure of communities forming at mutual development of forests and extra zonal steppes, correlation of phytocenoses with soils, as well as allowed to generate some forecasts. The profiles were designed with the aim to present all the diversity of phytocenoses and soils at the contact site of taiga and extra zonal steppe as completely as possible. The set of model communities reflects the whole spectrum of ecotopes conditions, the spatial variability, and dynamic trends of the modern vegetation in the changing climate of the region.

3. Results

Investigation history of the region's vegetation. The history of investigations into the vegetation of the basin of Lake Baikal was most thoroughly described (Galazy, Molozhnikov, 1982). The cited reference gives a detailed outline of all main stages of botanical studies in the region.

The characteristic features of the floristic and phytocenotic composition of vegetation were addressed by many workers engaged with the study of the vegetative cover of the region (Popov, 1953, 1957; Peshkova, 1962, 1972, 1985, 2001; Lukicheva, 1972; Malyshev, Peshkova, 1984; Molozhnikov, 1986; Belov, 1973, 1988,1990; Kasyanova, 1993; and others.). The vegetation structure in the studied area reflects some links with the history of environmental development in the whole Baikal region. During Tertiary, on the territory of modern Pre-Baikal there were broadleaf forests, in the valleys and dry cleavages herbaceous xerophytic communities dominated. Tectonic shifts and climate changes caused disappearance of heat-loving flora. Formation of nowadays landscapes in the Central Baikal and one of modern vegetation in the coasts of Lake Baikal are related to Holocene. Climate oscillations during Holocene determined the peculiarities of spatial variability and relationship dynamics between different vegetation types in the region, in particular, variability of areas occupied by forest and steppe phytocenoses during different Holocene periods. During last decades, climate in Pre-Baikal considerably varies. Average annual winter temperatures and average annual precipitation in summer increase. Many researchers consider steppes in taiga zones as relicts which remained since vegetation formation during xerothermic periods and believe that steppe communities (steppoids) formation is the reflection of regional topologic peculiarities on the environment in the spatial structure of the vegetation cover of a concrete territory. In their opinion, such communities are not native, and during neogenetic changes they are replaced by forest ones. It is in accordance all steppe islands (out of steppe zone) have a temporary character of their existence. The modern structural and dynamic organization of vegetation on the background of climate dynamics allows us to support a viewpoint concerning the formation of communities in the area studied as a result of climatogenic succession, secular dynamics and forests evolution with formation of taiga-steppe communities of the Lake Baikal' regionl.

Current structure of the region's vegetation. The main spatial structural-typological characteristics and dynamic attributes of the Prebaikalia's vegetative cover were represented on the small-scale map of vegetation for the southern part of Siberia. According to the scheme and principles of forest-vegetation regionalization of the mountain territories of Southern Siberia (The Types..., 1980, pp. 236-243), the forests of the study area were assigned to the Western Prebaikalia's mountainous forest-vegetation province of larch and pine forests, of the Primorsky district of sub-taiga-forest steppe pine (*Pinus sylvestris* L.) and mountain-taiga larch (*Larix sibirica* Ledeb.) forests. These forests occupy the Primorskaya and Baikalskaya (southern part) mountain systems. Here there is a pronounced Prebaikalia's sub-boreal dry type of zonality due to increased aridity of climate that is caused by the position of the territory in the systems of the Baikal region's mountains. The basis of the region's forest vegetation is formed by pine (*Pinus sylvestris* L.), shrub (*Rhododendron dauricum* Ledeb., *Duschekia fruticosa* (Rupr.) Pouzar.) and grass, green-moss forests of the lower parts of slopes, and shrub (*Rhododendron dauricum* Ledeb.) grass pine stands of the gentle southward slopes, in combination with shrub and foxberry (*Vaccinium vitis-idaea* (L.) - grass forests of slopes of different exposures. Shrub (*Rhododendron dauricum* L.) sedge-grass-moss larch stands develop in the lower and middle parts of slopes of different exposures. Along the bottoms of valleys between mountains, ridges and slopes of southward exposure there occur steppe-like grass larch stands. All of these forests are, to some extent, in contact with steppes to form ecotone features. Pine shrub (*Rhododendron dauricum* L.), green-moss grass and grass-steppe-like forests hold a central position, which - in combination with the steppes - develop along insolated slopes and can reach the sub-golets zone. The region's steppe vegetation reflects the traits inherent in the steppes of the South-Siberian formations that refer to the Mongolian-Chinese fratry of formations (The Vegetation..., 1972). The communities are dominates by grasses, in combination with steppe shrubs. The mountains of South Siberia are characterized by a combination of forests and steppes on slopes of eastward and southward exposures. This is typical of the mountains of Tuva, Altai, and Western Transbaikalia (Namzalov, 1994, 1996). Although the steppes of the western Prebaikalia are ascribed to the mountain-steppe zone, they have an island (azonal) character. The development of the steppes of the western Prebaikalia is associated with the character of their exposure and the stone composition of the substrate, the insufficiency of rainfall, and with strong winds that intensify transpiration in plants. Overall, all steppes of the Baikal region bear specific traits that reflect the evolution of the flora and vegetation of the region.

Current structure of the region's soils. Soils types characteristic for the steppes areas – mountain-chestnut colored with salinization cases together with grey forest soils occur in the area studied. A more detailed structure of soil cover is given in the papers by V. A. Kuz'min and V.A. Snytko (1988) determining soils types which were not reported for this region before. Ts.Kh. Tsybzhitov et al. (1999) give rather unambiguous soils characteristics, stating that the base of the soil cover consists of peat-humus taiga-permafrost gleys together with gley permafrost podzols, typical brown forest soil and acidulous taiga sod. In the paper by V.A. Snytko et al. (2001), soils are characterized from viewpoint of height and exposition heterogeneities of the relief on the territory considered. Lithogenic coarse-humus, brown forest soil, podzols; primitive organogenic-rubbly (taiga-lithogenic), sod-podzol and sod forest; sod lithogenic, sod forest and sod-carbonatic; sod-forest-steppe, mountain-steppe carbonate-free, mountain chernozem-like, mountain-steppe-chestnut-colored-like soils are determined. On the slopes of different expositions and watersheds organogenic rubbly taiga (forest) soils develop often jointly with brown soils, sod-forest ones with fragments of steppe carbonate-free ones and organogenic rubbly weakly developed ones. Steppe soils are underdeveloped and not always correlate with steppe communities; they are often developed under forests. On the sites of southern exposition slopes and on flattened surfaces with dense carbonatic rocks, a friable loamy-sandy humus grey horizon with unexpressed structure is characteristic. Such soils are related to humus carbo-petrozems, a subtype of dark-humus carbo-lithozems. Contrary to the opinion existing before on a wide distribution of chernozems and chestnut-colored soils, organogenic-rubbly, chernozem-like-carbonate-free grey forest and sod forest steppificated soils dominate in the region.

4. Spatial variability of the region's vegetation

Many years of studies of the region's vegetation revealed some structural and dynamic features of the plant communities that reflect the present tendencies of development of the vegetative cover in connection with the changing environmental conditions: an increase in moisture content in the summer season, and the rise of yearly mean winter temperatures. Communities that develop in conditions of contact of the forest and steppe types of vegetation in the region may serve as good indicators of such alterations. These communities are formed by plant species with different ecological amplitudes; they respond very rapidly to and visually clearly reflect changes in ecotope conditions at the topological and regional levels of organization of the natural environment. The presence of a particular plant species (or a group of plants) in the composition of a community of the transitional type between forest and steppe suggests that there are dynamic tendencies of the vegetation in connection with changes in the ambient environment. One of such model objects that accumulate the consequences of dynamic changes of the main parameters (rainfall, temperature) if the climate in the region does include the taiga-steppe communities. Occurring throughout the western Prebaikalia, such communities are representative models for monitoring the changes in the natural environment for the last 100 years. During the last several decades the trends of development of the region's vegetation in ever changing conditions (an increase in yearly mean summer rainfall and yearly mean winter temperatures) reflect an increasingly more gradual character of the forest to steppe transition thus smoothing away the boundaries between forest and steppe and reducing the size of territories occupied by steppe communities. In some cases it is difficult to draw a demarcation line between steppe and forest. In this connection, the problem of interrelationship between forest and steppes acquires a different aspect - the dynamics of climate at a local-regional level is becoming a decisive factor of development of the vegetation and, as a result, of the entire natural situation in the region. Along with a secular dynamics of the taiga where - as a consequence of the internal (coenotic) environment of phytocoenoses - there is occurring a change of forest-forming species. There are taking place spatial changes in the structure of communities, with an increasing predominance of mesophytes, or plants that demand increased moisture content of their habitats.

The work-maps, space photos, camera photos and tables for some key territories of investigation (Tunka valley, Barguzin valley, Selenga river basin and also camera photos for key territories – around Osinivka mountain, Lysaya mountain) putted as results and examples our research in Lake Baikal region (Fig. 2-12, Tables 1-3).

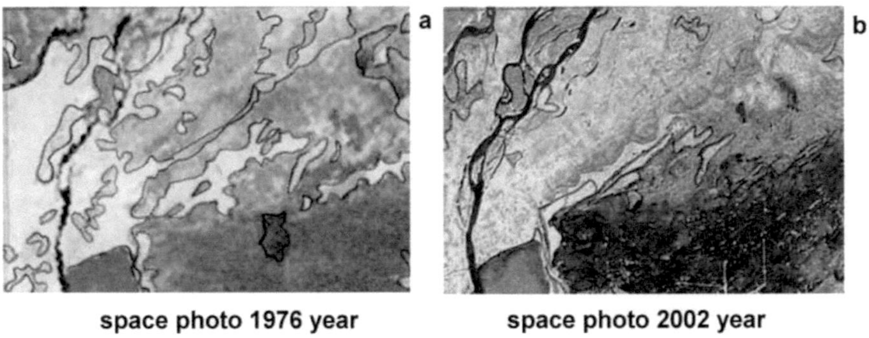

Figure 2. Space photo for key territories – Tunka valley, a – for 1976 year, b – for 2002 year

Pinus sylvestris L. forest in complex with steppe communities			
Woods species	**Shrubs**	**Herbs layer**	**Mosses**
Basic layer - *Pinus sylvestris* L., underwood – *Pinus sylvestris* L., underwoods very good developed and growing outside of canopy of forest, and between of steppe communities too.	*Spiraea media* Frans Scmidt., just a few one marked.	*Stipa krylovii* Roshev., *Bromopsis inermis* (Leyss.) Holub, *Poa botryoides* (Trin. ex Griseb.), *Artemisia frigida* Willd., *Galium verum* L., *Artemisia scoparia* Waldst. Et Kit., *Schizonepeta multifida* (L.) Briq., *Sanguisorba officinalis* L.	*Abietinella abietina* (Turn.) Fleisch., *Rhytidium rugosum* (Hedw.) Kindb, just marked under forest canopy, these species characteristic for polydominate forest for all valley

Table 1. The table of the basic composition of the plant species of the key territory – Tunka valley (a)

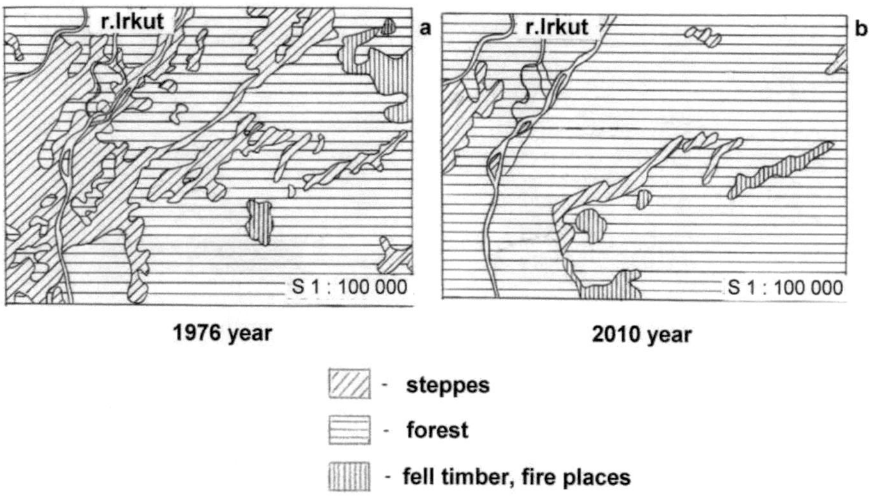

Figure 3. Work-map of the area investigation – Tunka valley, a – just for1976 year, b – for 2010 year.

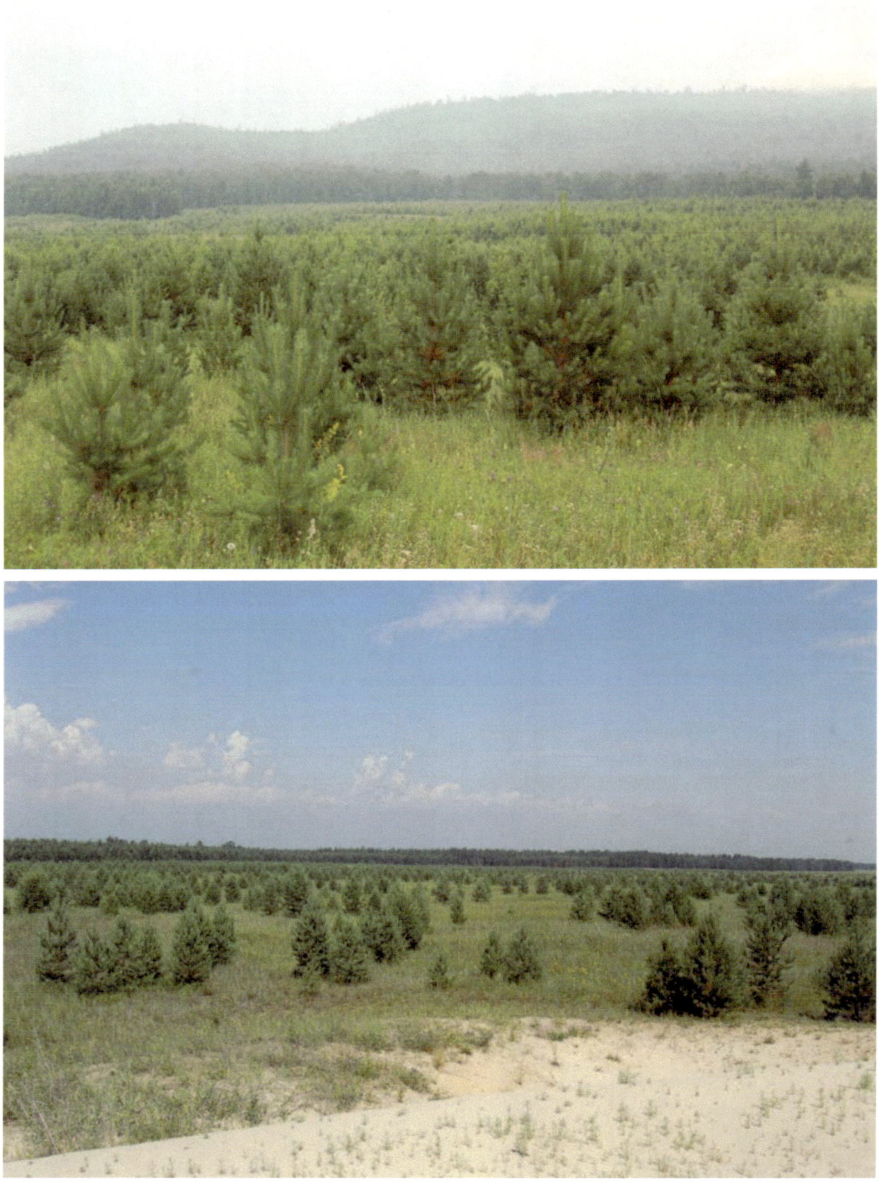

Figure 4. In the photos marked the processes of afforestation steppe land, key territories investigation – Tunka valley

Pinus sylvestris L. forest with complex steppe communities			
Woods species	**Shrubs**	**Herbs layer**	**Mosses**
Basic layer - *Pinus sylvestris* L., в underwoods – *Pinus sylvestris* L., underwoods very good developed and growing outside of canopy of forest, and between of steppe	*Rhododendron dahuricum* L., *Spiraea media* Franz Schmidt., *Rosa acicularis* Lindley	*Diantus versicolor* Fischer ex Link, *Veronica incana* L., *Allium tenuissimum* L., *Stipa krylovii* Roshev, *Artemisia frigida* L., *Galium verum* L., *Patrinia rupestris* (Pallas) Dufr., *Eletrigia repens* (L.) Nevski	*Abietinella abietina* (Turn.) Fleisch., *Rhytidium rugosum* (Hedw.) Kindb., just marked under forest canopy, these species characteristic for polydominate forest for all valley

Table 2. The table of the basic composition of the plant species of the key territory – Barguzin valley (b)

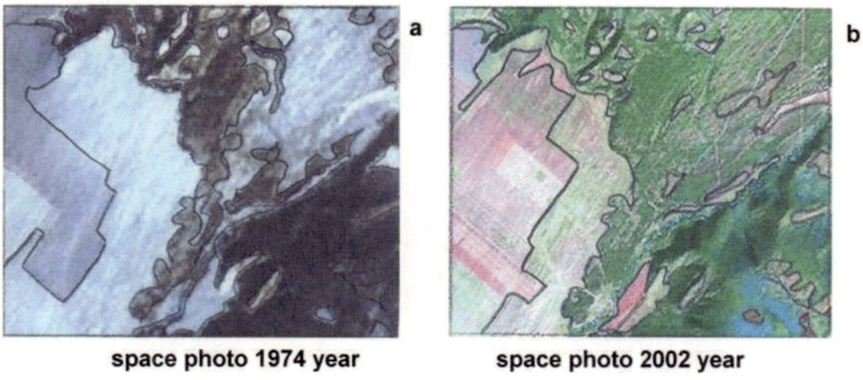

Figure 5. Space photo for key territories – Barguzin valley, a – for 1976 year, b – for 2002 year

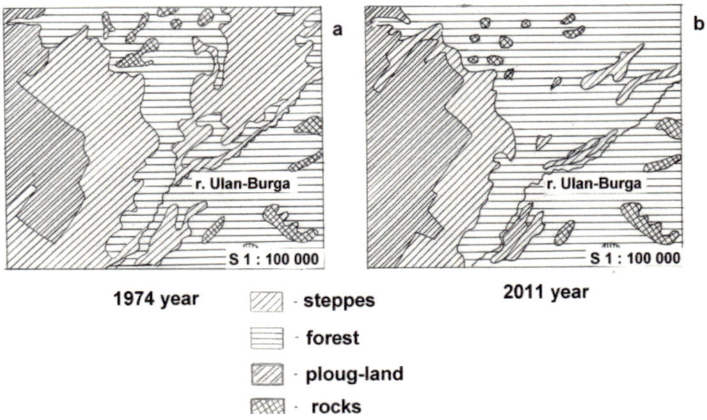

Figure 6. Work-map of the area investigation – Barguzin valley, a – just for1976 year, b – for 2011 year.

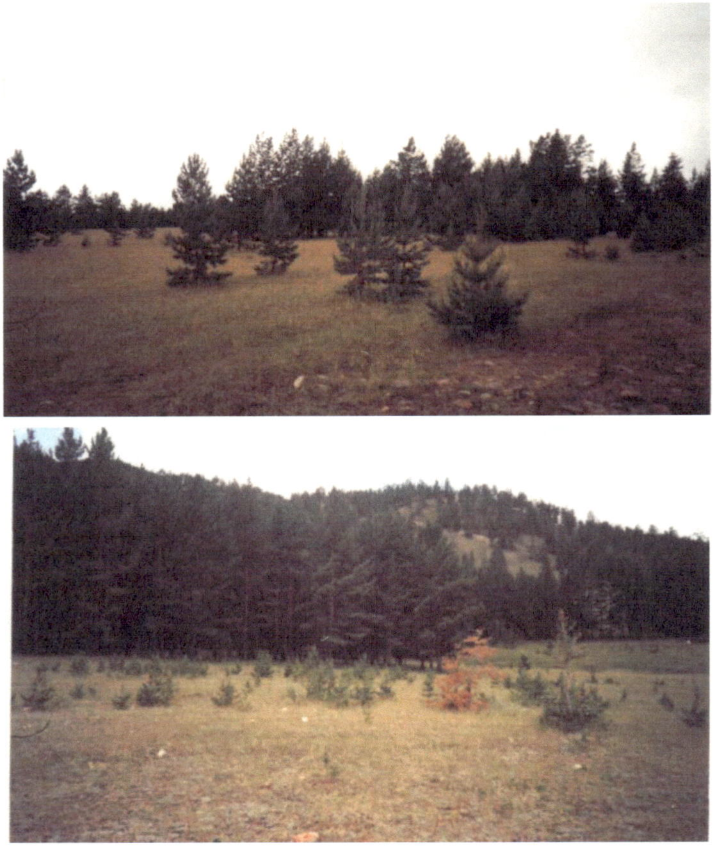

Figure 7. In the photos marked the processes of afforestation steppe land - key territories investigation – Barguzin valley

***Pinus sylvestris* L. forest in complex with shrubs and steppe communities**			
Woods species	**Shrubs**	**Herbs layer**	**Mosses**
Basic layer - *Pinus sylvestris* L., underwood - *Pinus sylvestris* underwoods very good developed and growing outside of canopy of forest, and between of steppe	*Spiraea media* Franz Schmidt, *Cotoneaster melanocarpus* Fischer ex Blytt, *Rosa acicularis* Lindley	*Carex pediformis* C.A. Meyer, *Carex macroura* Meinsh., *Pulsatilla patens* (L.) Miller, *Buphleurum sibiricum* Vest, *Scorzonera radiata* Fisch., *Crepis sibirica* L., *Thalictrum foetidum* L., *Phlomis tuberosa* L., Potentilla bifurca L., *Myosotis imitata* Serg., *Vicia cracca* L., *Poligala sibirica* L., *Dracocephalum ruyschiana* L., Equisetum sylvaticum	Very seldom - *Pleurozium schreberii* (Brid.) Mitt., *Abietinella abietina* (Turn.) Fleich, these species characteristic for polydominate forest for all valley

Table 3. The table of the basic composition of the plant species of the key territory – Selenga river basin (c)

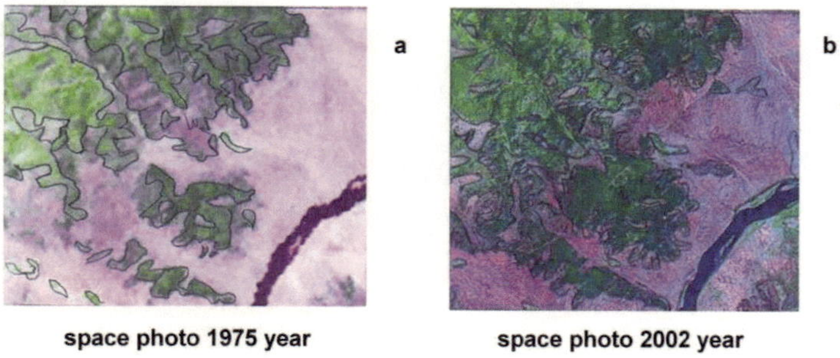

Figure 8. Space photo for key territories – Selenga river basin, a – for 1976 year, b – for 2002 year

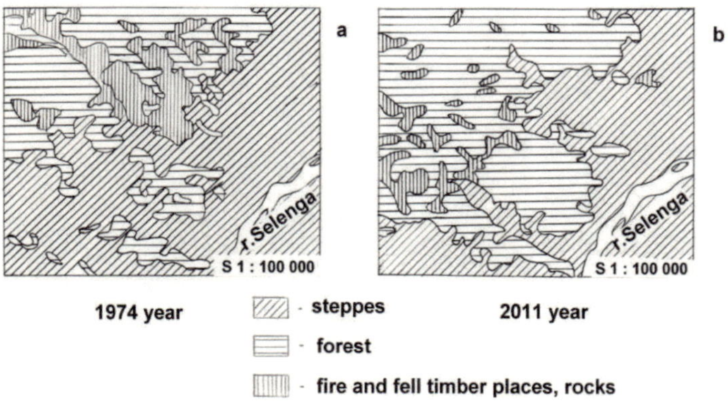

Figure 9. Work-map of the area investigation – Selenga river basin, a – just for1976 year, b – for 2011 year.

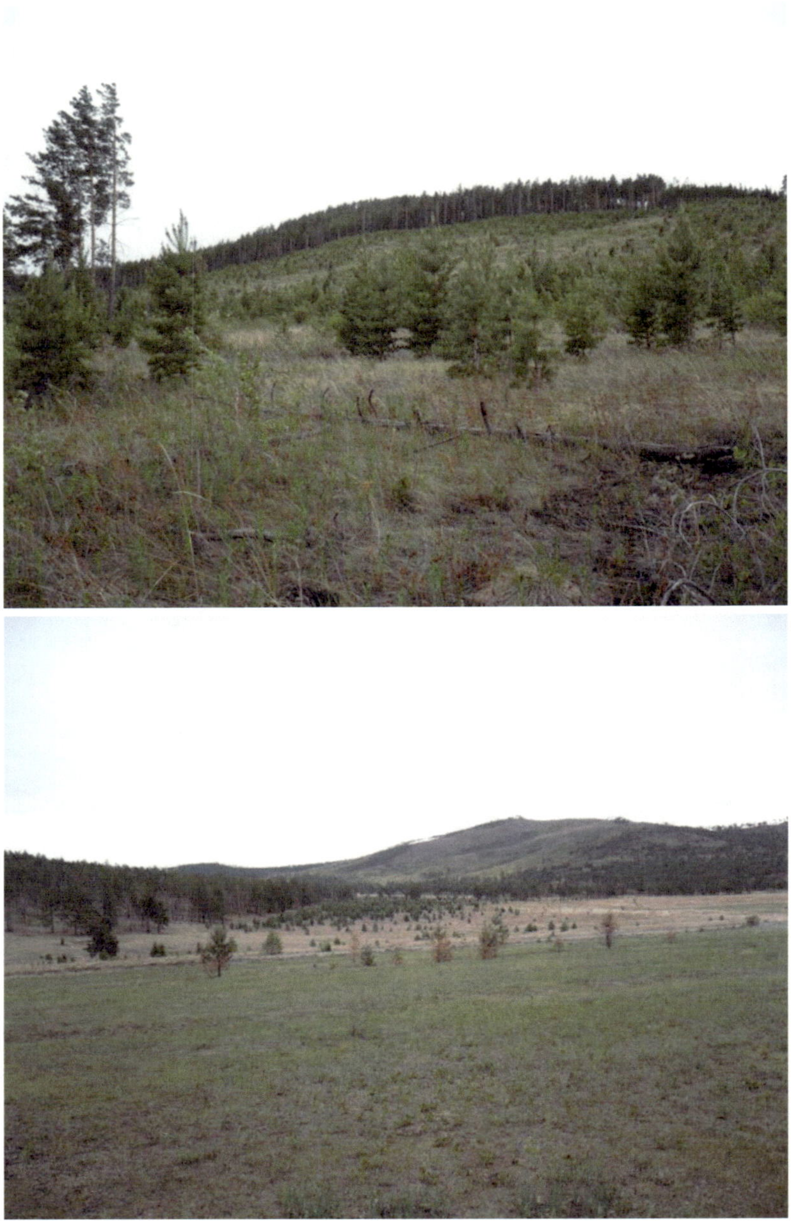

Figure 10. In the photos marked the processes of afforestation steppe land - key territories investigation – Selenga river basin

http://dx.doi.org/10.5772/55481

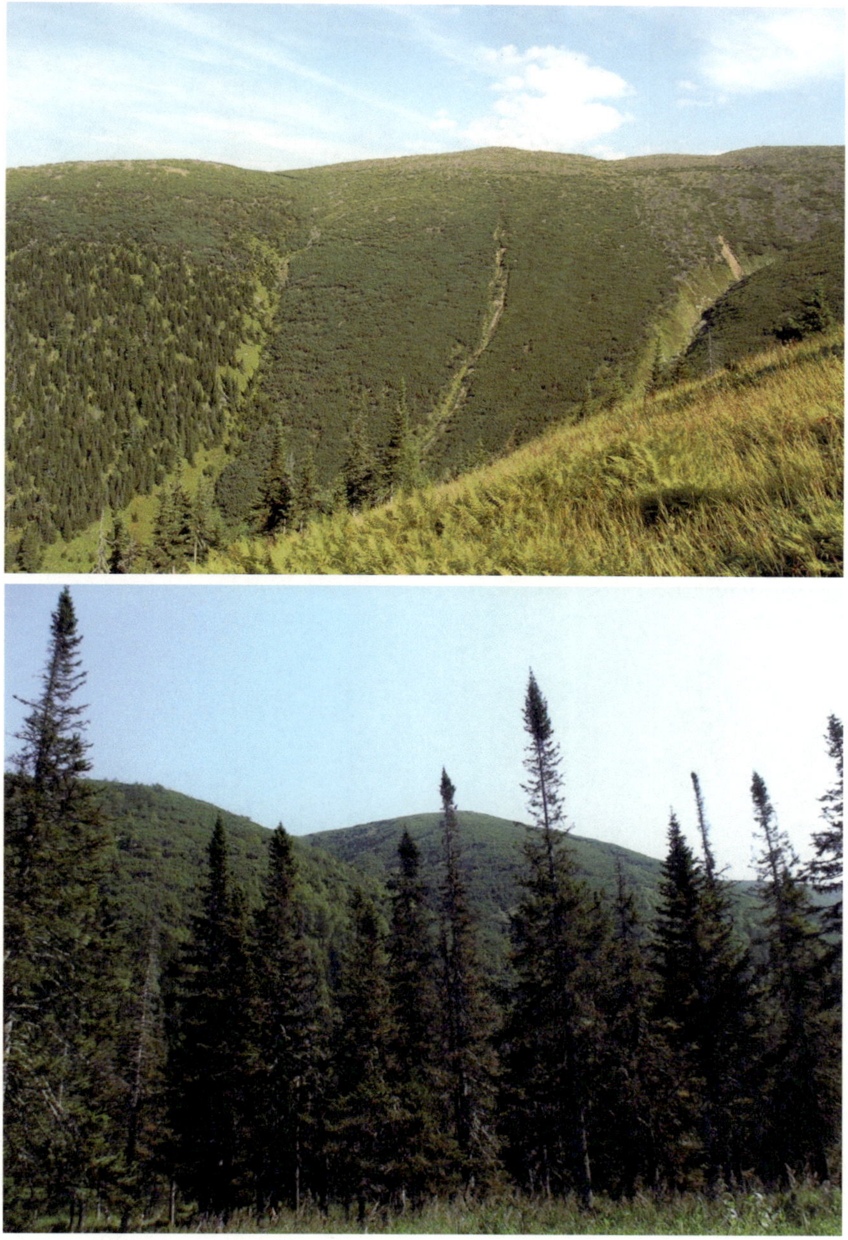

Figure 11. Key territories – around the Osinovka mountain (for 2011 year)

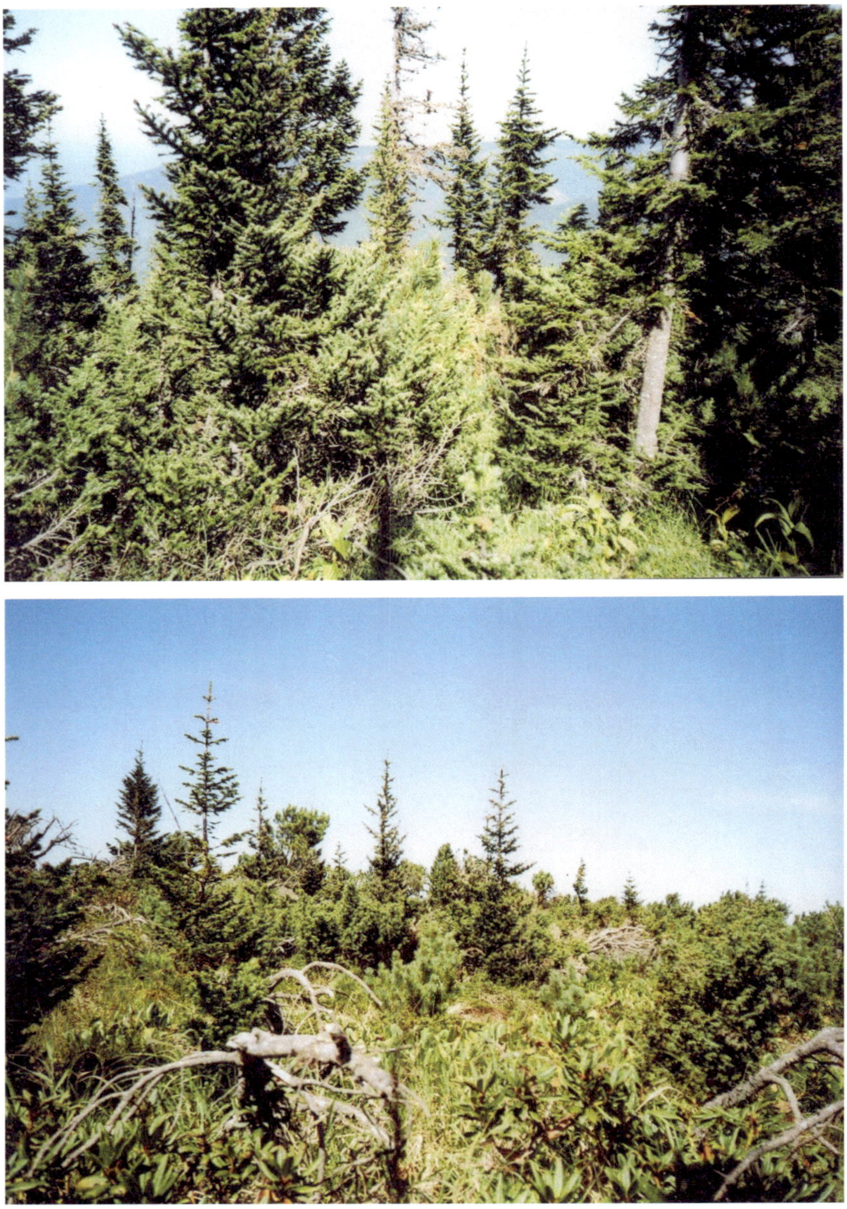

Figure 12. Key territories – around the Lysaya mountain (for 2011 year)

Tracing of soil-geobotanic profiles on the key sites reflecting the most diverse forms of forests and steppes contacts allowed to reveal the territorial diversity of the communities cenotically and typologically as well as cenoses correlation with the relief structure and with the conditions of communities habitats. The revealed character of alternation of forest and steppe communities under the conditions of extrazonality suggested that there are no clear floristic and cenotic links with edaphic conditions (mainly with soils) in the area studied in difference with zones or sub-zones (wooded steppe, sub-taiga). Here extra zonal effects are the most expressed in the vegetation development with manifestation of continuality (course) when there are in the communities species characteristic for dark-coniferous-light-coniferous taiga as well as xerophytic plants which make a base of cereal-motley grasses and petrophytic steppes. The occurrence of arboreal vegetation of different ages in steppe communities under the form of their gradual spatial expansion suggest mutual development and integrity of forest and steppe communities as of a united system. The formation of taiga (forest) soils here without a clear connection of steppificated soils with steppe communities shown by soil profiles combined with geobotanic ones confirms as well the opinion on the development of taiga-steppe communities specific for the area studied as on a peculiarity of the dynamics of forest type vegetation in the area studied.

5. Discussion

The structure of the taiga-steppe communities may be represented as a system where the coenoses consist of the tree layer dominated by *Pinus sylvestris* L. or *Larix sibirica* Ledeb. (depending on the genesis or on the recovery stage) of different age groups. The character of occurrence of *Betula platyphylla* Sukaczev and *Populus tremula* L. in tree stands is taken into account according to the genesis or recovery stage. Undergrowth is notable for an abundance of *Rhododendron dauricum* L. and *Duschekia fruticosa* (Rupr.) Pouzar. The soil cover includes the species composition of different variations, and often complexes of *Vaccinium vitis-idaea* L., *Bergenia crassifolia* (L.) Fritsch, sinuosities of *Pleurosium Schreberi, Dicranum polisetum* Sw., *Climacium dendroides* (Hedw.) Web. et Mohr., *Rhytidium rugosum* (Hedw.) Kindb., and for the involvement (predominance) of xerophytes, such as *Festuca lenensis* Drobov, *Thalictrum foetidum* L., *Artemisa frigida* Willd., *Chamaerthodos altaica* (Laxim.) Bunge, *Iris humilis* Georgi, and others. The taiga-steppe communities are characterized by the one- or two-age composition of tree species, and by the polydominance of the shrub zone and grass cover depending on the type of coenose habitat. Taiga-steppe communities are notable for dramatic restructurings of their vertical and spatial coenostructures. In addition to the development of stable young trees consisting of *Pinus sylvestris* L. and *Larix sibirica* Ledeb. in forest stands, tree ecobiomorphs are observed to actively penetrate into grass communities forming part of taiga-steppe communities in the form of curtains or isolated undergrowth aged 5-15 years. In recent years, the composition of grass communities, with xerophytes forming their basis, such as *Artemisa commutata* Besser, *Heteropappus altaicus* (Willd.) Kitam., *Phlomis tubirosa* L., *Poa attenuata* Trin., and *Agropyrom cristatum* L., revealed saplings of tree species, pine and larch. Also, the boundary is disappearing between forest and grass phytocoenoses. The composition of the soil cover shows an ever increasing predominance of forest species with a spatial increase of sinuosities of *Drepanocladus uncinatus* (Hedw.) *Warnst., Mnium cuspidatum* Hedw., *Dicranum polisetum* Sw., *Rhytidium rugosum* (Hedw.) Kindb., and *Vaccinium vitis-idaea* L.A central position in grass stands corresponds to *Astragalus versicolor* Pallas, *Galium verum* L., *Aster alpinum* L., *Trifolium lupinaster* L., *Potentilla tanacetifolia* Willd. ex., and *Campanuta glomerata* L., whereas steppe herbage: *Festuca lenensis* Drobov, *Koeleria cristata, Poa attenuata,* and *Agropyron cristatum,* are somewhat less abundant and are the stage of dynamics of the community during the growth period.

It is to notice thereupon that the spatial structure of the vegetation in the area studied is particular because forest (taiga) and steppe communities form often on the same soils quite uncharacteristic for zonal steppes. Modern processes of cryolithogenic humus formation due to modern environmental conditions, to the history of formation and to vegetation cover genesis suggest that the base of soils formation is a "forest type" with some specific features due to the situation of the territory studied in the mountain system of Lake Baikal basin.

E.g., pine with motley grasses, larch (*Larix sibirica* Ledeb.) – pine (*Pinus sylvestris* L.) motley grasses-cereal forests and steppe communities with cereals domination form on organogenic rubbly-taiga (forest) soils on the slopes of different expositions. On the same soils, larch-pine sparse grass forests and steppe polydominant communities, as well as larch-pine-rhododendron ones (*Rhododendron dauricum* L.) with *Dushekia fruticosa* (Rupr.) Pouzar, red bilberries (*Vaccinium vitis-idaea* (L.) Avrorin) with motley grasses ones from different habitats are developed. On chernozem carbonate-free soils, there form pine-larch forests and motley grass-steppe communities, as well as larch-pine rhododendron forests with *Spiraea media* Fr. Schmidt on the slopes of South-Western expositions. For organogenic-rubbly steppe soils from different slopes expositions, the presence of sparse larch groups with developed underwood expanding out of a canopy among motley grass steppe communities is characteristic. In a new soil of larch-pine-rhododendron forests and larch-motley grass forests developing on sod-forest and sod-brown soils a considerable role belongs to mosses characteristic for polydominant dark-coniferous-light-coniferous taiga. On regosols with rocks outcrops there form everywhere motley grassed sparse pine groups with underwood and steppe communities of petrophytic series. Motley grassed steppe communities with several pine-trees aged from 2 to 60 years, are found on podzol permafrost soils jointly with organogenic-rubbly taiga (forest) soils on the slopes of different expositions.

Similar structure-dynamic peculiarities of phytocenoses and of soils in the contact zone of larch forests and extra zonal steppe cenoses are found out also at other key site. Here the boundaries of links of taiga-steppe communities with edaphic conditions are more unclear independently on types of phytocenoses habitats.

6. Conclusions

The presence of undergrowth and pine and larch saplings in steppe grass communities is indicative of trends toward a spatial expansion of tree ecobiomorphs in connection with an increase in yearly mean precipitation in the Prebaikalia for the last 30 years. There has been a reduction of areas occupied by steppe communities, and an active penetration of mesophytes into steppe coenoses. There is a spatial expansion of mosses characteristic for the polydominant light-coniferous - dark-coniferous taiga. The appearance of undergrowth of *Pinus sibirica* (Du Tour) in the composition of light-coniferous forests is a further indication that the region undergoes a change of climate towards an increase of moisture content and temperature. This is also supported by structural changes in the composition of the region's dark-coniferous forests where the forests of *Pinus sibirica* (Du Tour) develop a stable canopy of tree species demanding more moisture content - *Abies sibirica* (Ledeb.), and *Picea obovata* (Ledeb.).

The sub-golets zone of the mountains surrounding Lake Baikal reveals individual *Pinus sibirica* (Ledeb.) trees, which indicates a change of the forest boundary, with a tendency towards an increase and forestation of the territories occupied by mountain-tundra plant groups. The spatial variability in the structure of the plant cover of the Prebaikalia reflects changes of the climate occurring during the last several decades in the Baikal region (Fig. 11, 12).

We can see camera photos which reflecting some processes of the spatial variability of vegetation different environment sites of the Baikal region (Fig. 4, 7, 10-12).

Soil-geobotanic studies in the region allowed to the reveal the peculiarities of phytocenoses dynamics reflecting present-day tendencies of vegetation cover development due to changing environmental conditions – humidity increase in summer and increase of average annual temperatures in winter. Good indicators of such changes are taiga-steppe communities of the Lake Baikal region manifesting the peculiarities of relationship in spatial variability of forests and of steppes communities. These communities formed by plants species with different ecological amplitudes respond very rapidly and reflect visually changes in ecotops conditions at topological and regional levels of environment organization. The presence of one or other plant species (or species group) in a concrete community allows to suppose dynamic tendencies of vegetation due to environmental changes. Taiga-steppe communities on all the of Lake Baikal region can be representative models reflecting peculiarities of structural-dynamic organization of the vegetation on the background of climate dynamics in the region during last decades.

The present-day tendencies of vegetation development reflect a transitional character of the steppes in the central part of the coasts with tendencies of disappearing of a boundary between forest and steppe communities. Thereupon the problem of finding out the character of relationship between forest and steppe communities is brought to the task to determine a way and dynamics of climatic factors at local-regional level under the conditions of changing of the environment as a whole. Along with secular dynamics of taiga, when due to changes in the internal (edapho-cenotic) environment of phytocenoses, forest-forming species change, and there are other changes in the spatial structure of the communities. On upper soil cover in the forests, spatial expansion of mosses synusia characteristic for a polydominant dark-coniferous-light-coniferous taiga occurs. Appearing of *Pinus sibirica* Du Tour underwood among light-coniferous forests can also suggest that in this region, along with recoverable vegetation dynamics, there occur change sin communities structure responding to changing climatic situation in this region. It is to notice thereupon that among the forests of Primorsky and Baikal'sky Ridges a stable canopy is forming of tree species more exigent to humidity – *Abies sibirica* Ledeb., *Picea obovata* Ledeb. Among mountain tundras there are some trees *Pinus sibirica* aged from 2 to 25 years.

Due to the peculiarities revealed among spatial-structural links of vegetation and soil cover in the area studied using combined soil-geobotanic profiles on the key sites, it is possible to make a conclusion that it is not so rightful to characterize the vegetation as forest and steppe types. In this very case, forest and steppe communities at environments contact site (taiga-steppe) are genetically united. Under the contrast conditions of the environment of the area studied, vegetation formation is due to climatogenic paragenesis as indicated by the results of our studies. The vegetative cover in this case serves as an indicator of the changing natural situation in the region. This would be reflected not only in the formation of the environmental conditions for the period of relative warming, as was the case at different stages of the Holocene, but also in the policy of economic development of the region as a whole.

Acknowledgements

This scientific work has been made by financial support of the Integration Parthenship Project of Russian Academy of Sciences (№ 69) and Russian Fond of Basic Research 12-04-09- 980013-p_siberia_a

Author details

A. P. Sizykh* and V. I. Voronin

*Address all correspondence to: alexander_sizykh@yahoo.com

Laboratory of Ecosystem Bioindication, Siberian Institute of Plant Physiology and Biochemistry, Siberian Branch of Russian Academy of Sciences, Irkutsk, Russia

References

[1] Alexander Sizykh, Victor Voronin, Michail Azovsky, Svetlana Sizykh. Paragenese of the vegetation in ecosystems contact zones (in Lake Baikal basin) // Natural Sciences. (2012). , 4(5), 271-275.

[2] Belov, A. V. (1973). The Map of the Vegetation of the South of East Siberia. Principles and Methods of Compilation. Geobotanical Mapping, Leningrad: , 16-30.

[3] Belov, A. V. (1988). A cartographic study of the vegetation of the Pribaikalsky National park. Recreation and Protected Areas. Proceedings of the. 5th Meeting on Applied Geography, Irkutsk, , 66-78.

[4] Belov, A. V. (1990). The Vegetation. Nature Management and Environmental Protection in the Baikal's Basin, Novosibirsk:, 147-154.

[5] Belova, V. A. (1975). The History of Development of Vegetative Depressions of the Baikal Rift Zone, Moscow.

[6] Belova, V. A. (1985). The Vegetation and Climate of the late Cainozoic in the South of East Siberia, Novosibirsk.

[7] Bezrukova, E. V. (1996). The Vegetation and Climate of the Prebaikalia in the Late Glaciation Era and Holocene. Author's Abstract of the Dissertation (Cand.Sc. Geogr.), Irkutsk.

[8] Bezrukova, E. V. (2002). The Vegetation and Climate of the South of East Siberia in the Late Neopleistocene and Holocene. Author's Abstract of the Dissertation (Cand.Sc. Geogr.), Irkutsk.

[9] Galazy, G. I, & Moloznikov, V. N. (1982). The History of Botanical Studies at Lake Baikal, Novosibirsk.

[10] Gustokashina, N. N. (2003). Long-Term Changes of the Main Climate Elements on the Territory of the Prebaikalia, Irkutsk.

[11] Grichuk, M. P. (1955). Toward the History of the vegetation in the Angara River basin. Dokl. AN SSSR. Nov. Ser. , 2, 335-338.

[12] Dylis, N. V, Reshikov, L. I, & Malyshev, L. I. (1965). The vegetation. In: The Prebaikalia and Transbaikalia, Moscow, , 225-281.

[13] Kapralov, D. S, Shiytov, S. G, Moiseev, P. A, & Fomin, V. V. Changes in the Composition, Structure and Altitudinal Distribution of Low Forests at the Upper Limit of Their Growth in the Northern Ural Mountains // Russian Journal of Ecology, (2006). , 37, 367-372.

[14] Kasyanova, L. N. (1980). Plant Ecology of the Steppes in the Olkhon Region, Novosibirsk

[15] Kuz'min V ASnytko V.A. (1988). Geochemical differences of soils in contrast landscapes within Pre-Baikal National Park. Soils geography and geochemistry of Siberian landscapes: , 41-55.

[16] Lukicheva, A. N. (1972). The regularities of vertical zonality of vegetation associated with terrain and rock characteristics (a case study of the Baikal ridge). Geobotanical Studies and Dynamics of Shores and Slopes at Baikal, Leningrad: , 3-70.

[17] Malyshev, L. I, & Peshkova, G. A. (1984). The Peculiarities and Genesis of the Flora of Siberia, Prebaikalia and Transbaikalia, Novosibirsk.

[18] Moloznikov, V. N. (1986). Plant Communities of the Prebaikalia, Novosibirsk.

[19] The Types of Forests in the South of East Siberia(1980). Novosibirsk: , 236-243.

[20] Namzalov, B. B. (1994). The Steppes of Southern Siberia, Novosibirsk-Ulan-Ude.

[21] Namzalov, B. B. (1996). The mountain forest-steppe of Southern Siberia landscape phenomenon of Central Asia. The Flora and Vegetation of Siberia and the Far East. Lectures in the memory of L.M.Cherepnin. Book of Abstracts of the nd All-Russia Conference, Krasnoyarsk: 215-217., 2.

[22] Peshkova, G. A. (1962). Forest-steppe relationship in the Angara region. Trans. East-Sib. Biol. Inst. , 1, 90-99.

[23] Peshkova, G. A. (1972). The Steppe Flora of Baikalian Siberia, Moscow.

[24] Peshkova, G. A. (1985). The Vegetation of Siberia, Prebaikalia and Transbaikalia, Novosibirsk.

[25] Peshkova, G. A. (2001). Florogenetic Analysis of the Steppe Flora of the Mountains in Southern Siberia, Novosibirsk.

[26] Popov, M. G. (1953). On the relationship of forest (taiga) and steppe in Middle Siberia. Bull. of Moscow Soc. of Naturalists, Biol. Dept. 58, 5: 81-85.

[27] Popov, M. G. (1957). The steppe and rock floras of the Baikal's western shore area. Trans. Baik. Limnol. st. , 15, 408-426.

[28] Savina, L. N. (1986). Taiga Forests of Northern Asia in the Holocen, Novosibirsk.

[29] Sizykh, A. P. Protection of the taiga-steppe ecosystems of the western shore of Lake Baikal // Journal of Design & Nature and Ecodynamics, UK, (2009). , 4, 66-71.

[30] Snytko, V A. Dan'ko L V, Kuz'min S B, Sizykh A Diversity of geosystems of taiga and steppe contact on the Western coast of Lake Baikal. Geography and Natural Resources: 61-68., 2001.

[31] ShiytovS. GTerent'ev M.M., Fomin V.V. Spatiotemporal Dynamics of Forest-Tundra Communities in the Polar Urals // Russian Journal of Ecology, (2005). , 36, 69-75.

[32] The Types of Forests in the South of East Siberia(1980). Novosibirsk: , 236-243.

[33] The Vegetation (South of East Siberia)(1972). Map 1: 1 500 000 (ed. by A.V.Belov), GUGK.

[34] Thomas, T. Veblen and Diane C. Lorenz. (1988). Recent vegetation changes along the forest/steppe ecotone of Northern Patagonia. Annals of the Association of American Geographers. , 78, 93-111.

[35] Tsybzhitov Ts KhTsybikdorzhiev Ts Ts, Tsybzhitov A I. (1999). Soils of Lake Baikal basin: 128.

[36] VoroninV. I Sizykh A. P Oskolkov V. A Voronin, Sheifer E.V. Structural-dynamics organization of the plant communities of the basic ecotones of the Lake Baikal // Environments- 2010, Russia, Tomsk, (2010). , 45-46.

Chapter 8

Historical and Ecological Factors Affecting Regional Patterns of Endemism and Species Richness: The Case of Squamates in China

Yong Huang, Xianguang Guo and Yuezhao Wang

Additional information is available at the end of the chapter

http://dx.doi.org/10.5772/55719

1. Introduction

Biogeography is closely tied to both ecology and phylogenetic biology and its main areas of interest are ecological biogeography, i.e. the study of factors influencing the present distribution, and historical biogeography, i.e. the study of causes that have operated in the past [1]. Ecological and historical biogeography therefore applies different concepts in order to explain the distribution of organisms. The former deals with functional groups of species and environmental constraints, whereas the latter focuses on taxonomic groups and historical biogeographical events [2]. Recently, the division between historical and ecological biogeography has been considered as an obstacle to the progress of biogeography and some authors have stressed the benefits of integrating these two points of view [1,3-4]. In this context, the present work attempts at integrating these two approaches to explore the regional patterns of endemism and species richness of the squamates(lizards and snakes) in China.

As summarized by Meng *et al.* [5], China has a relatively independent geological history. Six primary plates are involved in its tectonic history, namely the North China, Tarim, Yangtze, Cathaysian plates, and parts of the Siberia and Gondwana plates [6-7]. In the Pleistocene, seven collisions and integrations of these plates had united the ancient Siberian and European plates. With approximately 200 tectonic-facies, China has a complex topography, including towering mountains, basins of various sizes, undulating plateaus and hills, and fertile plains. As noted by Meng *et al.* [5], they are assigned to four different terraces in general. The highest terrace, the Qinghai-Tibetan Plateau – the 'roof of the world' – has an average elevation of over 4000 m. Tremendous differences in latitude (a span of more than 50°latitude), longitude (a span of more than 60°longitude), and altitude (a span of more than 88km) create the conditions for extremely diverse climate and a highly astounding heterogeneous landscape. Thus, a high degree of species richness and endemism in China as might have been expected in terms of squamates diversity. It is conservatively estimated that today there are about 422 squamates species in this country, belonging to 106 genera in 17 families and two suborders (see Appendix S1 in Supplementary Material).

It has long been recognized that geological complexity and history usually have a profound influence on the distributions of living organisms. China animal geography division was firstly put forward in 1959 [8]. Now based on the distributions of vertebrates, mainly mammals and birds, China was divided into seven major biogeographical regions and fifty-four provinces [9]. The Palaearctic realm includes North-eastern, Northern, Inner Mongolia-Xinjiang, and Qinghai-Tibetan China biogeographical regions, while the Oriental realm was divided into South-western, Central, and Southern biogeographical regions. The study on biogeographical divisions of China was both intriguing and challenging due to the complex topography and historical processes [9]. The zoogeographic division of China was explored into 30 units [10]. However, China's territory was divided into 124 basic units on the basis of comprehensive natural factors (including altitude, landform, climate, vegetation, water system, farm belt, and so on) by cluster analysis [11]. Recently, based on the distributional patterns of spiders, seven major biogeographical regions in China were investigated by PAE, not corresponding to any previous studies [5]. These studies played an important role in biodiversity conservation, planning and management in China. However, these divisions need further investigation due to primarily on basis of mammals and birds which are highly adapted to environment diversity and higher locomotion [12]. Thus, the ectothermic animals may act as a better indicator to determinate zoogeographical division than mammals and birds [12]. Although only a few studies on biogeographical patterns have been identified and emphasized their biogeographical complexity, data are still not enough to evaluate and compare directly for other taxa, such as squamates with limited dispersal abilities. It is necessary to compare patterns based on different groups of organisms to better understand their biogeography and infer a general pattern [13].

2. Compared biogeographical patterns of Chinese squamates based on parsimony analysis of endemicity (PAE) at different natural area units

2.1. Introduction

One of important goals of historical biogeography is to investigate convergent biogeographical patterns relying on different taxa [14]. These may assist in identifying priority areas or hotspots for biodiversity conservation, particularly today the issue of global concern biodiversity loss. A historical biogeographical method, parsimony analysis of endemicity(PAE), firstly proposed by Rosen [15] and further elaborated by Morrone [16], provided an insight to generate area cladograms to make inferences on historical patterns. PAE was originally used the most parsimony algorithm to reconstruct relations among sampling localities [15], then previously delimited areas [17] and quadrats [16]. Analogous to cladistic methods in phylogenetic analyses, PAE classifies areas (cf. taxa in cladistics) on the basis of the shared presence of taxa (cf. characters in cladistics) [15]. Using PAE, biogeographical studies can investigate biotic similarities between different geographical regions, give static or ecological interpretations [18], and estimate historical hierarchical congruence in target localities or geographical regions [19]. Although there is ongoing debate about the value of PAE [20-21], the PAE has been widely used in many biogeographical studies in recent years [5,22-23].

PAE has been applied to establish relationships among different areas units, for example localities, quadrats, areas of endemism, continents, islands, and so on [13]. The ideal organisms for using PAE are those with limited dispersal abilities and speciation in vicariant events [13, 19]. Although the same size and shape quadrats are not required in PAE and do not affect the analyses [24], the best PAE results were obtained with natural areas instead of quadrats [13]. Here, we used PAE to compare squamates biogeographical patterns at different natural area units with previously delimited biogeographic patterns obtained by Meng and Murphy [5] (Figure1), Zhang [9](Figure 2) and Xie *et al.* [11](Figure 3), in order to find areas of congruent distributional patterns in China.

2.2. Materials and methods

2.2.1. *Study area and operational geographical units*

For a comparable study area with previously provided optimal results in detecting the biogeographical patterns, we assumed the same operational geographic units (OGUs) as suggested by Meng and Murphy [5] (Figure 1), Zhang [9] (Figure 2) and Xie et al. [11] (Figure 3) defined, respectively. According to very similar climatic, geological characteristics, topographical characteristics and natural barriers to dispersal for neighbouring quadrats, 28 biological and physiographical similar areas were combined and divided as OGUs in PAE [5]. Zoogeographical divisions of China were classified into 54 biogeographical provinces based on the distribution of mainly mammals and birds [9]. The whole China was divided into 124 basic units using comprehensive natural factors, such as altitude, landform, climate, vegetation, water system, farm belt, and so on [11]. More details about the OGUS see these studies.

2.2.2. *Data sources and dataset*

The Squamates species catalogue and distributions were compiled from the most recent and comprehensive references, including specimens, exhaustive field surveys, monograph, published literature and expert reviews. All date Information from herbarium specimens was mainly obtained through Chengdu Institute of Biology, Chinese Academy of Sciences (CIB/CAS). Additional information was also obtained from HerpNET and a variety of published sources, for example *Fauna Sinica Reptilia, Vol.2 Squamates Lacertilia* [25], *Herpetology of China* [26], *Fauna Sinica Reptilia, Vol.3 Squamates Serpentes* [27], *Snakes of China (2 Volume set)* [28], *Zootaxa, Zoological Journal of the Linnean Society,Bonn Zoological Bulletin, Asian Herpetological Research, Zoological Research, Acta Herpetologica Information, Acta Herpetologica Sinica, Acta Zootaxonomica Sinica, Sichuan Journal of Zoology, Chinese Journal of Zoology*, and so on. For the taxonomic revisions and updated information recently, we follow the taxonomy of Fauna

Sinica Reptilia [26-27], Snakes of China [28] and the reptile database (http://www.reptile-database.org/). To reduce the sources of potential errors records, uncertain distributions and identifications, such as isolated distribution records, we checked again and removed erroneous records. If possible, we tried to overcome these difficulties by adding as many taxa as possible to the analyses. The distributional data with longitudes and latitudes were reviewed from museum databases or literature, and otherwise, we compiled coordinates from Google Earth. Finally, an initial data set of 422 Squamates with species names (see Appendix S1 in Supplementary Material) represented by a total of 50,749 records, of these, 61.0% records were lizards, while the remaining records were snakes.

2.2.3. Parsimony Analysis of Endemicity (PAE)

We used PAE to identify biogeographical patterns and followed the procedure modified by Morrone [16]. A taxon/area matrix for the basic PAE data set was built in which the absence of a species in an area was coded as '0' and presence as '1'. A hypothetical area coded '0' as an outgroup to provide a root for the final cladogram [13, 16]. We removed species that occurred in all areas, as well as those in only one area due to phylogenetically uninformative autapomorphies [15]. The taxon/area matrix were imported into PAUP * [29] to find the most parsimonious cladograms with a heuristic search of 1000 replicates and random sequence additions. We estimated relative support for each branch using bootstrapping, with 100 replicates and tree bisection–reconnection (TBR) swapping. All characters were weighted equally and a 50% majority consensus tree of the equally parsimonious trees was generated.

2.3. Results

2.3.1. Biological areas 28

The bootstrap 50% majority-rule consensus tree using 244"characters" in the analysis was shown in Figure 1(b). Our results were substantially different from the results of Meng *et al* [5]. The parsimony analysis obtained twelve most-parsimonious trees [Tree length = 676; Consistency index (CI) = 0.3609; Homoplasy index (HI) = 0.6391; Retention index (RI) = 0.6415]. Although two clear groups, D and E, were identified by the analysis, they did not support either the delimitation between palaearctic and oriental realms in China or the geographical barrier within the confines of the Qinling Mountains and Huai River, and east of the Hengduan Mountains [5]. The bootstrap value of group D (64%) was almost the same as that of group E (61%). The group D includes area 21 and area 23, which corresponded to the Tibetan Plateau and Taiwan Island in Map (Figure 1).

For Group E, it was very complex and ten clades were discovered. Subclade E1 as Sothern region (bootstrap 88%) corresponded to the clade C in [11], but major regions such as Central region (C2), Eastern Southern region (C3), Western Southern region (C4), and Central Southern region (C5) in [5] cannot be recognized. In subclade E1, A8 mainly representing Jiangsu was basal, followed by separation of A1 and the remaining areas in subclade E1. Areas A22, A24, A25, A26 and A27 formed a clade with a moderate support of 78%, corresponding to Southern China of zoogeographical division of [9] excluding Taiwan Island. Subclade E2 had a bootstrap support of 98%, including two sub-clades, A12 and A5 + A28. It corresponded to northeastern Tsaidam basin, Loess plateau and Alashan Plateau. Subclade E3 (A10 + A19) corresponded to the steppe and desert of north-western China, including Xinjiang and Inner Mongolia. Its bootstrap support value was 72%. Subclade E4 (A14 + A18) consists of the Xiao Xingan and Changbai mountains, with a bootstrap value of 86%. The Qinghai-Tibetan Plateau included A11+A21, however, subclade E6 (A11) was separated from A21 in the results with a bootstrap support value of 64%. The remaining subclades showed ambiguous.

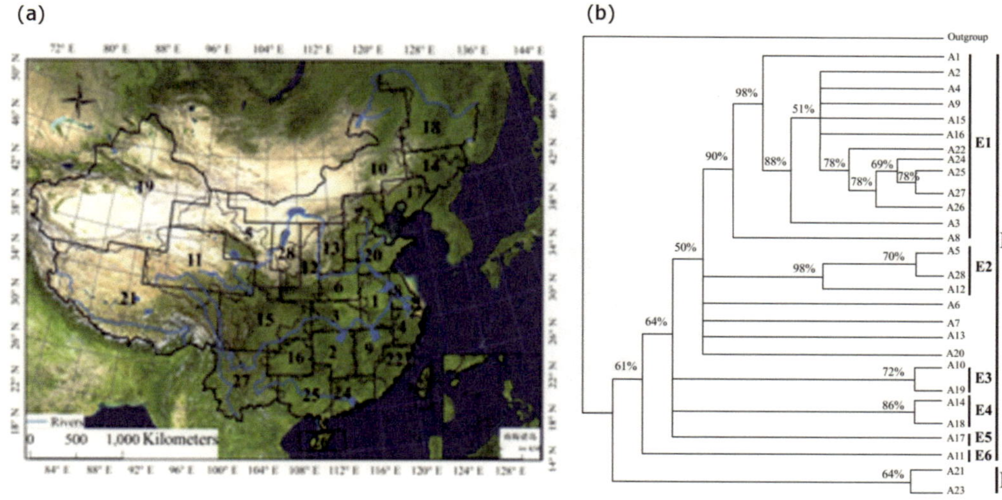

Figure 1. (a) The division of 28 areas (A01–A28) in China used in the PAE analysis. (b) 50 % majority consensus tree generated by PAE analysis. The terminals correspond to the OGUs shown in (a). Bootstrap values were shown above the branches

2.3.2. Biological areas 54

The 1507 most parsimonious cladograms of 930 steps with CI of 0.3172, HI of 0.6828, and RI of 0.6340 were found. The 50% majority-rule consensus tree using 295"characters" (Figure 2, b) showed a basal polytomy, but several clades emerged. Clade F consisted of areas A12, A13 and A14 with a bootstrap value of 57%, which corresponded to the Loess plateau subregion. Clade G had a weakly supported group containing areas A18, A19, A20, A21, A23 and A24 with a bootstrap proportion of 57%, which corresponded to Western desert subregion and Tian Shan mountains subregion of Mognolia-Xijiang China. Clade H had a well-support of 95%, including two sub-clades, A30 + A36 and A37, in response with the Himalaya mountains subregion of Southwestern China. Areas A40, A44, A45, A46, and A47 formed a clade I, including Eastern hills and plains subregion and Western mountains and plateau subregion of Central China, and coastal subregions of Guangdong and Fujian provinces of Southern China; its bootstrap value was 57%. Clade J consisted of areas A48 and A49 with a strongly support value of 100%, corresponding to Southern Yunnan mountains subregion of Southern China. Clade K corresponded to Hainan Island subregion of Southern China, consisting of areas A50 and A51 with 75% bootstrap value. Clade L contained Taiwan Island areas with similar Squamates faunas, areas A52 and A53; its well-supported value was 100%.

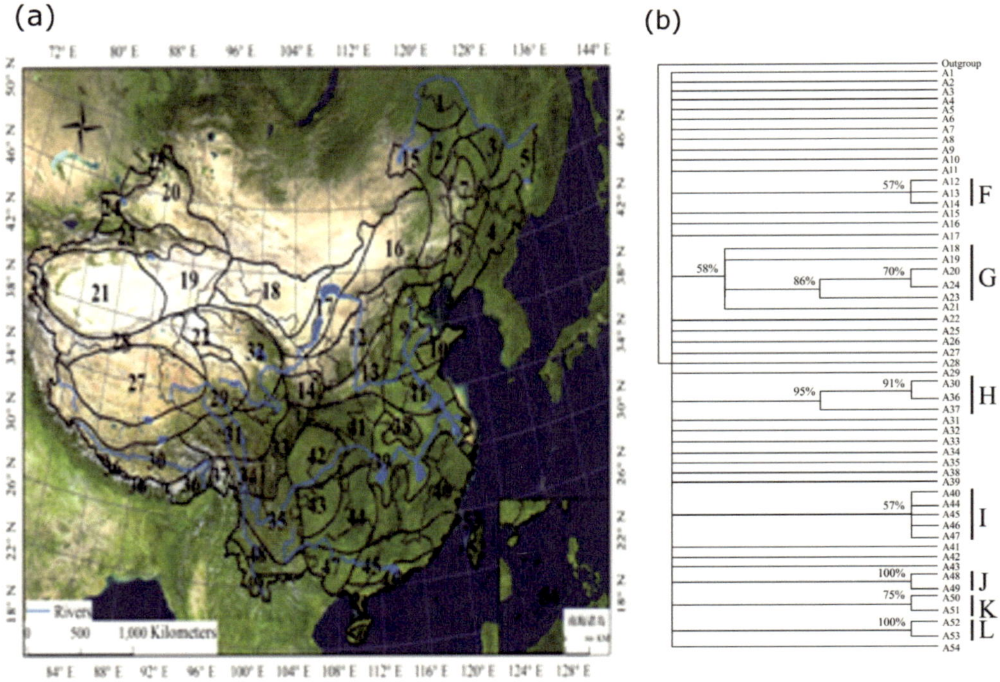

Figure 2. (a) The division of 54 areas (A01–A54) in China used in the PAE analysis. (b) 50 % majority consensus tree generated by PAE analysis. The terminals correspond to the OGUs shown in (a). Bootstrap values were shown above the branches

2.3.3. Biological areas 124

For OGUs of biological areas 124, the 1000 most parsimonious trees were obtained. The 50%-majority consensus tree using 294 characters (tree length = 1407, CI = 0.2090, RI = 0.7910) of the 1000 trees was shown in Figure 2 (b). Like the Figure 3, a basal polytomy were identified where only one of the branches contained a dicotomy in Figure 3. Clade M is moderately supported by Areas A10 and A14 with 88% bootstrap value. It corresponded to Yinshan mountains hill and Ordos Plateau. Areas (A21, ((A22, A23), A17)) formed the clade N with a week support value of 62%, corresponding to (Mountain front mesa, ((Liaodong Peninsula, Lower Liaohe Plain), Changbai mountains)) in Eastern Northeastern China. Clade O consisted of areas A29 and A32, including Southeast Shanxi plain and Western Henan mountains. Its bootstrap support proportion was 60%. Clade P contained areas (A101, (A37, A99)) with 68% bootstrap value, corresponding to the range of Qilian Mountain, Central Gansu incisive hill and Upper Yellow River incisive mountains. Areas A46 (Qinling mountains) and A47 (Daba–Micang mountains) in Central China formed clade Q with a moderate support value of 81%. Clade R was compose of Areas A58 and A63, corresponding to Xiangjiang valley hill and Honghe catchment montane basin; its support proportion was 80%. Clade S included Areas A61, A62 and A63 with a weekly support value of 51%, corresponding to Dalou Mountain mid-land valley, Miaoling hilly plain and Wujiang and Nanpanjiang catchments mid-land valley. Clade T was the largest clade including Areas A67, A68, A73, A74, A75 and A87 with 60% support value. It corresponded to Southeast Yunnan low-heat plateau, South central Yunnan low-heat valley, West Yunnan montane plain, Southwest Yunnan Plateau wide valley, South Yunnan wide valley and Salween and Lancang Rivers parallel valley. Areas A76 (West Guangdong and south Guangxi coastal mesa plain) and A79 (South Hainan montane hill) formed Clade U with 64% support value. Clade V had the greatest bootstrap value (98%), including areas A80, A81 and A83. It corresponded to Northwest subtropical hilly plain, Central subtropical mountain and East tropical coast in Taiwan Island. Clade W consisted of areas A92, A93, A94 and A95 with a bootstrap support of 73%, corresponding to areas in Himalayas mountains including Kangrigebu south wing mountains, Himalayas south wing mountains, Salween and Lancang Rivers incisive mountains and Brahmaputra Great Turn and upper Salween incisive mountains. Similarly, clade X consisted of areas A96, and A97, corresponding to areas in Himalayas mountains including Brahmaputra valley mountains and Himalayas central mountains; its bootstrap support value was 61%. Clade Y was compose of areas A104 and A105 with a week bootstrap support proportion of 59%. It corresponded to areas in Qinghai–Tibetan Plateau including South Qiangtang Plateau mountains and North Tibet plateau northwestern lake basin mountains. Clade Z included areas (A111, (A115, (A120, A122))), which corresponded to West Hexi Corridor, East Tianshan mountains, Central Tianshan mountains, Tarim Basin. Its bootstrap value was 57%. Areas A118 (Junggar Basin), A121 (Ili Valley), and A119 (Emin Valley) formed Clade AZ with a well support proportion of 97%.

2.4. Conclusion

Past major geological events have played important roles in shaping the biogeographic distribution of extant organisms. PAE originally aimed to find areas of congruent distributional patterns, and the best PAE results were obtained with natural areas (e.g. biogeographical provinces, ecoregions) instead of quadrats by increasing the absolute and relative numbers of synapomorphies [13]. If we compare the results of areas 28, 54 and 124, there seems to exist a trend to result in poor resolution of the resultant area cladograms as the size of OGU decreases. Although the samples within the regions are not uniform at different areas unit, in our area cladograms, biogeographic patterns of squamates distributions appear to have a hierarchical structure and general patterns for areas 28. Based on the above comprehensive squamates distributions patterns at different natural area units, seven major congruent biogeographic regions can be identified in China: Eastern Northern region, Tibetan Plateau region, Xinjiang and Inner Mongolia region, Loess plateau and Alashan Plateau region, Taiwan Island region and Southern region. However, there existed several unresolved areas relationships to one another, the uncertain position of certain areas or incongruence in the 'character' distributions. There may be basal problems with data themselves such as squamates distribution incomplete known. Sure, extinction, long-distance dispersal, isolation, or other undetected historical patterns may lead to incongruence in the distributions patterns [30].

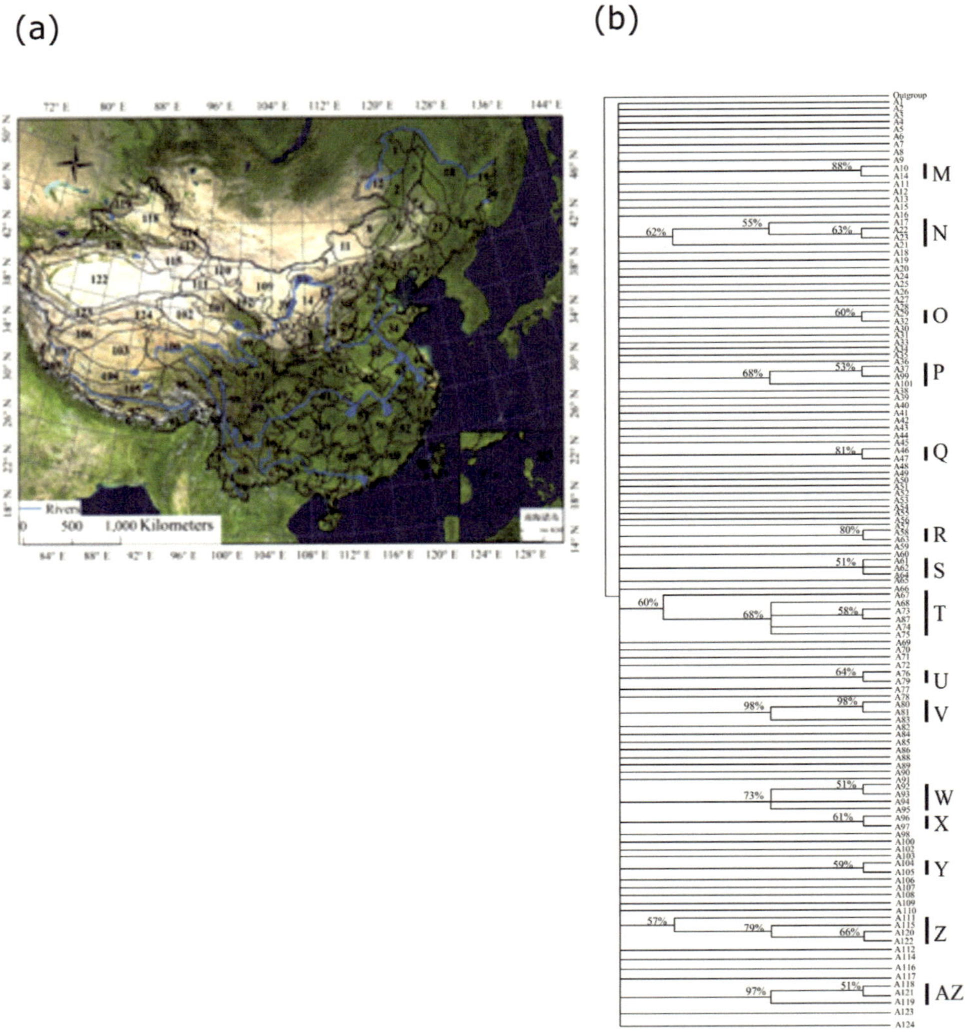

Figure 3. (a) The division of 124 areas (A01–A124) in China used in the PAE analysis. (b) 50 % majority consensus tree generated by PAE analysis. The terminals correspond to the OGUs shown in (a). Bootstrap values were shown above the branches

It is surely not coincidental that different organisms may share a general distribution pattern. A PAE area cladogram might contain areas related by shared ecologies or similar historical events (biotic divergence and isolation) [15]. Historical hypothesis, in other words, evolutionary history has recently been considered to be a driving force determining squamates regional species pools' differences in China. Geological complexity and history usually have a profound influence on the distributions of living organisms in China [5], though most of China has never been covered by ice sheets. Squamates species are followed this rule. For example, squamates were similar to spiders distributional patterns broadly corresponded to geological provinces

http://dx.doi.org/10.5772/55719

in China, such as Southern China geological province versus Southern regions, The Laurentian/Cathaysian Southern, South-western Margin geological province and Tibetan geological provinc vs Tibetan Plateau biogeographical region [9]. Furthermore, biotic and abiotic conditions are also important factors in determinative of the distribution of squamates species. Some correlations between species richness and reproductive modes with geography and ecological conditions have been reported [31-32]. The interpretations of those relationships have postulated that contemporary factors are the main regulatory force of the distribution of squamates taxa in China [33-35]. Thus, both history and ecology may well be inseparable and have a profound impact on not only the diversity of Squamates taxa but also their biogeographic patterns.

3. Distribution patterns in species diversity of lizards in China and their relationships to ecological factors

3.1. Introduction

Determining the causes of the great biodiversity variation across Earth has long been a major challenge for ecologists and biogeographers [36], ever since biotic diversity contrast between equatorial and polar latitudes was discovered two centuries ago [37]. Among the considerable number of hypotheses that aim to explain species richness patterns [36, 38], many ecological (environmental) hypotheses have been widely discussed and accepted [39].

Three alternative variants of ecological hypothesis, the species-energy, contemporary climate and habitat heterogeneity hypotheses, have received a great deal of attention as the primary determinants of species richness [39-43]. The species-energy hypothesis includes at least two versions, the ambient energy and productive energy hypotheses [38]. The ambient energy hypothesis, widely indicated by temperature or allied measures, argues that species richness was influenced by energy inputs into an area that affects the physiological tolerance of organisms [40, 44]. The productive energy hypothesis claims that animal species richness is limited by energy via food webs rather than by physiological requirements. The energy and water availability (i.e., energy–water dynamics) limits the total available plant productivity, which ultimately moves up the food chains [40, 45-47]. The contemporary climate hypothesis states that species richness correlates with contemporary climate conditions, and putative causal mechanisms are in terms of environmental stability, variability, favorability and harshness [40, 47-48]. The habitat heterogeneity hypothesis is measured either as the number of habitat types or the topographic relief (range in elevation) presented within an area [42, 50]. It assumes that high species richness is found in physically or biologically complex habitats, through higher speciation rates and providing more ecological niches [40-42].

However, the knowledge of the determinants of reptile richness remains insufficiently documented among terrestrial vertebrates [39, 51-82]. It is urgent to understand the drivers of reptile richness patterns due to global warming impact on species distribution and abundance [36, 52-53]. Lizards belong to Reptila and are good model systems to test these alternative hypotheses. Because their taxonomy is well resolved and distributional data are quite thorough. They are ectothermic and sensitive to environmental variables. In this study, we examine the correlation between lizard species richness and various environmental factors across China. Our objectives include (1) mapping distributions of Chinese lizards and describing any patterns, and (2) testing various ecological factors in determining species richness patterns.

3.2. Materials and methods

3.2.1. Data collection

We collected locality data for lizard species which occur in China from a variety of sources as above-mentioned. We excluded coastal grid cells with less than 96% land cover and all islands from the analysis in order to remove the effects of insularity. Finally, we built a database of 151 lizard with species names (see Appendix S1 in Supplementary Material) represented by a total of 3,391 records for unique point localities, with a range of 2–288 (mean = 22.5, standard deviation = 38.3).

3.2.2. Ecological niche modeling and species richness

For each of the 151 species, we used the Genetic Algorithm for Rule-set Prediction (GARP) (for free download see: http://www.nhm.ku.edu/desktopgarp/) [54] for reconstructing species distribution maps. GARP uses an evolutionary computing genetic algorithm to search iteratively for non-random correlations between species presence and environmental variables for localities using several different types of rules (i.e., atomic rules, range rules, negated range rules, logistic regression rules), and then creates ecological niche models for each species' predicted distribution, as contrasted with environmental characteristics across the overall study area [54]. GARP was found that it did not tend to be more sensitive to sampling bias than Maxent, and GARP is a very useful technique to estimate richness and composition of unsampled areas and have been tested to correctly predict the most of the species' distributional potential [48, 55-58], for example in applications to invasive species [57-58], tree species [59-60], squamate species [48, 61], and so on.

We included a total of eighteen environmental variables in the model. Variables for details, descriptions, and files for download are described in the following text. We set several optimization parameters while running the software following [48]. The parameters included: 20 runs, 0.001 convergence limit, and 1,000 maximum interactions; rule types: atomic, range, negated range, and logistic regression; best subset active, 5% omission error, 40% commission error, and 67% of points for training; omission measure = extrinsic, and omission threshold = hard; 10 models under hard omission threshold.

The estimation output of DesktopGarp produced in Arc/Info grid maps with 'zeros', where the species were not predicted to occur, and 'ones', where the species were predicted to occur. The area covered by the coincidence of at least seven out of the 10 models in the best subset selection (optimum models considering omission/commission relationships [62]) were used as the predicted distribution of each species. By doing so and by setting the commission error to 40%, this approach added a component of conservatism in predicting distribution by GARP, which might otherwise extrapolate too much and predict areas that are too far from where the species have previously been collected [48]. After generating such maps using the same criteria for all 151 species, we used ARCGIS software to overlay all species prediction maps into a composite map. This final map was used to create a girded of species richness map at a resolutions of 100 km (approximately equivalent to 1°at the equator) on an Albers Equal-Area Conic projection. Consequently, we used the occurrences of 151 lizard species within 827 grid cells to calculate species richness, summing the value of overlaid corresponding grid cells.

3.2.3. Environmental data

We used eighteen environmental variables. We selected these variables based on previous studies and the four associated hypotheses [40-43, 49]. All environmental variables for assessing hypothesized explanations of species richness were re-projected and re-sampled to the same equal-area cell as the species richness data in ARCGIS. The hypotheses and their related variables are:

1. Ambient energy—five variables are associated this hypothesis within each cell, including: mean annual potential evapotranspiration (PET) ([63], 30'resolution, available at http://www.grid.unep.ch/data/grid/gnv183.html); mean annual highest temperature (HT), and mean annual lowest temperature (LT) (data from 1961 to 1990 with 1 km^2 resolution, available at http://www.data.ac.cn/ index.asp); mean annual sum of effective temperature (≥0℃) (SET0) and mean annual sum of effective temperature (≥10℃) (SET10) (data from 1981 to 1996 with 500 m^2 resolution, available at http://www.geodata.cn/Portal).

2. Productive energy—three variables are used to account for productive energy hypothesis, including: mean annual remotely sensed Normalized Difference Vegetation Index (NDVI), obtained from Advanced Very High-Resolution Radiometer (AVHRR) record of monthly changes in the photosynthetic activity of terrestrial vegetation (data from 1998 to 2008 with 1 km^2 resolution, Data source: Environment and Ecology Scientific Data Center of western China, National Natural Science Foundation of China, available at http://westdc.westgis.ac.cn), mean annual actual evapotranspiration (AET)([60], 30' resolution, available at http://www.grid.unep.ch/data/grid/gnv183.html), and mean annual solar radiation (RAD) (data from 1950 to 1980 with 1 km^2 resolution, available at http://www.geodata.cn/Portal).

3. Contemporary climate hypothesis—eight variables are associated with this hypothesis within each cell, including: mean annual temperature (AT) (data from 1961 to 1990 with 1 km^2 resolution, available at http://www.data.ac.cn/index.asp); mean annual sunshine (SUN) (percent of daylength), mean annual diurnal temperature range (DTR) and mean annual frost-day frequency (FF) (data from 1961 to 1990 with 10' resolution [64]); and mean annual wind speed (WIND) (data from 1981 to 1996 with 500 m2 resolution, available at http://www.geodata.cn/Portal); mean annual precipitation (PRE) (data from 1961 to 1990 with 1 km^2 resolution, available at http://www.data.ac.cn/index.asp), mean annual wet-

day frequency (WET) (number days with >0.1 mm precipitation per month) and mean annual relative humidity (REH) (data from 1961 to 1990 with 10' resolution [64]).

4. Habitat heterogeneity—the count of 300 m elevation range within each quadrat (ELE) (HYDRO1 k data set for Asia, 1 km^2 resolution, available at http://eros.usgs.gov/) and the number of vegetation classes (VEG) (1 km^2 resolution, Data source: Environment and Ecology Scientific Data Center of western China, National Natural Science Foundation of China, available at http://westdc.westgis.ac.cn) as indicators of habitat heterogeneity.

3.2.4. *Statistical analyses*

In order to examine the potential predictors of lizard richness patterns in China, we first tested the relationship between lizard richness and environmental variables using a multiple regression analysis. We did not use all environmental variables employed to run GARP, because including many highly correlated variables in a multiple regression creates several theoretical and statistical problems, especially estimating partial regression coefficients [65]. We selected variables previously identified as affecting species richness and were not highly correlated ($r<0.80$) and there were one variable represented each hypothesis at least.

We used the eigenvector-based filtering, or spatial eigenvector mapping (SEVM) obtained by Principal Coordinates Neighbour Matrices (PCNM) to account for spatial autocorrelation [66]. Spatial autocorrelation is a potential problem when work with large-scale ecological data and explanatory variables [67-68]. Failure to account for spatial autocorrelation could result in inflating Type I error because model fitting may generate artificially narrow standard errors due to the lack of independence among residuals [67-68]. A truncation distance of 102.33 km, calculated in SAM—Spatial Analysis in Macroecology [69], was used to create the spatial filters. Eigenvector filters were chosen when their influence on species richness was both statistically significant ($P<0.05$) and had sufficient explanatory power ($r^2>0.02$). We selected eigenvector filters in an iterative process, by minimizing both the spatial autocorrelation among residuals and the number of filters used in regression. Moran's *I* coefficient were used to examine the model residuals of the spatial autocorrelation in reducing spatial autocorrelation [70]. These filters were then used as candidate predictor variables, together with other environmental predictors formed in the full model. In this way, the effects of environmental predictors are evaluated as partial effects, taking spatial factors into account explicitly [69]. The total explanatory power, r^2 values, was divided into three parts: a part explained by space, a part explained by environmental variables, and a part of shared explained variance.

To test which hypothesis best explains variation in lizard richness in China, we conducted separate regressions to fit each of the hypothesis, with an addition of mixed models using all variables associated with each hypothesis. The sample-size-corrected Akaike information criterion (AICc) was used to evaluate the goodness of model fit. The model with the lowest AICc score was considered the most parsimonious, therefore optimizing the tradeoff between bias and precision in model construction [71]. The difference between any candidate models and the best model (ΔAICc) was used to evaluate the relative model fit when their AICc scores were close. The larger the ΔAICc, the less possible is the fitted model as being the best approximating model in the given models set. In general, Models having $\Delta AICc \leq 2$ have substantial support (evidence), those in which 4 ≤ ΔAICc ≤7 have considerably less support, and models having ΔAICc≥10 have essentially no support [72]. Model-averaging of estimates using Akaike weights (wi) was used to confront model selection uncertainty [73].

Finally, to make a comparison between the actual available data and the lizard distributions predicted by ecological niche modeling, we mapped species locality points' data and calculated species richness at 100 km resolution (Figure 4a). This method allowed us to check whether a spatial sampling bias was shown in the final modeling map (i.e., areas that have more species collected coincide with the areas the model indicated as higher species richness) [48].

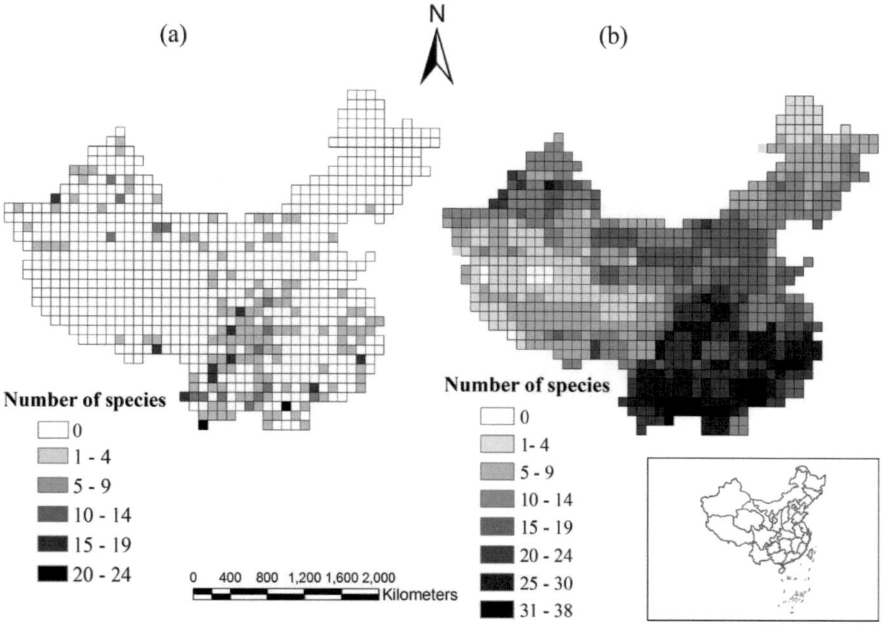

Figure 4. Number of species per grid cell based on (a) the raw data of museum collections, and (b) the ecological niche modeling of 151 species. The grid corresponds to the approximate area of China and the area of each cell is 100 km^2. Blank cells have no specimen based on the major collections [34].

3.3. Results

3.3.1. Patterns of species richness

Figure 4(b) shows the distribution map which summed all 151 lizard species richness in China. Lizard species richness varied between 1 and 38 species per cell (mean: 13 ± 8 SD) and displayed a consistent pattern that species number increased from higher latitudes to lower ones, and from west to east. The Highest species richness occurs in the Oriental Realm tropics, around the border between southern China and southwestern China, and around the Nanling Mountains, at the border between southern China and central China. Other areas with relative high richness included southwestern China, southern China, northwestern and eastern central

China of the Oriental realm (Figure 4b). The raw data map shows a slight sampling bias to the northwest central China and northeast southwestern China (Figure 4a), where the largest herpetological museum CIB/CAS in China are located. However, the niche modeling results are not highly influenced by this bias, since areas corresponding to the highest species richness in China do not overlay completely with the pattern. Furthermore, high richness areas were found by the niche modeling in the relatively poor sampling regions, such as the northwest Mongolia-Xinjiang China, west-south Qinghai-Tibet China areas (Figure 4b).

3.3.2. Species richness and environmental variables

The environmental models for the multiple regression analysis using SEVM with adding eigenvector spatial filters (PCNM), were sufficient to reduce autocorrelation in the residuals (filters data not shown). A spatial correlogram based on Moran's *I* index was used to evaluate the pattern of spatial autocorrelation in the residuals of the regression. The multiple regression model explained a total of 80.1% variance of lizard richness in China ($r^2 = 0.801$; $F = 203.47$; $P<0.001$). The total explanatory power explained by predictors alone was 17.0%, and explained by space alone was 5.4%, and the shared explained variance was 57.7%.

Based on the multiple regression analysis taking PCNM spatial filters into account, annual frost-day frequency (FF), elevation range (ELE), the number of vegetation classes (VEG), and wet-day frequency (WET) were the best predictors of species richness. FF was negatively correlated with lizard richness, while ELE, VEG, and WET, respectively, were positively correlated with lizard species richness. Based on model selection approach, the model with the lowest AICc value was the mixed model, which contained all variables related to the different hypotheses. It had an Akaike weight of 1.00. Other models had high ΔAICc values (>10, [69]) and low values of Akaike weights.

3.4. Conclusion

Our results indicate that mechanisms related to different ecological hypotheses might work together to account for lizard richness in China. It is important to consider the influence that environmental factors may have on shaping richness patterns [73]. The frost-day frequency, elevation range, vegetation and wet-day frequency were the most important environmental variable predicting lizard species richness in China. The current alternative hypotheses are not mutually exclusive and may work together and best explain patterns of lizard species richness in China. Based on results of the model selection, our conclusion is in concordant with several previous studies that multiple hypotheses may best account for species richness patterns [48, 66,74-75]. Clearly, a variety of factors works synergistically to determine species richness patterns. Our results indicate significant conservation implications, and habitat heterogeneity would be taken into account as an assessment of the threat to endemism from habitat loss in the future investigation. Lizards in China might have experienced large radiations and adapted to dramatic climatic fluctuations after the uplifting of the Tibetan Plateau in Pleistocene. For future studies, it is important to test species richness distribution in Asia at different spatial extent and sample resolution [76], as well as to explore other factors known to affect species richness, such as historical factors and biotic interactions (e.g., competition, predation, and parasitism).

4. Climate and history explain the origin and diversification for toad-headed agamas (genus *Phrynocephalus*) and racerunner lizards (genus *Eremias*)

Dramatic geologic events and climatic shifts are often considered to have significantly influenced the diversification and distributions of organisms. Central Asia has a long history of aridity, with the onset of desertification starting at least 22 million years ago (Ma) [77]. It is believed that the Miocene retreat of the Paratethys Sea, an epicontinental sea stretching over Eurasia 30 Ma, and the uplift of the Tibetan Plateau during the Oligocene–Miocene, played a major role in the shift of the Central Asian climate from oceanic to continental [78], leading to increasing levels of aridity. These climatic changes intensified in the Late Miocene and into the Plio-Pleistocene, as part of the global deterioration of the Cenozoic climates [77]. The Quaternary glaciations in the Qinghai-Tibetan Plateau (QTP) and the bordering mountains were the consequence of a combination between climate and local tectonic uplift. In particular, the Kunlun-Huanghe and Gonghe tectonic uplifts have played very important roles in triggering glaciations in high Asia [[79-81]. The dramatic geological and climatic histories on the Plateau during the Quaternary have a remarkable influence on regional and adjacent biogeographic patterns [82].

4.1. Toad-headed agamas (*Phrynocephalus*)

The genus *Phrynocephalus*, i.e., toad-headed agamas, are a modern group of lizards including about ~37 distinct species [83, but see 84]. They are typically grouped together with Asian Rock Agamas (*Laudakia*), *Bufoniceps*, and *Trapelus* in the subfamily Agaminae. Toad-headed agamas inhabit arid regions from northwestern China to the western side of the Caspian Sea, across the Tibetan Plateau, and southwest Asia to the Arabian Peninsula. They constitute one of the major components of the central Asian desert fauna and are highly adapted to sand dunes and desert environments. The reproductive biology of *Phrynocephalus* is notable in that there exist two reproductive modes: viviparity and oviparity. All six viviparous species are endemic to China and mainly restricted to high elevations in the Tibetan Plateau. Despite the progress that has been made in recent years for the systematics of certain *Phrynocephalus* groups, the large-scale pattern of their evolution in time and space remains open. Here, we review the origin and diversification of toad-headed agamas with their relationships to geological and climatic changes.

Until recently, our knowledge of the phylogenetic relationships and historical biogeography of *Phrynocephalus* was mainly based on anatomical studies [85-86]. Researchers usually agree that the broad distribution of *Phrynocephalus* may be explained by different hypotheses. Ananjeva and Tuniyev [87] speculated that there were two original centers for the *Phrynocephalus* species: Central Asia (a northern Tethys origin) and Middle Asia (a southern Tethys origin). They also inferred that diversification was related to geological events such as alpine orogenesis causing the isolation of valleys and basins and changes in the direction of river courses. Through a phylogenetic analysis of allozymes, Macey *et al.* [88] suggested that *Phrynocephalus* represents an old radiation that has been evolving in response to the Indian collision with Eurasia 35 Ma, and a clade in the former Soviet Union may have diverged as a result of internal Eurasian block movements in Afghanistan caused by the indenting Indian continent. Later, Arnold [86] proposed that *Phrynocephalus* originated in the Arabia-NW India area rather than in Central Asia, and achieved its current distribution by dispersal. However, Wang and Macey [89] initially considered the origin of the viviparous species group as a result of a vicariance event associated with the uplifting of the Tibetan Plateau, which was subsequently supported by Zeng *et al.* [90] and Pang *et al.* [91]. Meanwhile, Pang *et al.* [91] using mitochondrial DNA data, partial sequences of the mitochondrial genes (12S rRNA, 16S rRNA, cyt *b*, ND4-tRNA^{Leu}), corroborated the monophyly of the viviparous group for the first time, and hypothesized that the oviparous group achieved their current distribution by dispersal. Pang *et al.* [91]. also provided the first time estimate for the origin of Chinese *Phrynocephalus* at 6.2–3.1 Ma, using average evolutionary rates of rate-constant genes to apply a clock.

Most recent analyses use relaxed-clock methods, which allow evolutionary rates to vary among genes and lineages. Guo and Wang [92] re-analyzed the data of Pang *et al.* [91] by employing partition-specific modeling in a combined DNA analysis to clarify existing gaps in the phylogeny of Chinese *Phrynocephalus*. Using this phylogenetic framework, they inferred the genus' historical biogeography by using weighted ancestral-area analysis and dispersal-vicariance analysis in combination with a Bayesian relaxed molecular-clock approach. They drew three major conclusions: (i) the uplift of the QTP played a fundamental role in the diversification of viviparous *Phrynocepalus*; (ii) an evolutionary scenario combining aspects of vicariance and dispersal is necessary to explain the distribution of *Phrynocephalus*; (iii) Chinese *Phrynocephalus* originated at the Middle-Late Miocene boundary (12.78 Ma, 95% CI 17.61–8.25 Ma), and diversified from Late Miocene to Pleistocene from a center of origin in Central Asia, Tarim Basin, and Juggar Basin temperate desert.

A more recent study [93] using a ~1200 bp region of mitochondrial DNA (ND2-tRNA^{Tyr}) and a ~1200 bp nuclear gene (RAG-1) and samples across Central Asian agamids results in two well supported conclusions: (i) the onset of aridification in Central Asia during the Late Oligocene, resulting from the retreat of the Paratethys Sea and the intensified uplift of the Tibetan-Himalayan complex, appears to have played an important role in *Phrynocephalus* diversification and evolution; (ii) intensification of aridity and geologic events in the Plio-Pleistocene and Quaternary glacial cycling probably had a significant influence on intraspecific diversification patterns within *Phrynocephalus*. Melville *et al.* [93] generated age estimates using two data. One method relied on mtDNA data, while the other relied on nuclear DNA data. The mtDNA data suggests that the estimated age of the common ancestor for *Phrynocephalus* was at 28.9 million years ago (Ma) with a 95% credibility interval of 36.2-21.1 Ma, a finding that is consistent with previous estimates [88]. Using the nuclear gene RAG-1excluding *P. interscapularis*, the estimate for the age of the common ancestor was somewhat younger, 15.8 Ma (95% CI 23–11.8 Ma), in accord with estimates produced by Guo and Wang [92]. However, both the analysis of Guo and Wang [92] and RAG-1 analysis did not include the basal species *P. interscapularis*, which was included in the mtDNA analysis by Melville *et al.* [93]. From this analysis, Melville *et al.* [93] concluded that including *P. interscapularis*, the age of *Phrynocephalus* would probably be Late Oligocene or Early Miocene, which coincides with the onset of aridification in Central Asia. Thus, their findings are consistent with a scenario that *Phryncephalus* is an old radiation, rather than it being a more recent diversification associated with the global deterioration of the Cenozoic climates when aridification intensified in the Late Miocene and into the Plio-Pleistocene. In addition, the deep phylogenetic split between the Chinese and Central Asian lineages of the *P. alpherakii*/*P. guttatus*/*P. versicolor* species group is probably related to the uplift of the Altay and Tien-Shan Mountains [93]. It was also suggested that gradual intensification of orogenetic processes and caused by them progressive aridization in the Middle East and Central Asia served as one of the factors favoring the evolution and initial diversification of the species complex of *P. helioscopus* [94].

Dunayev *et al.* [95] pursued the evolutionary history of 35 *Prhynocepahlus* species from COI segments (600-750 bp), which is, so far, the phylogenetic study with the most comprehensive taxonomic coverage. This phylogeny shows that the clade of Iranian species (e.g. *P. scutellatus* and *P. maculatus*) is sister to the remaining taxa, which joins Middle-Asian and Central-Asian taxa. Within the latter clade the representatives of the subgenus *Megalochilus* form a monophyletic group (*P. mystaceus, P. interscapularis, P. sogdianus*) of probably Irano-Turanian origin. The monophyletic Tibeto-Himalayan subgenus *Oreosaura* joins viviparous species (*P. vlangalii, P. thebaldi, P. forsythia* etc.) and is grouped together with oviparous species of Central Asia. Within Middle-Asian taxa three main species groups can be distinguished: (i) the groups of sun-watcher agamas (*P. helioscopus, P. ersicus*), (ii) *P. ocellatus-P. strauchi* group and (iii) *P. guttatus-P. versicolor* group. They further inferred that various bigoegoraphic events might cause diversification of *Phrynocepahlus* in continental Asia: starting with orogenetic processes on the territory of present-day Iranian and Tibetan plateaus, transgressions of Paratethys as major factors for old-splits, and up to aridisation processes and dynamics of major river valleys as factors determining recent speciation processes.

The topographic variation of the Qinghai-Tibetan Plateau, coupled with cyclical climatic changes in the Pleistocene, and alternating glacial-interglacial periods exerted the greatest influence on the current spatial distribution and genetic structure of viviparous toad-headed lizards. Jin *et al.* [96] studied the phylogeographic patterns of the Qinghai toad-headed lizard *Phrynocephalus vlangalii* by analysing sequence data from Mitochondrial DNA (mtDNA) sequences (partial ND2, $tRNA^{Trp}$ and partial $tRNA^{Ala}$). The Qinghai toad-headed lizard is viviparous and lives at elevations of 2000–4500 m, and is the dominant terrestrial species in the QTP [26]. It is primarily distributed in the Qaidam Basin and surrounding area, with three major mountain chains, the Kunlun, the Arjin and the A'nyemaqen Mountains, in its range. With a thorough sampling across the entire distribution and a traditional phylogenetic analysis, five deeply diverged mtDNA lineages were recovered and geographical distribution of these lineages had almost no overlap [96]. Not only the spatial locations of the mountain chains coincided with the divisions of the lineages, but the times of the mountain uplift were also concordant with the times of mtDNA lineage divergence. Their NCPA analysis further demonstrated that the allopatric fragmentation resulted from historical vicariant events dominated the history of this species. Consequently, Jin *et al.* [96] concluded that the uplifts of the three major mountain chains formed the physical barrier that caused the initial vicariant events. They also inferred that populations from the Qaidam Basin appeared to have undergone major demographic and range expansions in the early Pleistocene (1.6 Ma), consistent with the colonization of areas previously covered by the huge Qaidam palaeolake, which desiccated at the onset of the Pleistocene [96].

Using data from 11 microsatellite DNA loci, Wang *et al.* [97] further supported the hypotheis of Jin *et al.* [96] that the uplift of the Arjin and the A'nyemaqen Mountains caused the initial vicariant events that led to the formation of the diverged lineages within *P. vlangalii*. Later, using a mitochondrial fragment ND4-tRNA^{Leu}, Guo *et al.* [98]confirmed that the uplift of the A'nyemaqen Mountains and glaciations since the mid-late Pleistocene, especially during the Kunlun Glaciation, are considered to have promoted the allopartric divergence of *P. vlangalii*. The diversification of *P. putjatia* may be triggered by the tectonic movement in the Huangshui River valley during the C phase of Qingzang Movement. Subsequently, the glacial climate throughout the Pleistocene may have continued to impede the gene flow of *P. putjatia*, eventually resulting in the genetic divergence of *P. putjatia* in the allopatric regions.

Jin and Liu [99] described the phylogeography of a unique endemic agamid lizard, *Phrynocephalus erythrurus* from the Qiangtang Plateau by analyzing sequence data from a mtDNA segment ND2- tRNA^{Ala}. *P. erythrurus* is viviparous and occupies the highest regions of any reptile on earth [26]. They found that (i) this species diverged into two major lineages/subspecies at 3.7 Ma corresponding to the Northern and Southern Qiangtang Plateau; (ii) the Northern Qiangtang lineage diverged into two subpopulations at 2.8 Ma separated by the Beilu River Region and Wulanwula Mountains [99]. Their NCPA analysis further demonstrated that the allopatric fragmentation and restricted gene flow were the most likely mechanisms of population differentiation. Their results also indicated the presence of at least three refugia since the Hongya glaciation. Consequently, Jin and Liu [99] concluded that the uplift of Tanggula Mountains movement and glaciations since mid-Pliocene have shaped phylogenetic patterns of *P. erythrurus*.

An aridification of the Tarim Basin and adjacent areas since middle Pleistocene has produced significant genetic structuring of the local fauna. Zhang *et al.* [100] compared the phylogeographic patterns, population structure and history of *Phrynocephalus axillaris* and *P. forsythii* using a mitochondrial fragment ND4-tRNA^{Leu}. They demonstrated that the two species might have experienced different evolutionary history throughout their current distribution. For *P. forsythii*, a vicariant event, as a consequence of geological isolation by the initiation of Quaternary folding at 2.1–1.2 Ma in the eastern Tien-Shan [101], and desert expansion, might have produced the significant divergence between the Tarim and the Yanqi populations. For *P. axillaris*, populations of the Yanqi, Turpan and Hami Basins might have been established through dispersal during demographic expansion. Climatic fluctuations caused alternate expansion and shrinkage of rivers and oases several times, which likely led to habitat fragmentation for both species. Interaction between vicariance, dispersal and habitat fragmentation produced the current distribution and genetic diversity.

4.2. Racerunner lizards (*Eremias*)

The lacertid genus *Eremias* Fitzinger 1834, is considered to comprise approximately 34 species, which inhabit sand, steppe, and desert regions from northern China, Mongolia, Korea, Central and Southwest Asia to Southeastern Europe. The reproductive biology of *Eremias* is notable in that there exist two reproductive modes: viviparity and oviparity. Most are oviparous, whereas the *Eremias multiocellata* complex (comprising 6 subspecies), *E. buechneri, E. kokshaaliensis, E. yarkandensis, E. quadrifrons,* and *E. przewalskii* are viviparous [102]. Despite the progress that has been made in recent years for the systematics of certain *Eremias* groups, the large-scale pattern of their evolution in time and space remains open. Here, we review the origin and diversification of racerunner lizards with their relationships to geological and climatic changes.

Until recently, our understanding of the phylogenetic relationships and historical biogeography of *Eremias* was mainly based on anatomical studies [103-105]. Boulenger [106] and FitzSimons [107] assigned most of the species now placed in *Pedioplanis* to the subgenus *Mesalina* within the large genus *Eremias*. Szczerbak [108] regarded *Eremias* sensu lato polyphyletic and considered *Eremias* (s. s.) endemic to Asia. Based on morphological characters and geographic distribution, Szczerbak [103] subdivided the inclusive genus *Eremias* (s. l.) into two distinct genera: the genus *Mesalina* as a north African and lowland Southwest Asian clade, and the genus *Eremias* (s. s.), which is endemic to Asia. Furthermore, Szczerbak [103] subdivided *Eremias* into five distinct subgenera: *Eremias* Fitzinger in Wiegmann, 1834 (group E. velox), *Rhabderemias* Lantz, 1928 (group *Eremias scripta–Eremias lineolata*), *Ommateremias* Lantz, 1928 (group *E. arguta*), *Scapteira* Fitzinger in Wiegmann, 1834 (group *Eremias grammica*), and *Pareremias* Szczerbak, 1973 (group *E. multiocellata*). The five subgenera were supported by Arnold (1986) on the basis of the hemipenial characters.

Wan *et al.* [109] made the first attempt to elucidate the phylogenetic relationships among the Chinese racerunner lizards on the basis of mitochondrial 16S rRNA data. They found that *E. brenchleyi* and *E. argus* formed a clade as the sister group of *E. multiocellata*. They further inferred that *E. arguta, E.grammica* and *E. velox* originated from Central Asia and the rest species in China originated from East Asia. However, these conclusions were tentative due to both limited taxa sampling as well as use of relatively short, partly nondiagnostic, gene fragment. On the other hand, one potential shortcoming of the analyses of Wan *et al.* [109] was that they did not incorporate secondary structural constraints of 16S rRNA into analyses.

Orlova *et al.* [110] studied the phylogeographic pattern of the steppe-runner lizard *Eremias arguta* by analyzing mtDNA cyt *b* gene sequences. The steppe-runner lizard inhabits steppes and semi-deserts of Eastern Europe and Middle Asia from Romania to Western Mongolia and China. They found an old split between *E. arguta uzbekistanica* and all other taxa, probably coming from the area of Ustyurt plateau. Consequently, Orlova *et al.* [110] inferred that this vicariant event is likely to have been caused by Paratethys regression.

More recently, a study [111 using combined DNA data sets (3925 bp) from two mitochondrial genes (cyt *b*, 12S rRNA) and one nuclear gene (RAG-1) and comprehensive taxonomic coverage resulted in three well-supported conclusions: (i) the species of the traditional genus *Eremias* form six clades; (ii) the Iranian plateau is the center of origin of the genus as a whole; (iii) genus *Eremias* should be divided into 4 distinct genera, and at least 14 new species should be described within these genera. Using a molecular clock calibrated with well dated paleological events as calibration, the average evolutionary rate for the mitochondrial genes was estimated as 1.3%-1.6% per million years. Based on the mitochondrial DNA data and using the globe molecular clock method, the origin time for the genus *Eremias* was dated to the early Miocene and the start of intrageneric divergence to the middle Miocene.

Another phylogenetic study [112] using mitochondrial 16S rRNA segment results in five major conclusions: (i) monophyly of *Eremias* and a clade comprising *Eremias, Acanthodactylus* and *Latastia* are recognized; (ii) monophyly of the subgenus *Pareremias* is corroborated, with *Eremias argus* being the sister taxon to *Eremias brenchleyi*; (iii) the first evidence that viviparous species form a monophyletic group was presented; (iv) *Eremias* probably diversified at about 9.9 million years ago (with the 95% credibility interval ranging from 7.6 to 12 Ma); (v) specifically, the divergence time of the subgenus *Pareremias* was dated to about 6.3 million years ago (with the 95% credibility interval ranging from 5.3 to 8.5 Ma), suggesting that the diversification of this subgenus might be correlated with the evolution of an East Asian monsoon climate triggered by the rapid uplift of the Tibetan Plateau approximately 8 Ma. A recent phylogeographic study [113] indicated that the Yellow River and Taihang Mountains may have acted as important barriers to gene flow in *Eremias brenchleyi.*

Rastegar-Pouyani *et al.* [114] explored the genealogical relationships and intraspecific differentiation of the rapid fringe-toed lizard *Eremias velox* by analyzing mtDNA cyt *b* and 12S rRNA gene sequences. The rapid fringe-toed lizard is widely distributed in the Iranian Plateau and Central Asia. In combination with molecular dating, they inferred that the *E. velox* complex originated on the Iranian Plateau in the Middle Miocene, which is in accordant with the result of Rastegar-Pouyani [115]. Another founding was that the northern Iranian clade diverged first some 11–10 Ma, caused by first uplifting of the Elburz Mountains in the late Miocene, and that the Central Asian lineages split from the northeastern Iranian lineage approximately 6 Ma, most likely as a result of uplifting of the Kopet-Dagh Mountains in the northern margin of the Iranian Plateau.

4.3. Conclusion

As exemplified with toad-headed agamas (genus *Phrynocephalus*) and racerunner lizards (genus *Eremias*), geomorphic and climatic changes in this big area definitely have remarkable influences on the regional and adjacent biogeographic patterns. Future comparative studies between *Eremias, Phrynocephalus* and other groups that distribute at the same area and inhabit similar habitat, can help to elucidate the origination, diversification and dispersion of these lizards, and test the link between speciation, adaptation, and historical changes in their biogeography. Specifically, further studies could search for differences in the ecological niches of species and clusters in order to assess ecological divergence among the several groups [116].

http://dx.doi.org/10.5772/55719

Appendix S1

List of the 422 squamates species.

Lacertilia:

Acanthosaura armata, A. lepidogaster, Alsophylax pipiens, A. przewalskii, Asymblepharus alaicus, A. ladacensis, A. sikimmensis, Ateuchosaurus chinensis, Calotes emma, C. medogensis, C. mystaceus, C. versicolor, Cyrtodactylus khasiensis, C. zhaoermii, Cyrtopodion dadunense, C. elongatum, C. medogense, C. stoliczkai, C. tibetanus, Dibamus bogadeki, D. bourreti, Dopasia gracilis, D. hainanensis, D. harti, D. ludovici, Draco blanfordii, D. maculatus, Eremias argus, E. arguta, E. brenchleyi, E. buechneri, E. grammica, E. kokshaaliensis, E. multiocellata, E. przewalskii, E. quadrifrons, E. stummeri, E. velox, E. vermiculata, E. yarkandensis, Eutropis longicaudata, E. multicarinata, E. multifasciata, Gehyra mutilate, Gekko auriverrucosus, G. chinensis, G. gecko, G. hokouensis, G. japonicas, G. kikuchii, G. melli, G. palmatus, G. reevesii, G. scabridus, G. similignum, G. swinhonis, G. taibaiensis, G. wenxianensis, Goniurosaurus bawanglingensis, G. hainanensis, G. lichtenfelderi, G. luii, G. yingdeensis, Hemidactylus aquilonius, H. bowringii, H. frenatus, H. garnotii, H. platyurus, H. stejnegeri, Hemiphyllodactylus typus, H. yunnanensis, Japalura andersoniana, J. batangensis, J. brevipes, J. brevicauda, J. dymondi, J. fasciata, J. flaviceps, J. graham, J. luei, J. kumaonensis, J. makii, J. micangshanensis, J. polygonata, J. splendida, J. swinhonis, J. tricarinata, J. varcoae, J. yulongensis, J. yunnanensis, J. zhaoermii, Lacerta agilis, Lamprolepis smaragdina, Laudakia badakhshana, L. himalayana, L. papenfussi, L. sacra, L. stoliczkana, L. tuberculata, L. wui, Leiolepis guttata, L. reevesii, Lepidodactylus lugubris, L. yami, Lygosoma bowringii, L. quadrupes, Mediodactylus russowii, Oriocalotes Paulus, Phrynocephalus axillaris, P. forsythia, P. guinanensis, P. guttatus, P. helioscopus, P. mystaceus, P. przewalskii, P. putjatai, P. roborowskii, P. theobaldi, P. versicolor, P. vlangalii, Physignathus cocincinus, Plestiodon capito, P. chinensis, P. elegans, P. liui, P. marginatus, P. popei, P. quadrilineatus, P. tamdaoensis, P. tunganus, Pseudocalotes brevipes, P. kakhienensis, P. kingdonwardi, P. microlepis, Ptyctolaemus gularis, Scincella barbouri, S. doriae, S. formosensis, S. huanrenensis, S. modesta, S. monticola, S. potanini, S. przewalskii, S. reevesii, S. schmidti, S. tsinlingensis, Shinisaurus crocodilurus, Sphenomorphus courcyanum, S. incognitus, S. indicus, S. maculatus, S. taiwanensis, Takydromus amurensis, T. formosanus, T. hsuehshanensis, T. intermedius, T. kuehnei, T. luyeanus, T. sauteri, T. septentrionalis, T. stejnegeri, T. sexlineatus, T. sylvaticus, T. viridipunctatus, T. wolteri, Teratoscincus przewalskii, T. roborowskii, T. scincus, T. toksunicus, Trapelus agilis, T. sanguinolentus, Tropidophorus berdmorei, T. guangxiensis, T. hainanus, T. sinicus, Varanus bengalensis, V. salvator, Zootoca vivipara.

Serpentes

Acalyptophis peronei, Achalinus ater, A. formosanus, A. hainanus, A. jinggangensis, A. meiguensis, A. niger, A. rufescens, A. spinalis, Acrochordus granulatus, Ahaetulla prasina, Aipysurus eydouxii, Amphiesma atemporale, A. bitaeniatum, A. boulengeri, A. craspedogaster, A. johannis, A. khasiense, A. metusia, A. miyajimae, A. modestum, A. octolineatum, A. optatum, A. parallelum, A. platyceps, A. popei, A. sauteri, A. stolatu, A. venningi, A. vibakari, Amphiesmoides ornaticeps, Archelaphe bella, Atretium yunnanensis, Azemiops feae, Blythia reticulata, Boiga cyanea, B. guangxiensis, B. kraepelini,

B. multomaculata, B. nigriceps, Bungarus bungaroides, B. fasciatus, B. multicinctus, Calamaria buchi, C. pavimentata, C. septentrionalis, C. yunnanensis, Calliophis maculiceps, Chitulia inornata, C. ornate, C. torquata, Chrysopelea ornate, Coelognathus radiates, Cyclophiops doriae, C. major, C. multicinctus, C. ruffus, Daboia siamensis, Deinagkistrodon acutus, Dendrelaphis biloreatus, D.hollinrakei, D. ngansonensis, D. pictus, D. subocularis, Dinodon flavozonatum, D. rosozonatum, D. rufozonatum, D. septentrionalis, Disteira stokesii, Elaphe anomala, E. bimaculata, E. carinata, E. davidi, E. dione, E. schrenckii, E. zoigeensis, Emydocephalus ijimae, Enhydris bennettii, E. bocourti, E. chinensis, E.enhydris, E. plumbea, Eryx miliaris, E. tataricus, Euprepiophis mandarinus, E. perlacea, Gloydius blomhoffii, G. brevicaudus, G. halys, G. intermedius, G. lijianlii, G. monticola, G. saxatilis, G. shedaoensis, G. strauchi, G. ussuriensis, Hemorrhois ravergieri, Hierophis spinalis, Hydrophis fasciatus, H. gracilis, H. parviceps, Kerilia jerdonii, Lapemis curtus, L. hardwickii, L. colubrine, L. laticaudata, Leioselasma cyanocincta, L. melanocephala, L. spiralis, Liopeltis frenatus, Lycodon capucinus, L. fasciatus, L. futsingensis, L. gongshan, L. laoensis, L. liuchengchaoi, L. ruhstrati, L. subcinctus, L. synaptor, Macropisthodon rudis, Naja atra, N. kaouthia, Natrix natrix, N. tessellate, Oligodon albocinctus, O. catenatus, O. chinensis, O. cinereus, O. cyclurus, O. eberhardti, O. formosanus, O. lacroixi, O. lungshenensis, O. melanozonatus, O. multizonatus, O. ningshaanensis, O. ornatus, O. taeniatus, Oocatochus rufodorsatus, Ophiophagus Hannah, Opisthotropis andersonii, O. balteata, O. cheni, O. guangxiensis, O. jacobi, O. kuatunensis, O. lateralis, O. latouchii, O. maculosa, O. maxwelli, Oreocryptophis porphyraceus, Orthriophis hodgsoni, O. moellendorffi, O. taeniurus, Ovophis monticola, O. tonkinensis, O. zayuensis, Paratapinophis praemaxillaris, Pareas boulengeri, P. carinatus, P. chinensis, P. formosensis, P. hamptoni, P. margaritophorus, P. monticola, P. nigriceps, P. stanleyi, Pelamis platura, Plagiopholis blakewayi, P. nuchalis, P. styani, P. unipostocularis, Polyodontognathus caerulescens, Praescutata viperina, Protobothrops cornutus, P. jerdonii, P. kaulbacki, P. mangshanensis, P. maolanensis, P. mucrosquamatus, P. xiangchengensis, Psammodynastes pulverulentus, Psammophis lineolatus, Pseudolaticauda semifasciata, Pseudoxenodon bambusicola, P. karlschmidti, P. macrops, P. stejnegeri, Ptyas carinata, P. dhumnades, P. korros, P. mucosa, P. nigromarginata, Python bivittatus, Ramphotyphlops albiceps, R. braminus, R. lineatus, Rhabdophis adleri, R. callichroma, R. chrysargos, R. himalayanus, R. leonardi, R. nigrocinctus, R. nuchalis, R. subminiatus, R. swinhonis, R. tigrinus, Rhabdops bicolor, Rhadinophis frenatus, R. prasinus, Rhynchophis boulengeri, Sibynophis chinensis, S. collaris, Sinomicrurus hatori, S. kelloggi, S. macclellandi, Sinonatrix aequifasciata, S. annularis, S. percarinata, S. yunnanensis, Thermophis baileyi, T. zhaoermii, Trachischium monticola, T. tenuiceps, Trimeresurus albolabris, T. gracilis, T. gramineus, T. gumprechti, T. medoensis, T. sichuanensis, T. stejnegeri, T. tibetanus, T. yunnanensis, Typhlops diardii, T. koshunensis, T. lazelli, Vipera berus, V. renardi, V. sachalinensis, V. ursinii, Xenochrophis flavipunctatus, X. piscator, X. hainanensis, X. unicolor.

Acknowledgements

Support was provided by National Science Foundation of China (30700062, 31272281) and Knowledge Innovation Program of the Chinese Academy of Sciences (KSCX2-EW-Q-6).

Author details

Yong Huang[1], Xianguang Guo[2] and Yuezhao Wang[2]

*Address all correspondence to: guoxg@cib.ac.cn

1 Guangxi Botanical Garden of Medicinal Plants, Nanning Guangxi, PR China

2 Department of Herpetology, Chengdu Institute of Biology, Chinese Academy of Sciences, Chengdu Sichuan, PR China

References

[1] Wiens JJ, Donoghue MJ. Historical biogeography, ecology, and species richness. Trends in Ecology and Evolution 2004; 19(12): 639-644. http://www.sciencedirect.com/science/article/pii/S0169534704002745

[2] Crisci JV, Sala OE, Katinas L, Posadas, P. Bridging historical and ecological approaches in biogeography. Australian Systematic Botany 2006; 19(1): 1–10. http://www.publish.csiro.au/view/journals/dsp_journal_fulltext.cfm?nid=150&f=SB05006

[3] Kent M. Numerical classification and ordination methods in biogeography. Progress in Physical Geography 2006; (3): 399-408. http://ppg.sagepub.com/content/30/3/399.full.pdf

[4] Posadas P, Crisci JV, Katinas L. Historical biogeography: A review of its basic concepts and critical issues. Journal of Arid Environments 2006; 66(3): 389-403. http://www.sciencedirect.com/science/article/pii/S0140196306000346

[5] Meng k, Li S, Murphy RW. Biogeographical patterns of Chinese spiders (Arachnida: Araneae) based on a parsimony analysis of endemicity. Journal of Biogeography 2008; 35(7): 1241-1249. http://onlinelibrary.wiley.com/doi/10.1111/j.1365-2699.2007.01843.x/pdf.

[6] Hsü KJ, Chen H. Geological Atlas of China: An Application of the Tectonic Facies Concept to the Geology of China. New York: Elsevier Science; 1999.

[7] Wan T. The Outline of Geotectonics of China. Beijing: Geological Publishing House; 2003.

[8] Chinese Academy of Sciences, Nature Division Committee. China Animal Geography Division and China Insect Geography Division (First Draft). Beijing: Science Press; 1959.

[9] Zhang R. Zoogeography of China. Beijing: Science Press; 1999.

[10] MacKinnon J, Meng S, Cheung C, Carey G, Zhu X, Melville D. A Biodiversity Review of China. Hong Kong: World Wide Fund for Nature International; 1996.

[11] Xie Y, Mackinnon J, Li D. Study on biogeographical divisions of China. Biodiversity and Conservation 2004; 13(7): 1391-1417. http://www.springerlink.com/content/p1355416n7h87706/

[12] Chen L, Song Y, Xu S. The boundary of Palaearctic and Oriental realms in western China. Progress in Natural Science 2008; 18(7): 833-841. http://www.sciencedirect.com/science/article/pii/S1002007108001457

[13] Morrone JJ, Escalante T. Parsimony analysis of endemicity (PAE) of Mexican terrestrial mammals at different area units: when size matters. Journal of Biogeography 2002; 29(8):1095-1104. http://onlinelibrary.wiley.com/doi/10.1046/j.1365-2699.2002.00753.x/full

[14] Humphries CJ, Parenti LR. Cladistic Biogeography, 2nd edn. Oxford Biogeography Series 12, Oxford: Oxford University Press; 1999.

[15] Rosen BR. From Fossils to Earth History: Applied Historical Biogeography. In: Myers AA, Giller PS. (eds). Analytical Biogeography: An Integrated Approach to the Study of Animal and Plant Distributions. London: Chapman and Hall; 1988. p437-481.

[16] Morrone JJ. On the identification of areas of endemism. Systematic Biology 1994; 43(3): 438-441. http://www.jstor.org/stable/2413679

[17] Cracraft J. Patterns of diversification within continental biotas: hierarchical congruence among the areas of endemism of Australian vertebrates. Australian Systematic Botany 1991; 4(1): 211-227. http://www.publish.csiro.au/paper/SB9910211.htm

[18] Trejo-Torres JC, Ackerman JD. Biogeography of the Antilles based on a parsimony analysis of orchid distributions. Journal of Biogeography 2001; 28(6): 775-794. http://onlinelibrary.wiley.com/doi/10.1046/j.1365-2699.2001.00576.x/full

[19] Ron SR. Biogeographic area relationships of lowland Neotropical rainforest based on raw distributions of vertebrate groups. Biological Journal of the Linnean Society 2000; 71(3): 379-402. http://onlinelibrary.wiley.com/doi/10.1111/j.1095-8312.2000.tb01265.x/pdf

[20] Brooks DR, van Veller MGP. Critique of parsimony analysis of endemicity as a method of historical biogeography. Journal of Biogeography 2003; 30(6): 819-825. http://onlinelibrary.wiley.com/doi/10.1046/j.1365-2699.2003.00848.x/full

[21] Nihei SS. Misconceptions about parsimony analysis of endemicity. Journal of Biogeography 2006; 33(12): 2099-2106. http://onlinelibrary.wiley.com/doi/10.1111/j.1365-2699.2006.01619.x/full

[22] Contreras-Medina R, Vega IL, Morrone JJ. Application of parsimony analysis of endemicity to Mexican gymnosperm distributions: grid-cells, biogeographical provin-

ces and track analysis. Biological Journal of the Linnean Society 2007; 92(3): 405-417. http://onlinelibrary.wiley.com/doi/10.1111/j.1095-8312.2007.00844.x/full

[23] Melo Santos AM, Cavalcanti DR, da Silva JC, Tabarelli M. Biogeographical relationships among tropical forest in north-eastern Brazil. Journal of Biogeography 2007; 34(3): 437-446. http://onlinelibrary.wiley.com/doi/10.1111/j.1365-2699.2006.01604.x/full

[24] Posadas P. Distributional patterns of vascular plants in Tierra del Fuego: a study applying parsimony analysis of endemicity (PAE). Biogeographica 1996; 72: 161-177.

[25] Zhao E, Zhao K, Zhou K. Fauna Sinica, Reptilia, Vol. 2. (Squamates, Lacertilia). Beijing: Science press; 1999.

[26] Zhao E, Adler K. Herpetology of China. Oxford: Ohio: Society for the Study of Amphibians and Reptiles in cooperation with Chinese Society for the Study of Amphibians and Reptiles; 1993.

[27] Zhao E, Huang M, Zong Y. Fauna Sinica Reptilia, Vol.3 Squamates Serpentes. Beijing: Science press; 1999.

[28] Zhao E. Snake of China. Hefei: Anhui Science and Technology Publishing House; 2006.

[29] Swofford DL. PAUP*. Phylogenetic Analysis Using Parsimony (*and Other Methods). Version 4. Sinauer Associates, Sunderland, MA; 1998. http://www.sinauer.com/detail.php?id=8060

[30] Glasby CJ, Álvarez B. Distribution patterns and biogeographic analysis of Austral Polychaeta (Annelida). Journal of Biogeography 1999; 26(3): 507–533. Http://onlinelibrary.wiley.com/doi/10.1046/j.1365-2699.1999.00297.x/pdf

[31] Ji X, Brana F. Among clutch variation reproductive output and egg size in the wall lizard (*Podarcis muralis*) from a lowland population of Northern Spain. Journal of Herpetology 2000; 34(1): 54-60. http://www.jstor.org/stable/1565238

[32] Ji X, Du W. Effects of thermal and hydric environments on incubating eggs and hatchling traits in the cobra, *Naja naja atra*. Journal of Herpetology 2001; 35(2): 186-194. www.jstor.org/stable/1566107

[33] Fu C, Wang J, Pu Z, Zhang S, Chen H, Zhao B, Chen J, Wu J. Elevational gradients of diversity for lizards and snakes in the Hengduan Mountains, China. Biodiversity and Conservation 2007; 16(3): 707-726. http://www.springerlink.com/article/10.1007%2Fs10531-005-4382-4

[34] Huang Y, Dai Q, Chen Y, Wan H, Li J, Wang Y. Lizard species richness patterns in China and its environmental associations. Biodiversity and Conservation 2011; 20(7): 1399-1414. http://www.springerlink.com/ article/10.1007/s10531-011-0033-0#

[35] Cai B, Huang Y, Chen Y, Hu J, Guo X, Wang Y. Geographic patterns and ecological factors correlates of snake species richness in China. Zoological Research 2012; 33(4): 343-353. http://www.zoores.ac.cn/EN/abstract/abstract3193.shtml#

[36] Gaston KJ. Global patterns in biodiversity. Nature 2000; 405(6783): 220-227. http://www.nature.com/nature/journal/v405/n6783/pdf/405220a0.pdf

[37] von Humboldt A. Ansichten der Natur mit wissenschaftlichen Erlauterungen. Germany: J. G. Cotta, Tübingen; 1808.

[38] Hawkins BA, Field R, Cornell HV, Currie DJ, Guegan JF, Kaufman DM, Kerr JT, Mittelbach GG, Oberdorff T, O'Brien EM, Porter EE, Turner JRG. Energy, water, and broad-scale geographic patterns of species richness. Ecology 2003; 84(12): 3105-3117. http://www.esajournals.org/doi/full/10.1890/03-8006

[39] Terribile LC, Olalla-Tárraga MÁ, Morales-Castilla I, Rueda M, Vidanes RM, Rodríguez MÁ , Diniz-Filho JAF. Global richness patterns of venomous snakes reveal contrasting influences of ecology and history in two different clades. Oecologia 2009; 159(3): 617-626. http://www.springerlink.com/article/10.1007%2Fs00442-008-1244-2

[40] Currie DJ. Energy and large-scale patterns of animal- and plant-species richness. The American Naturalist 1991; 137(1): 27-49. http://www.jstor.org/stable/2462155

[41] Kerr JT, Packer L. Habitat heterogeneity as a determinant of mammal species richness in high-energy regions. Nature 1997; 385(6613): 252-254. http://www.nature.com/nature/journal/v385/n6613/abs/385252a0.html

[42] Kerr JT, Southwood TRE, Cihlar J. Remotely sensed habitat diversity predicts butterfly species richness and community similarity in Canada. Proceedings of the National Academy of Sciences of the United States of America 2001; 98(20): 11365-11370. http://www.pnas.org/content/98/20/11365.full.pdf+html

[43] Rahbek C, Graves GR. Multiscale assessment of patterns of avian species richness. Proceedings of the National Academy of Sciences of the United States of America 2001; 98(8):4534-4539. http://www.pnas.org/content/98/8/4534.full.pdf+html

[44] Turner JRG, Gatehouse CM, Corey CA. Does solar energy control organic diversity? Butterflies, moths and British climate. Oikos 1987; 48(2): 195-205. http://www.jstor.org/stable/3565855

[45] Hawkins BA, Porter EE. Water-energy balance and the geographic pattern of species richness of western Palearctic butterflies. Ecological Entomology 2003; 28(6): 678-686. http://onlinelibrary.wiley.com/doi/10.1111/j.1365-2311.2003.00551.x/full

[46] Mittelbach GG, Steiner CF, Scheiner SM, Gross KL, Reynolds HL, Waide RB, Willig MR, Dodson SI, Gough L. What is the observed relationship between species richness and productivity? Ecology 2001; 82(9): 2381-2396. http://www.esajournals.org/doi/full/10.1890/0012-9658%282001%29082%5B2381%3AWITORB%5D2.0.CO%3B2

[47] Wright DH. Species–energy theory: An extension of species–area theory. Oikos 1983; 41(3): 496-506. http://www.jstor.org/stable/3544109

[48] Costa GC, Nogueira C, Machado RB, Colli GR. Squamate richness in the Brazilian Cerrado and its environmental-climatic associations. Diversity and Distribution 2007; 13(6): 714-724. http://onlinelibrary.wiley.com/doi/10.1111/j.1472-4642.2007.00369.x/pdf

[49] Tognelli MF, Kelt DA. Analysis of determinants of mammalian species richness in South America using spatial autoregressive models. Ecography 2004; 27(4): 427-436. http://onlinelibrary.wiley.com/doi/10.1111/j.0906-7590.2004.03732.x/full

[50] Hortal J, Triantis KA, Meiri S, Thébault E, Sfenthourakis S. Island species richness increases with habitat diversity. The American Naturalist 2009; 174(6): E205-E217. http://www.jstor.org/stable/10.1086/645085

[51] McCain CM. Global analysis of reptile elevational diversity. Global Ecology and Biogeography 2010; 19 (4): 541–553. http://onlinelibrary.wiley.com/doi/10.1111/j.1466-8238.2010.00528.x/pdf

[52] Qian H, Wang XH, Wang SL, Li YL. Environmental determinants of amphibian and reptile species richness in China. Ecography 2007; 30(4): 471-482. http://onlinelibrary.wiley.com/doi/10.1111/j.0906-7590.2007.05025.x/full

[53] Pounds JA, Fogden MPL, Campbell JH. Biological response to climate change on a tropical mountain. Nature 1999; 398(6728) : 611-615. http://www.nature.com/nature/journal/v398/n6728/full/398611a0.html

[54] Stockwell D, Peters D. The GARP modelling system: problems and solutions to automated spatial prediction. International Journal of Geographical Information Science 1999; 13(2): 143-158. http://www.tandfonline.com/doi/abs/10.1080/136588199241391

[55] Pearson RG, Raxworthy C, Nakamura M, Peterson AT. Predicting species' distributions from small numbers of occurrence records: A test case using cryptic geckos in Madagascar. Journal of Biogeography 2007; 34(1): 102-117. http://onlinelibrary.wiley.com/doi/10.1111/j.1365-2699.2006.01594.x/full

[56] Peterson AT, Papefl M, Eaton M. Transferability and model evaluation in ecological niche modeling: A comparison of GARP and Maxent. Ecography 2007; 30(4): 550-560. http://onlinelibrary.wiley.com/doi/10.1111/j.0906-7590.2007.05102.x/full

[57] Peterson AT, Robins CR. Using ecological-niche modeling to predict barred owl invasions with implications for spotted owl conservation. Conservation Biology 2003; 17(4): 1161-1165. http://onlinelibrary.wiley.com/doi/10.1046/j.1523-1739.2003.02206.x/full

[58] Peterson AT, Papeß M, Kluza DA. Predicting the potential invasive distributions of four alien plant species in North America. Weed Science 2003; 51(6): 863-868. http://www.bioone.org/doi/full/10.1614/P2002-081

[59] Ferreira de Siqueira M, Durigan G, de Marco Ju´nior P, Peterson AT. Something from nothing: using landscape similarity and ecological niche modeling to find rare plant species. Journal for Nature Conservation 2009; 17(1): 25-32. http://www.sciencedirect.com/science/article/pii/S1617138108000484

[60] Menon S, Choudhury BI, Khan LM, Peterson AT. Ecological niche modeling and local knowledge predict new populations of Gymnocladus assamicus a critically endangered tree species. Endangered Species Research 2010; 11: 175-181. http://www.int-res.com/articles/esr2010/11/n011p175.pdf

[61] Raxworthy C, Martínez-Meyer E, Horning N, Nussbaum R, Schneider G, Ortega-Huerta M, Peterson AT. Predicting distributions of known and unknown reptile species in Madagascar. Nature 2003; 426(6968): 837-841. http://www.nature.com/nature/journal/v426/n6968/full/nature02205.html

[62] Anderson RP, Lew D, Peterson AT. Evaluating predictive models of species' distributions: criteria for selecting optimal models. Ecological Modelling 2003; 162(3): 211-232. http://www.sciencedirect.com/science/article/pii/S0304380002003496

[63] Ahn CH, Tateishi R. Development of a global 30-minute grid potential evapotranspiration data set. Journal of the Japan Society Photogrammetry and Remote Sensing 1994; 33(2): 12-21.

[64] New M, Lister D, Hulme M, Makin I. A high-resolution data set of surface climate over global land areas. Climate Resarch 2002; 21: 1-25. http://www.int-res.com/articles/cr2002/21/c021p001.pdf

[65] Tabachnick BG, Fidell LS. Using Multivariate Statistics, 4th edn. Boston: Allyn and Bacon, MA; 2000.

[66] Diniz-Filho JAF, Bini LM. Modelling geographical patterns in species richness using eigenvectorbased spatial filters. Global Ecology and Biogeography 2005; 14(2): 177-185. http://onlinelibrary.wiley.com/doi/10.1111/j.1466-822X.2005.00147.x/full

[67] Legendre P. Spatial autocorrelation—trouble or new paradigm. Ecology 1993; 74(6): 1659-1673. http://www.jstor.org/stable/1939924

[68] Legendre P, Dale MRT, Fortin MJ, Gurevitch J, Hohn M, Myers D. The consequences of spatial structure for the design and analysis of ecological field surveys. Ecography 2002; 25(5): 601-615. http://onlinelibrary.wiley.com/doi/10.1034/j.1600-0587.2002.250508.x/full

[69] Rangel TF, Diniz-Filho JAF, Bini LM. SAM: A comprehensive application for spatial analysis in macroecology. Ecography 2010; 33(1): 46-50. http://onlinelibrary.wiley.com/doi/10.1111/j.1600-0587.2009.06299.x/full

[70] Diniz-Filho JAF, Bini LM, Hawkins BA. Spatial autocorrelation and red herrings in geographical ecology. Global Ecology and Biogeography 2003; 12(1): 53-64. http://onlinelibrary.wiley.com/doi/10.1046/j.1466-822X.2003.00322.x/full

[71] Burnham KP, Anderson DR. Model Selection and Inference: A Practical Information Theoretic Approach. New York: Springer-Verlag; 1998.

[72] Burnham KP, Anderson DR. Multimodel inference—understanding AIC and BIC in model selection. Sociological Methods and Research 2004; 33(2): 261-304. http://smr.sagepub.com/content/33/2/261.full.pdf+html

[73] Powney GD, Grenyer R, Orme CDL, Owens IPF, Meiri S. Hot, dry and different Australian lizard richness is unlike that of mammals, amphibians, and birds. Global Ecology and Biogeography 2010; 19(3): 386-396. http://onlinelibrary.wiley.com/doi/10.1111/j.1466-8238.2009.00521.x/full

[74] Andrews P, O'Brien EM. Climate, vegetation, and predictable gradients in mammal species richness in southern Africa. Journal of Zoology 2000; 251(20): 205–231. http://onlinelibrary.wiley.com/doi/10.1111/j.1469-7998.2000.tb00605.x/pdf

[75] Bohning-Gaese K. Determinants of avian species richness at different spatial scales. Journal of Biogeography 1997; 24(1): 49-60. http://onlinelibrary.wiley.com/doi/10.1111/j.1365-2699.1997.tb00049.x/pdf

[76] Willis KJ, Whittaker RJ. Species diversity–scale matters. Science 2002; 295(5558): 1245-1248. http://www.sciencemag.org/content/295/5558/1245.full

[77] Guo Z, Ruddiman WF, Hao Q, Wu H, Qiao Y, Zhu R, Peng S, Wei J, Yuan B, Liu T. Onset of Asian desertification by 22 Myr ago inferred from loess deposits in China. Nature 2002; 416(6877): 159-163. http://www.nature.com/nature/journal/v416/n6877/full/416159a.html

[78] Ramsetin G, Fluteau F, Besse J, Joussaumes S. Effect of orogeny, plate motion and land-sea distribution on Eurasian climate change over the past 30 million years. Nature 1997; 386: 788-795. http://www.nature.com/nature/journal/v386/n6627/abs/386788a0.html

[79] Shi Y, Zhao J, Wang J. New Understanding of Quaternary Glaciations in China. Shanghai: Shanghai Popular Science Press; 2011.

[80] Zhao J, Shi Y, Wang J. Comparison between Quaternary glaciations in China and the marine oxygen isotope stage (MIS): An improved schema. Acta Geographica Sinica 2011; 66(7): 867-884.

[81] Zhou S, Li J, Zhao J, Wang J, Zheng J. Quaternary Glaciations: Extent and Chronology in China. In: Ehlers J, Gibbard PL, Hughes PD. (eds) Quaternary Glaciations-Extent and Chronology, Volume 15: A closer look (Developments in Quaternary Science). Amsterdam: Elsevier Press; 2011. p981-1002. Available from http://www.sciencedirect.com/science/article/pii/B9780444534477000702

[82] Yang S, Dong H, Lei F. Phylogeogrpahy of regional fauna on the Tibetan Plateau: A review. Progress in Natural Science 2009; 19(7): 789–799. http://www.sciencedirect.com/science/article/pii/S1002007109000513

[83] Barabanov AV, Ananjeva NB. Catalogue of the available scientific species-group names for lizards of the genus *Phrynocephalus* Kaup, 1825 (Reptilia, Sauria, Agamidae). Zootaxa 2007; 1399: 1-56. http://www.mapress.com/zootaxa/2007f/z01400p068f.pdf

[84] Uetz P. The Reptile Database, http://www.reptile-database.org (accessed Aug 3, 2012).

[85] Whiteman RS. Evolutionary history of the lizard genus *Phrynocephalus* (Lacertilia, Agamidae). Master of Art thesis. California State University, Fullerton; 1978.

[86] Arnold EN. Phylogenetic relationships of toad-headed lizards (*Phrynocephalus*, Agamidae) based on morphology. Bulletin of the British Museum (Natural History) Zoology 1999; 65: 1-13.

[87] Ananjeva NB, Tuniyev BS. Historical biogeography of the *Phrynocephalus* species of the USSR. Asiatic Herpetology Research 1992; 4: 76-98. http://www.asiatic-herpetological.org/Archive/Volume%2004/04_12.pdf

[88] Macey JR, Ananjeva NB, Zhao E, Wang Y, Papenfuss TJ. An allozyme-based phylogenetic hypothesis for *Phrynocephalus* (Agamidae) and its implications for the historical biogeography of arid Asia. In: Zhao E, Chen B, Papenfuss TJ. (eds.) Proceedings of the First Asian Herpetological Meeting. Beijing: China Forestry Press; 1993.

[89] Wang Y, Macey JR. On the ecological-geographic differentiation of Chinese species of the genus *Phrynocephalus*. In: Zhao E, Chen B, Papenfuss TJ. (eds.) Proceedings of the First Asian Herpetological Meeting. Beijing: China Forestry Press; 1993.

[90] Zeng X, Wang Y, Liu Z, Fang Z, Wu G, Papenfuss TJ, Macey JR. Karyotypes of nine species in the genus *Phrynocephalus*, with discussion of karyotypic evolution of Chinese *Phrynocephalus*. Acta Zoologica Sinica 1997; 43(4): 409-418.

[91] Pang J, Wang Y, Zhong Y, Hoelzel AR, Papenfuss TJ, Zeng X, Ananjeva NB, Zhang YP. A phylogeny of Chinese species in the genus *Phrynocephalus* (Agamidae) inferred from mitochondrial DNA sequences. Molecular Phylogenetics and Evolution 2003; 27(3): 398-409. http://www.sciencedirect.com/science/article/pii/S1055790303000198

[92] Guo X, Wang Y. Partitioned Bayesian analyses, dispersalvicariance analysis, and the biogeography of Chinese toad-headed lizards (Agamidae: *Phrynocephalus*): A re-evaluation. Molecular Phylogenetics and Evolution 2007; 45(2): 643-662. http://www.sciencedirect.com/science/article/pii/S1055790307002175

[93] Melville J, Hale J, Mantziou G, Ananjeva NB, Milto K, Clemann N. Historical biogeography, phylogenetic relationships and intraspecific diversity of agamid lizards in the Central Asian deserts of Kazakhstan and Uzbekistan. Molecular Phylogenetics and Evolution 2009; 53(1): 99-112. http://www.sciencedirect.com/science/article/pii/S1055790309001754

[94] Solovyeva EN, Poyarkov NA, Dunayev EA, Duysebayeva TN, Bannikova AA. Molecular differentiation and taxonomy of the sunwatcher toad-headed agama species

complex *Phrynocephalus* superspecies *helioscopus* (Pallas 1771) (Reptilia: Agamidae). Russian Journal of Genetics 2011; 47(7): 842-856. http://www.springerlink.com/content/h245501257785793/

[95] Dunayev EA, Ivanova N, Poyarkov NA, Borisenko A, Dujsebayeva T, Hebert PD. Molecular perspective on the evolution and barcoding of toad-headed agamas (genus *Phrynocephalus*, Agamidae) in Middle Asia. Programme and Abstracts of 14th European Congress of Herpetology and SHE Ordinary General Meeting, 19-23 September 2007, Porto (Portogal); 2007.

[96] Jin Y, Brown RP, Liu N. Cladogenesis and phylogeography of the lizard *Phrynocephalus vlangalii* (Agamidae) on the Tibetan plateau. Molecular Ecology 2008; 17(8): 1971-1982. http://onlinelibrary.wiley.com/doi/10.1111/j.1365-294X.2008.03721.x/pdf.

[97] Wang Y, Zhan A, Fu J. Testing historical phylogeographic inferences with contemporary gene flow data: population genetic structure of the Qinghai toad-headed lizard. Journal of Zoology 2009; 278(2): 149-156. http://onlinelibrary.wiley.com/doi/10.1111/j.1469-7998.2009.00564.x/full

[98] Guo X, Liu L, Wang Y. Phylogeography of the *Phrynocephalus vlangalii* species complex in the upper reaches of the Yellow River inferred from mtDNA ND4-tRNA^{Leu} segments. Asian Herpetology Research 2012; 3(1): 52-68. http://www.ahr-journal.com/index.php?module=case&act=List&ClassID=19

[99] Jin Y, Liu N. Phylogeography of *Phrynocephalus erythrurus* from the Qiangtang Plateau of the Tibetan Plateau. Molecular Phylogenetics and Evolution 2009; 54(3): 933-940. http://www.sciencedirect.com/science/article/pii/S1055790309004503

[100] Zhang Q, Xia L, He J, Wu Y, Fu J, Yang Q. Comparison of phylogeographic structure and population history of two *Phrynocephalus* species in the Tarim Basin and adjacent areas. Molecular Phylogenetics and Evolution 2010; 57(3): 1091-1104. http://www.sciencedirect.com/science/article/pii/S1055790310004094

[101] Fu B, Lin A, Kano K, Maruyama T, Guo J. Quaternary folding of the eastern Tian Shan, northwest China. Tectonophysics 2003; 369(1-2): 79-101. http://www.sciencedirect.com/science/article/pii/S0040195103001379

[102] Szczerbak NN. Guide to the Reptiles of the Eastern Palearctic. USA: Krieger Publishing Company, Malabar, Florida; 2003.

[103] Szczerbak NN. Yashchurki Palearktiki (*Eremias* lizards of the Palearctic). Axadeimiya Nauk Ukrainskoi USSR Institut Zoologii. Naukova Dumka, Kiev; 1974.

[104] Arnold EN. The hemipenis of lacertid lizards (Reptilia: Lacertidae): structure, variation and systematic implications. Journal of Natural History 1986; 20: 1221-1257. http://www.tandfonline.com/doi/abs/10.1080/00222938600770811#preview

[105] Arnold EN. Towards the phylogeny and biogeography of the Lacertidae: relationships within an Old-World family of lizards derived from morphology. Bulletin of

the British Museum (Natural History) Zoology 1989; 55(2): 209-257. http://biostor.org/reference/107021

[106] Boulenger GA. Monograph of the Lacertidae, vol. II. London: Trustees of the British Museum of Natural History; 1921.

[107] Fitzinger L. Systema Reptilium. Vienna: Fasciculus Primus; 1843.

[108] Szczerbak NN. Taxonomy of the genus *Eremias* (Sauria, Reptilia) in connection with the focuses of the desert-steppe fauna development in Paleoarctic. Vestnik Zoologii 1971; 2: 48-55.

[109] Wan L, Sun S, Jin Y, Yan Y, Liu N. Molecular phylogeography of the Chinese lacertids of the genus *Eremias* (Lacertidae) based on 16S rRNA mitochondrial DNA sequences. Amphibia-Reptilia 2007; 28(1): 33-41.. http://www.ingentaconnect.com/content/brill/amre/2007/00000028/00000001/art00005

[110] Orlova VF, Poyarkov NA, Chirikova M, Dolotovskaya S.I. Preliminary molecular phylogeography of wide-spread steppe-runner lizard – *Eremias arguta* (Lacertidae) and considerations on its subspecific structure. Programme and Abstracts of 14th European Congress of Herpetology and SHE Ordinary General Meeting, 19-23 September 2007, Porto (Portogal); 2007.

[111] Rastegar-Pouyani E, Joger U, Wink M. A molecular phylogeny of the genus *Eremias* (Reptillia, Lacertidae) based on the mitochondrial and nuclear DNA sequences. Programme and Abstracts of 15th European Congress of Herpetology and SHE Ordinary General Meeting, 28 September-02 October 2009, Kuşadasi, Turkey; 2009.

[112] Guo X, Dai X, Chen D, PapenfussTJ, Ananjeva NB, Melnikov DA, Wang Y. Phylogeny and divergence times of some racerunner lizards (Lacertidae: *Eremias*) inferred from mitochondrial 16S rRNA gene segments. Molecular Phylogenetics and Evolution 2011; 61(2): 400-412. http://www.sciencedirect.com/science/article/pii/S1055790311003113

[113] Zhao Q, Liu HX, Luo L, Ji X. Comparative population genetics and phylogeography of two lacertid lizards (*Eremias argus* and *E. brenchleyi*) from China. Molecular Phylogenetics and Evolution 2011; 58(3): 478-491. http://www.sciencedirect.com/science/article/pii/S1055790310004987

[114] Rastegar-Pouyani E, Noureini SK, Joger U, Wink M. Molecular phylogeny and intraspecific differentiation of the *Eremias velox* complex of the Iranian Plateau and Central Asia (Sauria, Lacertidae). Journal of Zoological Systematics and Evolutionary Research 2012; 50(3): 220-229. http://onlinelibrary.wiley.com/doi/10.1111/j.1439-0469.2012.00662.x/pdf

[115] Rastegar-Pouyani E. A Phylogeny of the *Eremias velox* complex of the Iranian Plateau and Central Asia (Reptilia, Lacertidae): molecular evidence from ISSR-PCR finger-

prints. Iranian Journal of Animal Biosystematics 2009; 5(1): 33-46. http://www.sid.ir/en/VEWSSID/J_pdf/116420090105.pdf

[116] Warren DL, Glor RE, Turelli M. Environmental niche equivalency versus conservatism: quantitative approaches to niche evolution. Evolution 2008; 62(11): 2868-2883. http://onlinelibrary.wiley.com/doi/10.1111/j.1558-5646.2008.00482.x/full

Chapter 9

In vitro Propagation of Critically Endangered Endemic *Rhaponticoides mykalea* (Hub.-Mor.) by Axillary Shoot Proliferation

Yelda Emek and Bengi Erdag

Additional information is available at the end of the chapter

http://dx.doi.org/10.5772/55599

1. Introduction

Turkey is one of the richest countries in variability of flora. It has nearly 9000 plant species about 3000 of which are endemic [1]. *Asteraceae,* is represented by 50 species in Turkey with an endemism of nearly 54% [2]. *Rhaponticoides mykalea* (Hub.-Mor.) M.V. Agab. & Greuter which belongs to the *Asteraceae* family, falls within the CR (Critically Endangered) category in the Red Data Book of Turkey [1]. While *R. mykalea* (Hub.-Mor.) was classified under the section *Centaurea* as *Centaurea mykalea* (Hub.-Mor.) before now. Today it has been separated from the section Centaurea [3]. It spreads very scarce in Kuşadası (Aydın), Muğla and Isparta, and faces with the danger of extinction. *R. mykalea* that has very limited number of individuals is under strong anthropogenic pressure such as the gradually increase in ongoing urbanization due to rapid developments of tourism sector, the conversion of natural habitats into human dominated lands, the over-grazing and collecting capitula of *R. mykalea* by local people for food. The species has already been under the threat of extinction and the situation above will increase the risk of extinction of this species even more [4]. For this reason, local protection measures and global conservation strategies are necessary [5].

Nowadays, the conservation of wild plant genetic resources is very important for preventing a decrease in genetic variability. Conservation of the endemic or threatened plants is carried out using different strategies. *In vitro* culture is an efficient method for *ex situ* conservation of plant diversity [6,7], because many endangered species can be quickly propagated and preserved from a minimum of plant material with low impact on wild populations with this technology [8]. In recent years, there has been an increased interest in *in vitro* techniques that offer powerful tools for germplasm conservation and the mass multiplication of many threatened plant species [9]. Especially *in vitro* propagation of endangered plants can offer considerable benefits for the rapid cultivation of at risk species that have a limited reproductive capacity and exist in threatened habitats [5].

Micropropagation constitutes a powerful tool for *ex situ* conservation programs of threatened plants, especially for species with very reduced populations or low seed production [6,7]. This technique facilitates the rapid establishment of a large number of stock plants, from a minimum of original plant material, thus imposing minimum impact on the endangered wild populations. Axillary shoot proliferation typically results in average tenfold increase in shoot number per monthly culture passage. In a period of 6 months, it is feasible to obtain as many as 1 000 000 propagulesor plants, starting from a single explant [10].With this technology various endemic and endangered species have been successfully propagated; such as and *Centaurea paui* [8], *Anthemis xylopoda* O.Schwarz [11], *Centaurea spachii* [12], *Centaurea zeybek*ii [13], *Centaurea junoniana* [14], *Astragalus chrysochlorus* [15], *Centaurium rigualii* [16] and *Syzygium alternifolium* [17].

However, during our literature search, no report concerning *in vitro* regeneration of *R.mykalea* by axillary shoot proliferation was found.

The objective of the present study was to establish an efficient *in vitro* method for the rapid propagation via axillary shoot propagation of *R.mykalea,* a critically endangared endemic plant species. The shoots that were obtained from *in vitro* germinated mature embryos were used for axillary shoot proliferation. For that reason, the most appropriate cytokinin type and concentration were determined.

2. Material and methods

2.1. Plant material and explant source

Capitula of *Rhaponticoides mykalea* were collected from a wild population in Aydın-Turkey (Samsun mountain, localities: N 37 º 47.01 " ; E 027º 19.16 ") during summer period (July and August -2008) before seed dormancy period (Figure 1).

R. mykalea has been propagated from seed in the past [18]. However, researchers have explained that the seed is not suitable explant for *in vitro* propagation of *R. mykalea* due to strong seed dormancy and low germination frequency even after dormancy period. Therefore, embryos isolated from achenes which have not yet crossed dormancy periods were used as initial explant.

The achenes isolated from capitula were sterilised, and mature zygotic embryos that were dissected out from achene were used as initial explant. Mature zygotic embryos were dissected out from achenes and cultured on Murashige and Skoog (MS) [19] basal medium for germination. The shoots that were obtained from *in vitro* germinated mature embryos were used for axillary shoot proliferation.

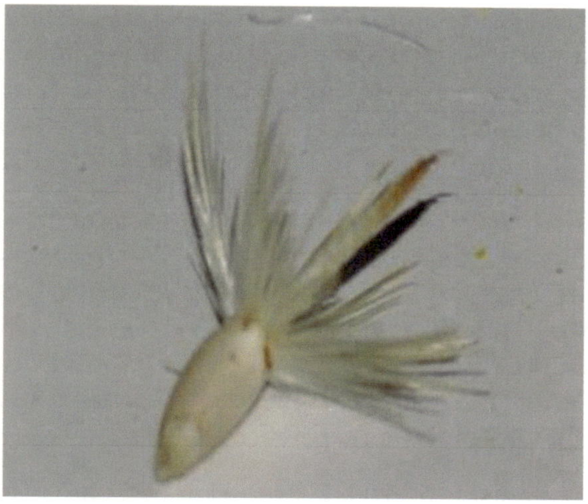

Figure 1. Achene containing mature embryo (before dormancy).

2.2. Achene viability

Achene viability was subjected to tetrazolium test.Tetrazolium test is based on reduction of colourless solution 2,3,5–tripheniltetrazolim chloride or bromide into insoluble 2,3,5– triphenilformazan red in colour. This solution acts as an indicator for detection of reduction processes that take place in living parts of the seed. Inside the seed, tetrazolium intakes hydrogen from dehydrogenase. By hidrogenization of tetrazolium a red, stable substance called formazan, which dyes living parts of the seed, is formed in the living cells.Tissue of many plant species must be removed to introduce the dye into the tissue. Tissue removal can be done by pilling the seed coat off, punching, and longitudinal or cross-cutting of unessential seed parts. Prepared seed is submerged into 0,5 – 1% tetrazolium solution. Seed must be completely covered with solution, and not exposed to direct light. After the time needed for dyeing expires (it depends on plant species) the estimation of dyeing is approached. All tissue (necessary for normal seedling development) of a viable seed should be dyed. Except completely dyed, viable seeds, and completely undyed, unviable seeds, a partly dyed seeds may also be found. Depending on the species, small undyed spots of some parts of these tissues may be accepted. Location, size of undyed areas, and sometimes intensity of dyeing, determine whether some seed is considered as viable or not [20].

To determine achene viability of *R. mykalea*, longitudinally-halved seeds were treated in tetrazolium solution (TTC, 1%) for 2 h at room temperature. After that time, red staining embryos were evaluated as alive.

2.3. Seed sterilisation, media preparation and culture conditions

In order to determine proper sterilisation procedure, achenes isolated from capitula were washed thoroughly under running tap water for 30 mins. Subsequently at various times, achenes were put in 70% (w/v) ethanol and 4.5% (w/v) sodium hypochlorite containing 2 drops of wetting agent (Tween-80); afterwards, the achenes were rinsed three times (5 mins each) with sterile distilled water in a laminar flow hood. After sterilisation, zygotic embryos were isolated from achenes and cultured on PDA (Potato Dextrose Agar) to determine early contamination. PDA cultures were maintained at 24 ± 2 ºC for 3 days. At the end of this period, observations were made in order to determine the appropriate sterilisation time.

All the experiments were maintained on semi-solid basal medium supplemented with or without various concentration of plant growth regulators. Basal medium contained Murashige and Skoog (MS) [19] mineral salts, 100 mgl^{-1} myo-inositol, 2 mgl^{-1} glycine, 0.5 mgl^{-1} nicotinic acid, 0.5 mgl^{-1} pyridoxine-HCl, 0.1 mgl^{-1} thiamine-HCL, 3% (w/v) sucrose, 8 gl^{-1} agar (Agar-agar), various concentration of plant growth regulators $^{1}N^{6}$- Benzyladenine (BA) and Kinetin (KIN), indole-3-butyric acid (IBA), indole-3-acetic acid (IAA) or naphthalene acetic acid (NAA) were used in experiments depending on experimental objectives.

The pH of media was adjusted to 5.8 with 1M NaOH or HCl prior to autoclaving at 105 kPa and 121° C for 15 min. Culture vessels were 190 ml glass jars containing 30 ml of medium.

2.4. Axillary shoot proliferation

Mature embryos that were isolated from achenes were cultured on MS basal medium to obtain sterile seedlings (unpublished data). After eight weeks, seedlings (~2-3 cm), were separated from primary roots and transferred to MS medium containing different concentrations of BA or KIN (0.1, 0.5, 1.0 and 2.0 mgl^{-1}) for axillary shoot propagation. A control treatment without cytokinins was also included. At the end of the 3 subculture, the number of shoots per explant and average shoot length was evaluated for each cytokinin type and concentration.

Axillary shoot proliferation experiments were conducted with 15 replications consisting of one explant per jar and were repeated three times. Cultures were incubated at 24 ± 2 °C under a light regime of 16 h photoperiod by cool-white fluorescent lamps. The cultures were subcultured to fresh medium of the same composition at an interval of 4 weeks.

2.5. Shoot rooting and acclimatization of plantlets

After three subcultures, elongated shoots (~4 cm) were excised stock cultures and transferred to MS and half strength MS medium (½ MS) with or without different concentrations (0.5, 1.0, 2.0 and 5.0 mgl^{-1}) of auxins (IBA, IAA or NAA) for rooting. The results of rooting experiments were expressed in percentage after 6 weeks of culture initiation.

Rooting experiments were conducted with 15 replications consisting of one explant per jar and were repeated three times. Cultures were incubated at 24 ± 2 °C under a light regime of 16 h photoperiod by cool-white fluorescent lamps. The cultures were subcultured to fresh medium of the same composition at an interval of 4 weeks.

After 8 weeks of rooting *in vitro*, the plantlets were removed from the culture jars then the agar was carefully washed off the rooted plantlets to minimize pathogen attack. The plantlets were planted into 10 cm diameter plastic pots containing garden soil and kept in the growth chamber under 24 ± 2°C and 16-h light photoperiod. After 4 weeks the plantlets kept at normal laboratory conditions.

2.6. Statistical analyses

Means of shoot number per explant, shoot lenght and frequency of rooting were analyzed by one-way analysis of variance (ANOVA, SPSS for Windows v.9., SPSS, USA). Differences were analyzed by analysis of variance and the means compared using Duncan's multiple range test at $p< 0.05$. Data giving in percentages were subjected to $x' = \text{arcsine} \sqrt{(x/100)}$ transformation [21].

3. Results and discussion

The viability percentage of achenes was 80% according to Tetrazolium test. According to our results, the most suitable sterilisation procedure of achenes is as follows: The achenes are washed thoroughly under running tap water for 30 mins. After this process, seeds must be exposed to 70% (w/v) ethanol for five mins and then to 4.5% (w/v) sodium hypochlorite containing 2 drops wetting agent (Tween-80) for eight mins. Finally, seeds are rinsed three times with sterilised distilled water (5 mins each). Sterile cultures are than obtained in high proportion (100%).

Four-week-old sterile seedlings obtained from mature zygotic embryos were used as explant for axillary shoot proliferation experiments. At the end of the experiments, the most appropriate cytokinin type and concentration were determined (Figure 2). Axillary shoot propagation of *R. mykalea* was obtained in all media without or with cytokinin. Cytokinins are generally recognized as critical for the production of shoot primordia under *in vitro* conditions. Both cytokinins induced healthy shoots in our study. However, it is shown that BA is more effective cytokinin than KIN. The maximum shoot number per explant were obtained in 0.5 mgl^{-1} BA added MS medium (5.8 shoot/explant) (Figure 2 and 3).

A decrease in the number of shoots were observed at both higher (1 and 2 mgl^{-1}) and lower concentrations of BA (0.1 mgl^{-1}). Similar results were also reported for axillary shoot proliferation of *Centaurea spachii* [12] and *Centaurea zeybekii* [13]. BA was also reported as an effective cytokinin for other endemic and threatened *Centaurea* species [14, 16]. However, BA was evaulated as an effective cytokinin for shoot multiplication in many species of *Asteraceae*; such as *Centaurea junoniana* [14], *Gerbera jamesonii* hybrida [22], *Centaurium rigualii* [16], *Syzygium alternifolium* [17] and *Anthemis xylopoda* [11].

MS medium supplemented with 0.1 mgl^{-1} Kinetin (KIN) was determined as the most suitable medium for the maximum shoot length (7.35 cm) (Figure 4). While BA is more effective cytokinin on shoot multiplication, KIN is more effective on shoot lenght. In spite of the increased number of shoots on media containing cytokinin, the shoot length is decreased. A negative correlation between the shoot number and their length has been observed. This kind of negative correlation was reported in *Centaurea paui* by using inflorescence stalk as explant [8] and *C. zeybekii* by axillary shoot proliferation [13].

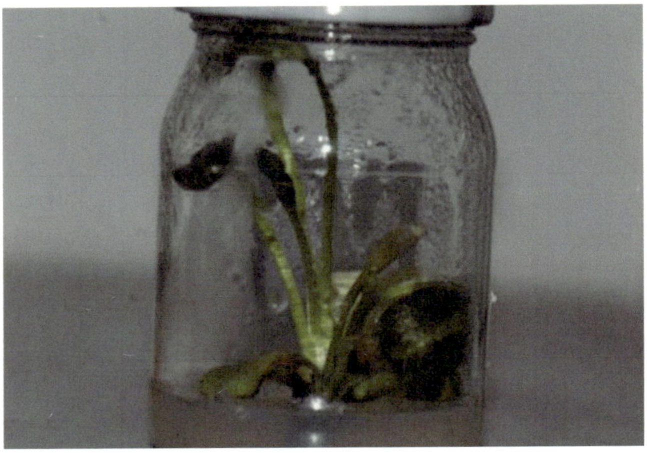

Figure 2. Axillary shoot proliferation on MS medium added 0.5 mgl^{-1}BA.

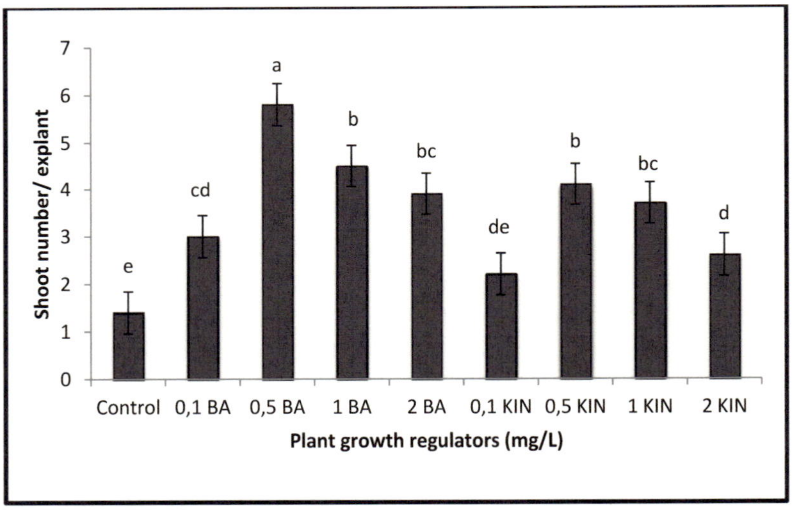

Means by different letters in each column and capital letters in each row are significantly different ($p < 0.05$), according to Duncan Multiple Range Test.

Figure 3. Cytokinin effects on axillary shoot multiplication of *R.mykalea*.

After three subculturing, solitary shoots excised from multiple shoot cultures were transferred to MS and ½ MS media containing IAA, IBA and NAA at various concentrations for rooting. Rhizogenezis was not occured MS and ½ MS medium without plant growth regulators. Auxin is necessary for *in vitro* rooting of *R.mykalea* axillary shoots. Generally, ½ MS medium added auxin is more effective than MS medium added auxin for rooting. The maximum rooting rate was obtained with half-strength MS medium supplemented with 0.5 mgl^{-1} IBA (55%) (Figure 5 and 6).There are many of reports about IBA is

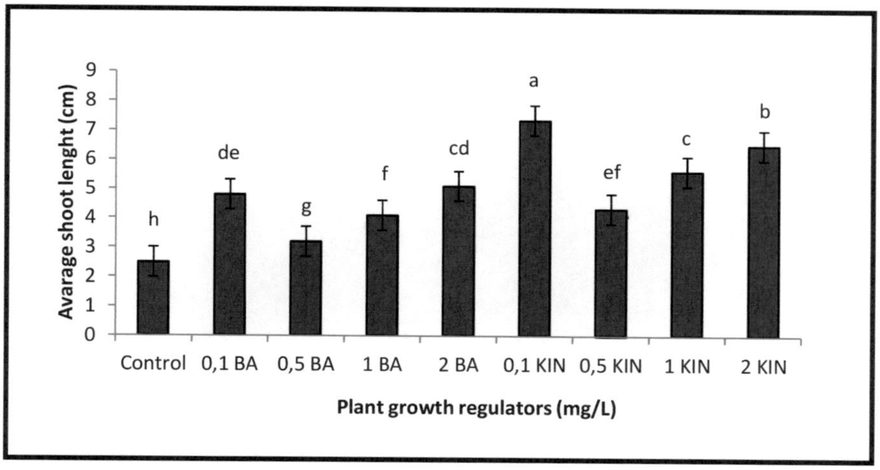

Means by different letters in each column and capital letters in each row are significantly different ($p < 0.05$), according to Duncan Multiple Range Test.

Figure 4. Average shoot lengths of axillary shoots dependent on cytokinin type and concentration.

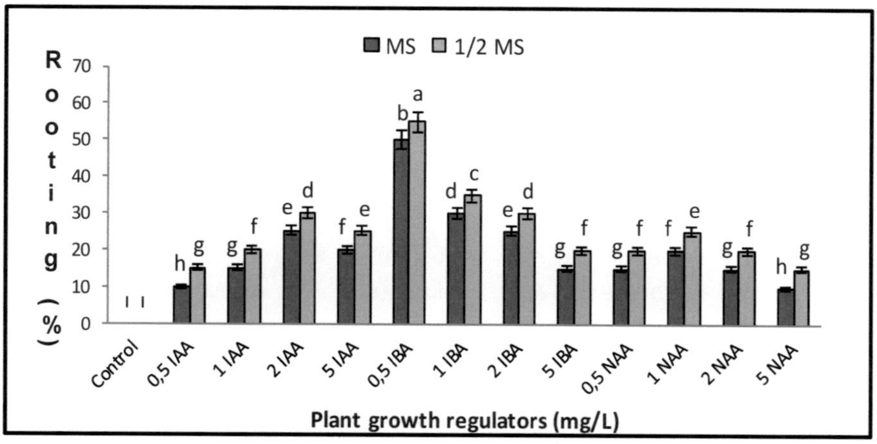

Data were subjected to $x' = \text{arcsine}\sqrt{(x/100)}$ transformation and used analysis. Means by different letters in each column and capital letters in each row are significantly different ($p < 0.05$), according to Duncan Multiple Range Test.

Figure 5. Rooting of *R.mykalea* axillary shoots.

more effective than other auxins on rooting for Asteraceae such as *Anthemis xylopoda* [11, 23] , *Centaurea spachii* [12], *Centaurea ragusina* [24], *Centaurea zeybekii* [25] and *Saussurea obvallata* [26].

There was a statistically significant difference between MS and ½ MS medium on rooting. ½ MS medium is more effective than MS medium on rooting in all experiments. Also, there was a statistically significant difference on rooting of *R. mykalea* between auxin type and concentration.

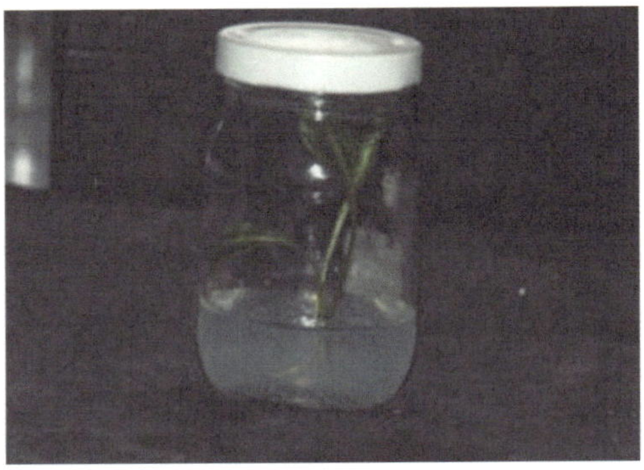

Figure 6. Rooting plantlets on ½ MS medium added 0.5 mgl^{-1} IBA.

In this study, we described a successful and rapid propagation techniques to regenerate critically endangered *R.mykalea* the first time by *in vitro* tissue culture techniques. Mature zygotic embryos isolated from achenes were used as starting material. The shoots that were obtained from *in vitro* germinated mature embryos were separated from primary roots and used for axillary shoot propagation. The highest axillary shoot number per explant was obtained on MS medium supplemented with 0.5 mgl^{-1} BA (5.8 shoot/explant). MS medium supplemented with 0.1 mgl^{-1} KIN was determined as the most suitable medium for the maximum shoot length (7.35 cm). Solitary shoots, removed from stock cultures, were transferred onto half-strength MS (½ MS) or MS media supplemented with various concentrations of auxins. The maximum rooting rate was obtained with half-strength MS medium supplemented with 0.5 mgl^{-1} IBA (55%). Rooted plantlets were transferred to external environment step by step.

The plantlets with well devoloped root were transferred to *ex vitro* conditions (Figure 7). Percentage of survival of shoots was approximately 60%. The appearance and growth of these plantlet were also normal.

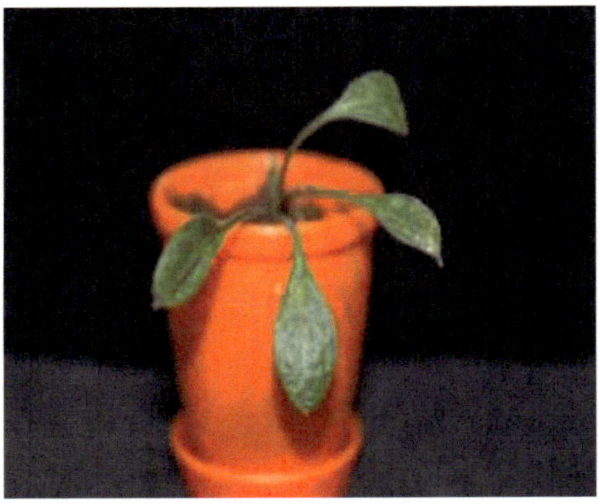

Figure 7. Acclimatized plantlets.

4. Conclusions

In conclusion, the present work presents a simple and successful procedure for the *in vitro* propagation of *Rhaponticoides mykalea* (Hub.-Mor.) M. V. Agab. & Greuter, a critically endangered endemic plant species.

To date there is no report on micropropagation of *R. mykalea*. This study is the first report on micropropagation of this species using seedlings from *in vitro* germinated embryos and aims to contrubute ongoing *ex situ* conservation programs. Additionally, this outlined protocol can be utilized as an aid in the local conservation programs to preserve this species, and it will lead for further studies on conservation and propagation of this rare and critically endangered endemic plant.

Acknowledgements

The authors are thankful to University of Adnan Menderes for financial support (Project no: FEF-07012)

Author details

Yelda Emek* and Bengi Erdag

*Address all correspondence to: yelda@adu.edu.tr

Department of Biology, Faculty of Arts & Science, Adnan Menderes University, Aydın, Turkey

References

[1] Ekim, T, Koyuncu, M, Vural, M, Duman, H, Aytaç, Z, & Adigüzel, N. Red Data Book of Turkish Plants (Pteridophyta and Spermatophyta). Ankara-Turkey: Turkish Association for the Conservation of Nature; (2000).

[2] Davis, P. H. Flora of Turkey and East Aegean Islands. Edinburg, U.K.: University Press; (1975).

[3] Hellwig, F. H. Centaureinae (Asteraceae) in the Mediterranean-history of ecogeographical radiation. Plant Systematics and Evolution (2004)., 246-137.

[4] Emek, Y, & Erdag, B. Observations on Kuşadası Population of *Rhaponticoides mykalea*, Resarch Journal of Biology Sciences (2010)., 3(2), 169-174.

[5] Fay, M. F. Conservation of Rare and Endangered Plants Using *In Vitro* Methods. *In Vitro* Cellular Development Biology (1992)., 28-1.

[6] Krogstrup, P, Baldursson, S, & Norgaard, J. V. *Ex Situ* Genetic Conservation by Use of Tissue Culture. Opera Botany (1992)., 113-49.

[7] Fay, M. F. In What Situation Is *In Vitro* Culture Appropriate to Plant Conservation? Biodiversity Conservation (1994)., 3-176.

[8] Cuenca, S, Marco, J. B, & Parra, R. Micropropagation From Infloresсense Stems of the Spanish Endemic Plant *Centaurea paui* Loscos ex Wilk. (Compositae). Plants Cell Reports (1999)., 18-674.

[9] Murch, S. J. KrishnaRaj S, Saxena PK. Phytomaceuticals: Mass Production, Standardization and Conservation. Scientific Review of Alternative Medicine (2000)., 4-39.

[10] Phillips, G. C, & Hubstenberger, J. F. Micropropagation by Proliferation of Axillary Buds. In: Gamborg OL., Phillips GC. (ed) Plant Cell Tissue and Organ Culture. Fundemental Methods. Germany: Springer-Verlag Berlin-Heidelberg; (1995)., 46-54.

[11] Erdag, B, & Emek, Y. *In Vitro* Micropropagation of *Anthemis xylopoda* O.Schwarz, a Critically Endangered Species from Turkey. Pakistan Journal of Biologicial Sciences (2005)., 8(5), 691-695.

[12] Cuenca, S, & Marco, J. B. *In Vitro* Propagation of *Centaurea spachii* From Inflorescence Stems. Plant Growth Regulation (2000)., 30-99.

[13] Kurt, S, & Erdag, B. *In Vitro* Germination and Axillary Shoot Propagation of *Centaurea zeybekii*. Biologia (2009)., 64(1), 97-101.

[14] Hammatt, N, & Evans, P. K. The *In Vitro* Propagation of an Endangered Species: *Centaurea junoniana* Svent. (Compositae). The Journal of Horticultural Science and Biotechnology (1985)., 60-93.

[15] Hasançebi, S. Turgut Kara N, Çakır Ö,Arı Ş. Micropropagation and Root Culture of Turkish Endemic *Astragalus chrysochlorus* (Leguminosae). Turkish Journal of Botany (2011)., 35-203.

[16] Iriondo, J. M, & Perez, C. Micropropagation and *In Vitro* Storage of *Centaurium rigualii* Esteve (*Gentianaceae*). Israel Journal of Plant Sciences (1996)., 44-115.

[17] Sha Valli Khan PSPrakash E, Rao KR. *In Vitro* Micropropagation of an Endemic Fruit Tree *Syzygium alternifolium* (Wight) walp. Plant Cell Reports (1997)., 16-325.

[18] Emek, Y, & Erdag, B. Researchs on *In Vitro* Seed Germination of The Critically Endangered Endemic Plant *Rhaponticoides mykalea* (Hub.-Mor.) Journal of Nevsehir University of Science and Technology Institute (2012)., 2-46.

[19] Murashige, T, & Skoog, F. A Revised Medium For Rapid Growth And Bioassays With Tobacco Tissue Cultures. Physiologia Plantarum (1962)., 15-473.

[20] Miloševic, M, Vujakovic, M, & Karagic, D. Vigour Tests as Indıcators of Seed Viability. Genetika (2010). , 42(1), 103-118.

[21] Fowler, J, & Cohen, L. Practical Statistics for Field Biology. Buckingham: Open University Press; (1990).

[22] Ruffoni, B, & Massabo, F. Tissue Culture in *Gerbera jamesonii* hybrida. Acta Horticulturae (1991). , 289-147.

[23] Erdag, B, & Emek, Y. Adventitious Shoot Regeneration and *In Vitro* Flowering of *Anthemis xylopoda* O. Schwarz, a Critically Endangered Turkish Endemic.Turkish Journal of Biology (2009). , 33(4), 319-326.

[24] Pevalek, K. B. *In vitro* germination of *Centaurea ragusina* L., a Croatian Endemic Species. Acta Biologica Cracoviensia Series Botanica (1998). , 40-21.

[25] Kurt, S. Researchs on *In Vitro* Seed Germination of The *Centaurea zeybekii* Wagenitz. PhD thesis. Adnan Menderes University Turkey; (2005).

[26] Dhar, U, & Joshi, M. Efficient Plant Regeneration Protocol Through Callus for *Saussurea obvallata* (DC.) Edgew. (Asteraceae): Effect of Explant Type, Age and Plant Growth Regulators. Plant Cell Reports (2005). , 24-195.

Section 2

Biosciences, Genetics and Health

Chapter 10

Some Observations on Plant Karyology and Investigation Methods

Feyza Candan

Additional information is available at the end of the chapter

http://dx.doi.org/10.5772/56081

1. Introduction

Karyology deals with the structure of cell nuclei, especially chromosomes. Cytology dealing with the study of cells in terms of structure also, function is known nowadays to mean only the study of chromosomes or nucleus and made synonymous with karyology wrongly. Cytotaxonomy means the application of cytological data to taxonomy. Cytotaxonomy studies the morphological and cytological characteristics of the organism along with their chromosome numbers and structures (karyotype)[1, 2]. It is a secondary discipline that reinforces the principles of plant and animal taxonomy by abiding to the phylogenetic kinships. In classical taxonomy, the plants are categorized through determining their natural kinships in accordance with their morphological characteristics. Especially, the taxonomists are advisable in connection with chromosomes. So, often chromosome number is assumed to be the all important, if not the only, chromosome character of interest to taxonomists, but size, shape, and behavior of chromosomes may throw more light on a taxonomic problem than their number alone.

F. Ehrendorfer, in an erudite essay on Cytologie, Taxonomie und Evolution bei Samenpflanzen [Cytology, taxonomy and evolution in seed plants], gives a detailed outline of these developments in cytogenetics since 1900 that have had a bearing on problems of taxonomy. Examples of taxonomic corrections based on chromosome studies include the removal of *Yucca* and *Agave* from the Amaryllidaceae to the Agavaceae and a number of rearrangements of species and genera in the Gramineae, Liliaceae, Compositae and other families; warnings are sounded against an uncritical use of chromosome pairing as a criterion of affinity, secondary pairing being dismissed altogether. A concrete example of the use of morphological and cytological considerations in deciding questions of relationships and evolution is given for the Dipsacaceae, where two distinct lines of phylogenetic development are traced: one of bushy species with clear polyploid series and the other of annuals with diploid series and a strong tendency towards structural chromosome differentiation [1].

In addition, findings about the status of the karyotypes, the chromosome numbers, the chromosome structures, sizes and enlightening data about the controversial situations of the members of the genus such as *Pandanus, Typha, Sparganium, Funcia, Polyantes* [2]. As it can be seen, karyological studies were helpful in classification considering the cytological characteristics. Today, palinogical and micromorphological characteristics detected with a scanning electron microscope (SEM) and the DNA sequence analysis are helpful in classification along with the karyological studies. However, in plant taxonomy, the emergence and geographical diffusion of cytotaxonomic new karyotypes continues to be an important problem. The study of karyotypes is important for cell biology and genetics, and the results may be used in evolutionary biology and medicine [2, 3]. Karyotypes can be used for many purposes; such as to study chromosomal aberrations, cellular function, taxonomic relationships, and to gather information about past evolutionary events.

In recent years numerous plants have been published in the field of cytotaxonomy which have been concerned with the cytological aspects of many species. For example, the morphological, anatomical and molecular biological studies and the cytological examinations carried out have caused modifications to be made on the classification of algaes [4].

There are two types of cell division for high plants; mitosis and meiosis. Mitosis is the type of division required for the plants to grow, develop and for the plant parts to be ingenerated. Mitosis is observed at the cambium, root tips and the somatic cells of other growth points. Mitosis allows for the genetic content of a cell to be transferred to the new generations without being distorted. Because, mitosis process of the haploid and diploid cells takes place after the chromosome duplication process.

Plant cells contain 3 genomes; in the nucleus, in the mitochondria and in plastids. During mitosis, the main cell doubles the chromosomes and its organelles such as mitochondria and chloroplast which proceed from the prokaryotic cells and membranes. Prokaryotes are multiplied with the method of binary fission. Mitochondria and chloroplast are organelles which are multiplied by division, as their ancestors. First the DNAs of these organelles are doubled. The small chromosomes produced, hold on to the inner membrane of the organelles. As the organelles grow in length, these two chromosomes move away from each other. At this stage, the membrane collapses inwards reciprocally at one point and it becomes narrower. As a result, two small organelles are produced.

In Eukaryotic cells, the cell cycle is consisted of the constant repetition of consecutive processes. The cell cycle includes the time period between the beginning of one cell division and the beginning of the following cell division. The cell division is divided into two stages; one long interphase and a short division stage. The division stage, or the M stage, includes the nucleus division (mitosis) and the cytokinesis (the division of the cytoplasm). The interphase takes place before the mitosis and cytokinesis. Interphase is the stage where the cell members are synthesized and the active growth occurs. Replication (DNA replication) and the duplication of chromosomes (doubling) occur in the interphase stage. The interphase is consisted of G1, S and G2 stages. G is the abbreviation for the word 'gap' and S is the abbreviation for the word 'synthesis'. G1 is the stage where the molecules and the intracellular elements are intensively synthesized. In the S stage, replication of DNA takes place. G2 stage is where the required preparations for cell division are completed [3].

As the prophase progresses, the length of the chromosomes are contracted. As the contraction increases, it can be observed that the chromosomes are consisted of two chromotids and that they are connected to each other at the centromere. Although in some sources, centromere and kinetochore are used as synonyms, they have differences. Centromere has a special DNA sequence which is present in every chromosome and which connects the chromosome to mitotic fibers. Kinetochore, on the other hand, is a special protein complex formed by each chromotid in the centromere. The mitotic fibers consisted of microtubes emerge at the end of the prophase stage. The nucleus and the nuclear membrane are dissolved at the end of the prophase [3, 5].

During metaphase, the chromosomes are lined through the equator of the mitotic fibers. The kinetochores are connected at the equator level to the ends of the cell which is thought to be the + end of the microtubes. The - ends of the microtubes are on the polar side. When a kinetochore is connected to the microtubes, the chromosome begins to move towards the polar side to which the microtube is extended. As all the chromosomes are aligned reciprocally at the equator level, the anaphase ends. The sister chromotids are separated from each other at the anaphase stage [3].

The nucleuses of the plant cells which do not divide are generally close to the cell walls. The nucleus takes place at the center of the cell before the division. Cytokinesis begins in the telophase stage. Phragmosome is produced firstly in the section where the cell is to be divided into two. Later, after the division of nucleus, the cell wall and fragmoplast allows for the cytoplasm to be portioned in two small cells. During the telophase, fragmoplast and the cell wall are visible.

As it is seen, if the division of the full-length of the chromosomes in mitosis did not occur equally, the new cells coming into existence as a result of the cell division would be very different from each other. If the number of chromosomes was not divided equally to both cells, large, immoderate and excessive cells would originate. In this case, the cells originated would not be able to perform fully.

Sometimes the chromosome number can be doubled without cell or nucleus divisions. The increase in the chromosome numbers of antipode nucleuses provides a good example for this situation [6, 7]. If the chromotids produced with endomitosis are separated from each other to form independent chromosomes, this is called endopolyploidy.

As it is in other organisms, the number and the morphology of chromosomes vary in plants. The number of chromosomes in a plant does not provide information with regard to its development level. For example, *Ophioglossum petiolatum*, which belongs to Pteridophyta, has 2n=2000 chromosomes, whereas *Allium cepa* (onion), which is a monocotyle has 2n=16 chromosomes. Also, one of the two plants which have equal chromosomes may be more developed than the other. For example, the number of chromosomes of *Acetabularia mediterranea*, which is a green algae is equal to the number of chromosomes *Zea mays* (corn) has 2n=20. As it can be seen, the important point is the data included in the chromosomes.

Some studies have shown that the changes in the number of chromosomes of the same species affect the flower sizes [8]. Also the idea that the chromosome number variety observed in the same species is related to the changes in the morphological characteristics of the plant was proposed [9, 10]. In reference [10], the differences seen in the number of chromosomes among the problematic genus such as the *Crocus* which is a monocotyle or among the problematic species such as the *Crocus chrysanthus* can be related to the differences in the morphological characteristics of the plant, such as the color of the anther, tepal or throat of the flower. This also constitutes a good example regarding the reflection of the karyotype differences on the phenotype (Figure 1). In references [10-15], the researcher even claims that these differences are indications of new taxa.

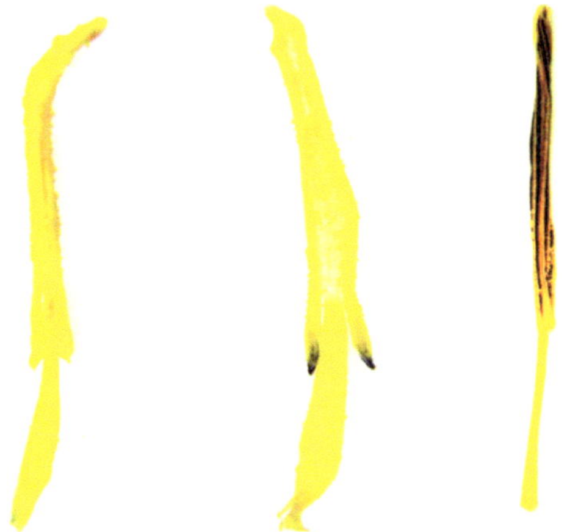

Figure 1. Three different anther types (wholly yellow, blackish lobed, blackish lined) of *Crocus chrysanthus* with different chromosome numbers [10]

Each chromosome includes a single DNA molecule in the form of a chain and in the length of thousands of nucleotides. DNA includes one nucleotide chain. Adenine (a), Guanine (g), Thymine (t) and Cytosine (c), which are the bases in the nucleotides which contain nitrogen, only connect to deoxyribose. The spine of the nucleotide chain is held together with the chemical bonds of sugar deoxyribose and phosphate groups. Chromosomes carry the genes coded for the synthesis of genetic proteins. Genes are units of genetic data.

Prokaryotes contain the smallest amount of DNA. Mycoplasma, which is a bacterium, is one of the organisms known that consist the minimal amount of DNA. Eukaryotes, as opposed to prokaryotes, contain greater amounts of DNA. However, approximately 90% of the DNA of eukaryotes do not code any proteins. 20-40% of the DNA in eukaryotes are consisted of unnecessary repetition series and their functions are unknown. Introns, which interrupt the protein coding series are an another example for DNAs which do not carry any coded data. Prokaryotes do not have any introns. Exons are regions which code a certain protein. The data coded in mRNA are transformed into proteins in the ribosome. A protein includes 300-400 amino acids in average. In order to code this amount of amino acids, 1,000 base pairs are required unknown [3]. According to this view, it can be said that the Zea *mays* with 4,500,000 base pairs contain 4,500-5,000 coded proteins.

Arabidopsisthaliana species have a small amount of DNA. Its small size, its short reproduction period, the scarcity of the number of the chromosomes it contains, its availability for cross breeding experiments and the high production of seeds are required for an experimental organism and because of these characteristics, this plant is preferred by plant geneticists. The studies conducted have revealed that the DNA of the plant *Arabidopsis thaliana* is similar to many plants used by humans [3].

Trillium sp., which is a flower that blossoms in spring, is the plant with the greatest genome known. The DNA of this plant contains 100 billion base pairs. The reason this plant needs that many DNA is unknown [3].

Meiosis is the cell division that allows for the male and female gametes to originate in order to ensure the continuity of developed plants. During meiosis, one main cell produces 4 daughter cells with halved chromosome numbers after two consecutive divisions. In meiosis, there are two stages; reduction, which reduces the chromosome number in half and mitosis, which preserved the halved number. If mitosis takes place first and is followed with reduction division, it is called postreduction. If reduction takes place first and is followed with mitosis, it is called prereduction [6, 7].

Cytokinesis is the division of cytoplasm into two young cells after the division of nucleus. In plants, following the production of the young nucleuses, with cytokinesis, 4 cells (gons) are produced [6-8]. The microspore main cell produces 4 microspores. The group formed by these 4 microspores is called a tetrad. Later, these microspores are separated from each other and each form a pollen as they develop. The pollens are produce in the anthers. *Anemone coronaria* var. *coccinea* anthers show this structure clearly (Figure2, 3) [16].

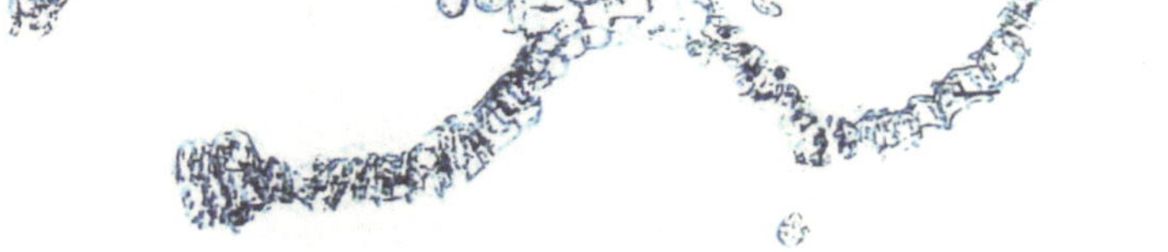

Figure 2. Anther cross section of *Anemone coronaria* var. *coccinea* (P:pollen, E:endotesium) [16]

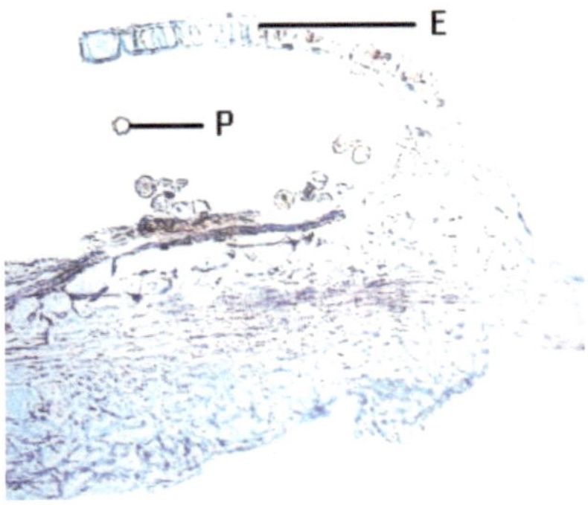

Figure 3. Anther transversal section of *Anemone coronaria* var. *coccinea* (P:pollen, E:endotesium) [16].

Proteins exist on the intine and exine layers of the pollen wall (Figure 4). These proteins are especially concentrated around the germination pores and the exine dents. The proteins in the intine have a gametophytic origin, whereas the proteins in the exine have a saprophytic origin. Following the contact of the pollens to the humid surface of the stigma, the proteins in the intine and exine are rapidly released and are diffused on the contact surface [17, 18]. The first significant stage of this interaction between the stigma and pollen is the pollen tube produced as a result of the intine stemming out of the germination pore (Figure 5).

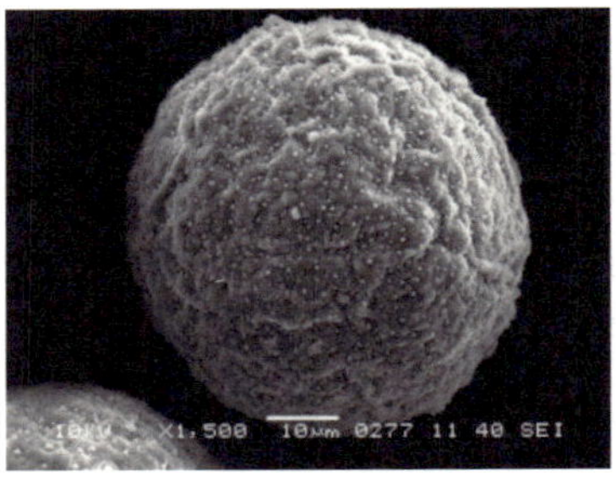

Figure 4. *Crocussieheanus* pollen exine layer (SEM photograph) [10]

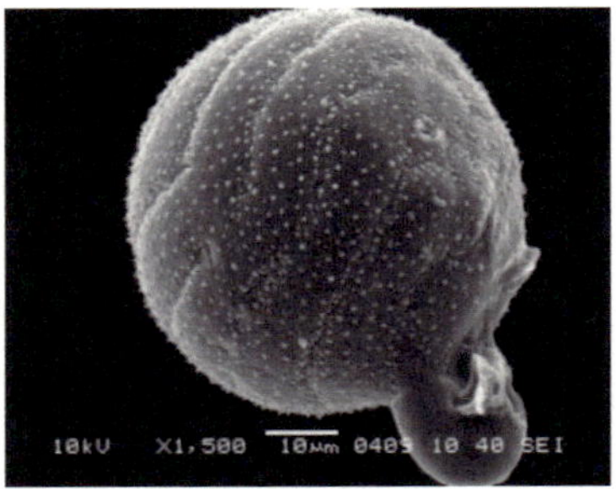

Figure 5. *Crocus ancyrensis* pollen with pollen tube (SEM photograph) [10]

Different fertility values may be observed as a result of the studies carried out on the pollen grains obtained from the stamens of male and female flowers of the same plant. The fertility values obtained from the male flowers are generally higher. If the fertility value of the female flower is also high, the plant will be able to self-fertilize, because the stamens are rich in pollens and that they almost cover the stigma. Thus, the main typical characteristics are often preserved. For example, Turkey constitutes a great variation center for the species, *Cucumis melo*. It is known that especially in the Eastern Anatolia region, gene exchanges are made and as a result of natural cross-breeding of the cultural and wide forms of this species [19].

Tissue culture studies generally use mitosis and meiosis divisions basically. The plant tissue culture, is the production of new tissue, plant or herbal products (such as metabolites) from a complete plant or plant parts such as cells (meristematic cells, suspension or callus cells), tissues (various plant parts=explants) or organs (apical meristem, root, etc.). Explant is the plant parts which can be collected from various sections of the plant and which can be used for culture. Creating new species and causing variability in the existing species can be regarded as the main purposes of tissue culture. For this reason, plant tissue cultures are important with regard to genetic optimization studies. Also various tissue culture methods are used for the preservation of endangered species and the reproduction of the species which are not easily reproduced [20].

The main method used in plant tissue culture processes and genetic optimizations is the regeneration capability of plants. Plant regeneration can be assessed in three parts with regard to the characteristics of the cultured cells: 1) regeneration from the somatic tissue consisting of organized meristematic cells, 2) regeneration from the somatic tissue consisting of non-meristematic cells, 3) regeneration from the gametic cells divided with meiosis. The first kind of regeneration consists of the reproduction of plants from the apical and lateral meristems. This is called clone reproduction with meristem culture method. The cells obtained look exactly like the donor plant. The second kind of regeneration is the formation of an embryo or a complete plant by the constant division of a somatic cell (direct somatic embryogenesis) or the formation of organs and then a complete plant by the division of some of the certain somatic cells on the cut surfaces of a plant explants, generally caused by plant growth regulators (especially auxins and cytokinins) and the organization of these divided cells (direct organogenesis). Also, both situations can occur following a certain callus, proto-callus or cell suspension generation phase (indirect regeneration). Some genetic or temporary variations can occur in the plants produced. Lastly, plants can regenerate directly or indirectly from the cells which include half the number of chromosomes it should normally have. With this method it is possible to reproduce haploid plants which are generally sterile and have half of the chromosomes the donor plant has [20, 21].

Explant should be chosen carefully with regard to tissue culture studies. Younger tissue is more easily dividable and has a higher capacity to form a callus. Cells should be actively dividable and they should not have the tendency to get in a dormancy period [22].

Comparative genomics, the study of the similarities and differences in structure and function of hereditary information across taxa, uses molecular tools to investigate many notions that long preceded identification of DNA as the hereditary molecule. Over the past two decades, multiple investigations of many additional taxa have delivered two broad messages:(1) In most plants, the evolution of the small but essential portion of the genome that actually encodes the organism's genes has proceeded relatively slowly; as a result, taxa that have been reproductively isolated for millions of years haveretained recognizable intragenic DNA sequences as well as similar arrangements of genes along the chromosomes. (2) A wide range of factors, such as ancient chromosomal or segmental duplications, mobility of DNA sequences, gene deletion, and localized rearrangements, has been superimposed on the relatively slow tempo of chromosomal evolution and causes many deviations from colinearity [23].

2. Chromosome morphology

Prokaryotes have one chromosome and haploid genomes. The chromosomes of prokaryotes have an annular structure. The DNA of eukaryotes is consisted of long and linear shaped molecules to form distinctive and different chromosomes, as opposed to the annular chromosomes mentioned.

Every chromosome of eukaryotic cells is found in pairs and they have a diploid (2n) structure. Thus, diploid organisms carry two copies of each gene. Every member of the chromosome pairs are the homologue chromosomes of each other (Figure 6). The chromosomes are found metacentrically, submetacentrically, acrocentrically and telocentrically in the cell. Haploid cells (n) have one complete set of chromosomes. Chromatin is a mass of uncoiled DNA and associated proteins called histones. A small segment of DNA that contains the information necessary to construct a protein or part of a protein (polypeptide) is called a gene. Genes are the unit of inheritance.

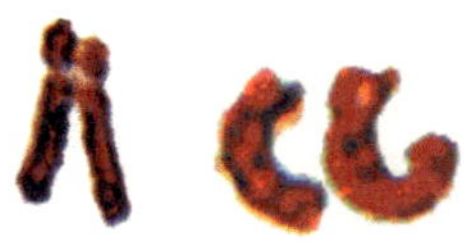

Figure 6. Two chromosome pairs of submetacentric homologue chromosomes [10]

Karyogram: Chromosomes are cut or taken from the photos as regards metaphase stages of an individual, in which chromosomes can be observed clearly. Chromosomes which are morphologically, which similar have the similar or the same length are placed in juxtaposition in the horizontal axis. The karyograms allow for the chromosome characteristics of the individual to be in comparison in themselves, and it helps to present the relation between different individuals with regard to different chromosome properties. According to references [9, 10, 24, 25], performed karyograms for various *Crocus* taxa and compared them to each other. In reference [10], samples of the problematic species *Crocus chrysanthus* have been grouped up, which have different morphological structures and examined

http://dx.doi.org/10.5772/56081

them with respect to their cytological, palinogical and micromorphological properties during and after her doctorate thesis. Consequently, she compared the karyograms of the samples (Figure 7, 8) she has examined and stated that their cytological properties differ as well as their other characteristics [10]. Then, she suggested a new identification key for 7 new taxa of *Crocus chrysanthus* [11-15].

Ideogram: Some cells can be observed in the right metaphase stage; however, since the chromosomes are small, these are not in the size to be made a karyogram with. In these cases, ideograms are prepared with chromosomes. The chromosomes are examined with a microscope and the drawings of chromosomes are made with camera lucida or another photographic computer program. Later, drawings of the chromosomes are made by beginning from the longest chromosome as straight lines which determine the average branch lengths. First the lower branch is drawn, than 1 mm space is left for the centromere and the short branch is drawn on it. Later, other chromosomes are drawn on the same axis by leaving 4-5 mm space in between. Thus the ideogram is prepared.

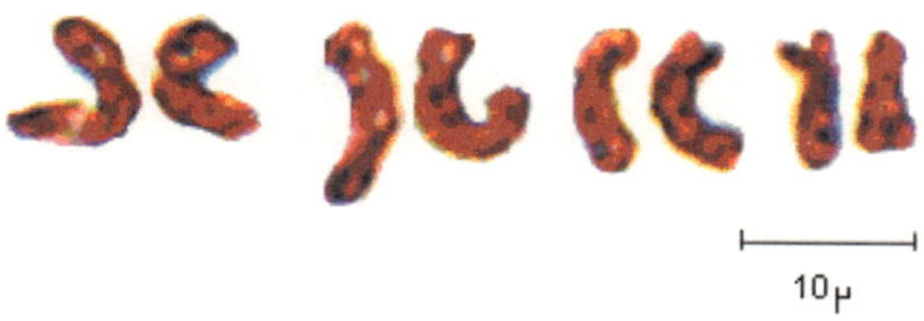

Figure 7. Karyogram of the *Crocus chrysanthus* sample which is suggested as a new taxon, 2n=8 [10, 15]

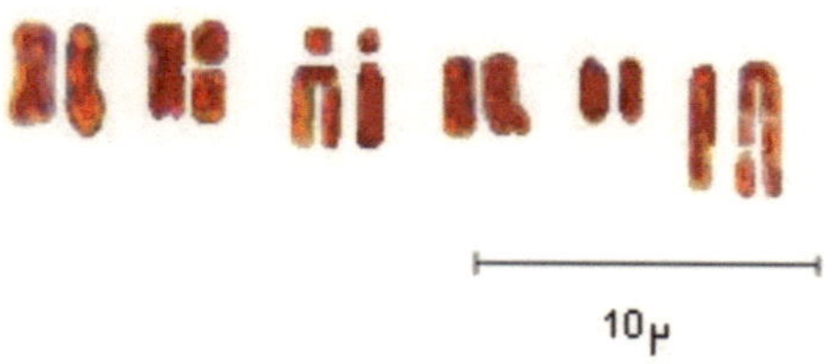

Figure 8. Karyogram of the *Crocus chrysanthus* sample which is suggested as a new taxon, 2n=12 [10, 15]

Sometimes the karyotype analysis are made by measuring the lengths of the chromosomes of the species similar to each other and the letters J and V are used in order to facilitate the comparison. The capital and lower case letters are used to determine the sizes of the chromosomes and each chromosome is classified in two types depending on the position of the centromere. If the centromere of the chromosome is close by 1/3 of the total length, this chromosome is represented with the letter J or j in the karyotype formula. According to this representation, the centromere is called subterminal or terminal. If the centromere of the chromosomes is near to the center or at the center, the chromosome is represented with the letter V or v. The centromere is called metacentric or submetacentric. In V type chromosomes the ratio between the length of the short branch and the total

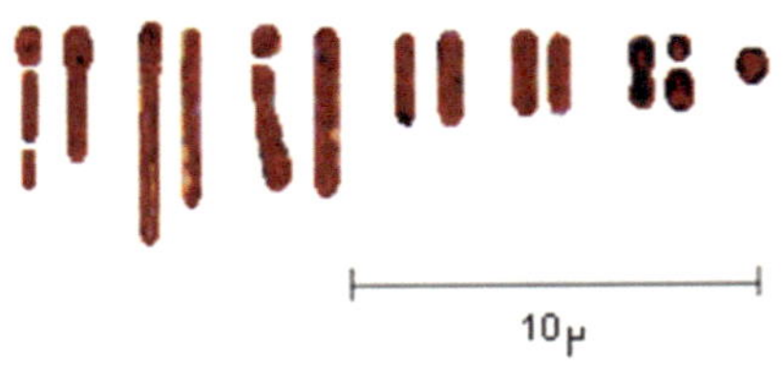

Figure 9. Karyogram of the *Crocus ancyrensis*, 2n=12+1B [10]

chromosome length is more than 33.3%, and in J type chromosomes this ratio is less than 33.3%. On the other hand, if the length of the chromosome is more than half the length of the longest chromosome, it is represented with V or J and if it is less than half the length of the longest chromosome, it is shown with v or j [26, 27].

2.1. B Chromosomes

B chromosomes can be observed in plants and animals. The chromosomes which are part of the genome and carry the essential genetic data are known as the 'A' chromosomes. The organism does not need the 'B' chromosomes for survival. For this reason, they are called as 'B' chromosomes. If an organism has many B chromosomes, its development (phenotypic defects), fertilization and its capacity to produce effective seeds (differences in pollen sizes, sterile seeds or seeds which include different genetic data) are negatively affected. B chromosomes are not observed in polypoid plants. It can be observed in monocotyles, particularly in herbaceous dicotyles and in primitive plants such as bryophytes. B chromosomes may exist on the individuals of a species. It may also be observed in the pollen mother cells of an individual, even if its root cells do not consist of B chromosomes.

B chromosomes may be observed in monocotyles and dicotyles in the populations of the same species, which have been subject to differentiation, and to ensure the adaptation to the environmental conditions. For example, some samples of *Crocus ancyrensis,* which is an endemic species with 2n=12 chromosomes [28], were observed to have 2n=12+1B chromosomes (Figure 9). The fact that there were some individuals of *Crocus ancryensis* species with B chromosomes and that no individuals of the subspecies *Crocus flavus* subsp. *flavus* and *Crocus flavus* subsp. *dissectus* with B chromosomes were observed, has led us to believe that the environmental adaptation capability of *Crocus ancryensis* is stronger, when compared to the species *Crocus flavus* [10].

B chromosomes were observed in the samples collected from different populations, as seen in the samples of the species *Crocus chrysanthus* with 2n=20+2B chromosomes (Figure 10). In reference [15], the researchers have observed during their field studies and herbarium examinations that these samples, which also have a different morphology and blackish lined anthers (Figure 1), are differentiated within the species and they proposed for them to be accepted as a subspecies.

B chromosomes are not observed in all of the cells of a certain plant. It only can be observed in some of its cells. Smaller numbers of B chromosomes in a plant (1-3, sometimes 4) may be

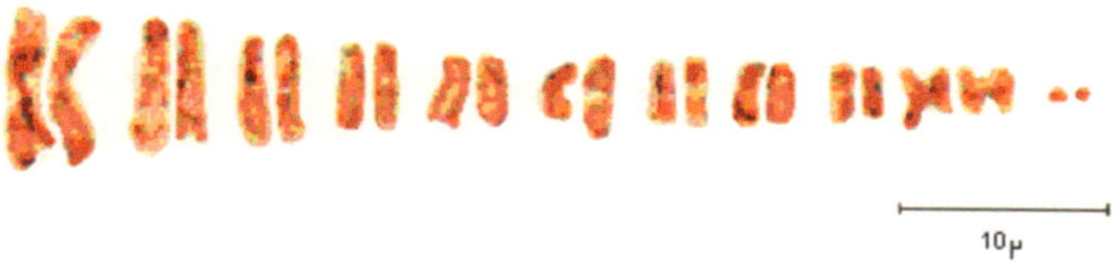

Figure 10. Karyogram of the *Crocus chrysanthus* samples with balckish lined anthers suggested as a new subspecies, 2n=20+2B [10]

accepted as an indicator of a good adaptive capability. For a study conducted, which was related to B chromosomes, the samples of the *Secale cereale* with 2n=14, 2n=14+1B, 2n=14+2B, 2n=14+3B and 2n=14+4B chromosomes were compared with regard to the growth rate of the pollen tube. The results revealed that the pollen percentage and the pollen tube length of the sample with 2n=14+2B chromosomes was higher than the other samples. The second in ranking was the sample with 2n=14 chromosomes [29, 30].

The studies performed revealed that when there are more than two B chromosomes, multivalents produces. The B chromosomes in the mother pollen cells sometimes replicate themselves and they are observed in all the cells produced with the division. Sometimes, in meiosis, it is observed that when there is one B chromosome in the cell, this chromosome remains out of the equatorial level. In this case, the B chromosome is an underdeveloped chromosome. It is not observed in the other nucleuses. However, this chromosome may exist as a micronuclei in 80-85% of the mother pollen cells at the end of the meiosis stage [30, 31].

2.2. Chromosome enormity

The chromosome enormity is regarded as an indicator of primitiveness. Small chromosomes have been differentiated throughout evolution as a result of chromosome disassociations. If all the chromosomes are metacentric, the karyotype will be symmetrical. The differences in sizes of the chromosomes and the existence of acrocentric chromosomes show that the karyotype is asymmetrical. Excess asymmetry of the karyotype may point out that the species is at a more advanced level with regard to evolution. In other words, between the similar species, the one with metacentric chromosomes is regarded more primitive than the species which include submetacentric chromosomes in majority. Thus, the species with submetacentric chromosomes in majority is a more recent flora element than the other. The chromosome enormity may be regarded as a reliable characteristic in the phylogenetic aspect, if similar species are being compared. During evolution, the karyotype may transform from being asymmetrical when it is symmetrical and chromosomes may have disassociate. With an advanced specialization, even polyploidy may emerge. In similar taxa it can be said that the ones with smaller chromosomes are more specialized than the ones with larger chromosomes [32, 33].

Different environment factors cause ecotypes to emerge. Ecotypes can be examined under 5 categories; climatic ecotypes, edaphic ecotypes, culture ecotypes, physiologic ecotypes and chemotypes [33]. It would be imperfect to state that the chromosome number, size and form of a species will be constant. Because of ecological properties and edaphic factors, the total size of the chromosomes of the members of the same species grown in different places. For this reason, it is natural for a plant with edaphic ecotypes such as *Lythrum salicaria*, which is grown in clayed, sandy and salty soil, to have different chromosome lengths in different soils.

For example, it was determined that the chromosomes of *Allium cepa* grown in an environment rich in phosphate, are twice the size of the ones grown in environments with less phosphate [30]. In reference [10], the researcher has determined the chromosome sizes on the karyograms as regards the samples collected from two different populations of *Crocus flavus* subsp. *flavus* and has resulted that the chromosome lengths of these two populations are different from each other (Figure 11). It is stated that this difference is caused by the differences in the chemical content of the soil [10, 34].

Enormous chromosomes are most generally found in animal cells. Also, if the chromotides emerging with endomitosis stay stuck to each other, they may form enormous chromosomes which consist of chromotide packs. This is called polyteny.

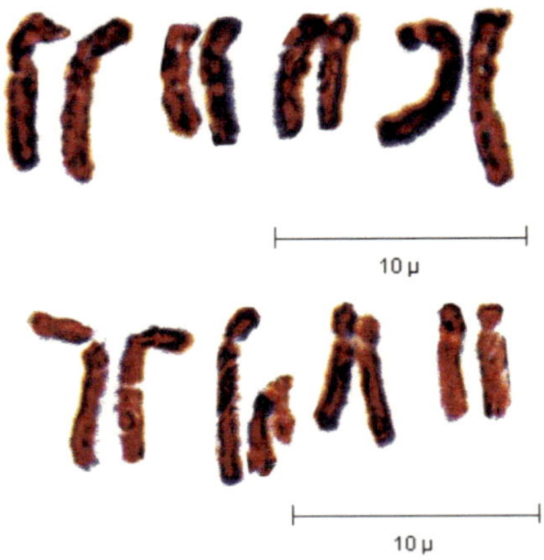

Figure 11. Karyograms of *Crocus flavus* subsp. *flavus* collected from different localities [10]

3. Procurement of the material, the first treatment and fixation

Root tips obtained from the plant grown in land or in a pot, root tips from the seed germinated in petri dish, tips of very young leaves, flower primordiums, growth points of the buds of lateral branches, very young petals, glumes of some monocotyle plants can be used for the examination of somatic chromosomes. Root tips are the most commonly used part among all these, when conducting a mitosis examination.

In order for the chromosomes to be examined quantitatively and structurally in the somatic sense in detail, first, the material needs to be pretreated. The pretreatment allows for the chromosomes to remain at the metaphase level, to decrease in length by increasing the number

http://dx.doi.org/10.5772/56081

of spirals and to be observed clearly. The pretreatment solutions alter the viscosity of the plasma in the cell, the chromosomes diverge from each other and this allows for them to be observed separately. In addition to this, all pretreatment solutions insure the coagulation of proteins in organelles of the cell and perform the fixation process at a certain level. The cleanness and the pH and oxygen levels of the pretreatment solution are extremely important. If the root tips are collected from the land or a field, they should be decontaminated of soil particles and dirt before being rested in the pretreatment solution. The most practical method when cleaning root tips is to use water. However, they should be wiped with a blotting paper before being put in the pretreatment solution. If the root tips are placed in the pretreatment solution without being cleaned or with water drops on them, the concentration of the solution may change and it may not perform well. Also, the bottle which holds the pretreatment solution should be left in an airy environment with its lid open at least one day before the treatment, so that it would aerate. There are several pretreatment solutions. It may be necessary to use different kinds of pretreatment solutions for different kinds of plants. Also, the periods of the samples are to be rested in the solutions differ according to each plant. Thus, it would be beneficial to collect many samples and perform many trials.

Generally, the most commonly used pretreatment solutions are iced water, monobromonaphthalene (α-bromonaphthalene), colchicine, 8-hydroxyquinoline, coumarin, paradiclorobenzene, acenaphtene. Samples should not be rested for a long time in pretreatment solutions such as 8-hydroxyquinoline or α-bromonaphthalene. Each sample should be tested for the resting duration and the duration which gives good results should be determined. For example, it was observed that if Fabaceae and Poaceae family members are rested in α-bromonaphthalene, at +4 ^{0}C for 16 hours or at room temperature for 1 hour, the results would be satisfactory [30]. It would be sensible to use this solution with plants which have large chromosomes. Also, it works when 0.01% colchicine is applied on the root tips of the plants for 3 hours [33, 35]. Applying 2% colchicine on the young leaf tips is also a good solution. The root tips are rested in 8-hidroxyquinoline at 10-18 ^{0}C for 3-6 hours. In references [10, 15, 24, 25], the root tips are rested in 8-hidroxyquinoline at room temperature for 4 hours during the cytological studies conducted on the *Crocus* species and the results were satisfactory. 8-hidroxyquinoline pretreatment can also be applied to the root tips on the plant. It can be prepared with the slide taken from the root tip in 8-hidroxyquinoline. However, it would be more convenient if the slide is prepared after being dyed with aseto-orcein and after maceration is employed. When the root tips are being rested in this liquid, the excess temperature of the room may cause the root tips to get stuck to each other. The coumarin application suggests for the root tips to be rested in solution at 16 ^{0}C for 2-3 hours and this application facilitates the examination. The water saturated solution of coumarin (2%) should be used. If the coumarin is used with chloral hydrate, paradiclorobenzene sulphanilamide and bromonaphthalene combinations, better results will be obtained. If paradiclorobenzene will be used for the examination of somatic chromosomes, the root tips are rested in the saturated solution of paradiclorobenzene in pure water (1-2%) for 1-4 hours. For example, if the root tips as regards members of Poaceae and Cyperaceae are heated in the acid solution and dyed with aceto-orcein, after being rested in this solution at 12-16 ^{0}C for 3 hours, satisfactory results will be obtained [33]. With the application of paradiclorobenzene the images of many plants with 120 or more chromosomes were obtained in the metaphase where the chromosome length is reduced. Acenaphtene was used in the karyotype studies of pollen tube chromosomes. This liquid was not regarded as the appropriate solution for the karyotype examinations of root tips [36].

After the pretreatment, the sample should be put to fixation. There are many kinds of fixatives. The most important ones among all are; alcohol, acetic alcohol (1 measure of glacial acetic acid: 3 measures of absolute alcohol), Carnoy's fixative (1 measeure of glacial acetic acid:3 measures of chloroform:6 measures of absolute alcohol or 1 measure of chloroform:3 measures of acetic acid:6 measures of absolute alcohol), Helly's fixative and Navaschin's fixative. In reference [10], the root tips have been collected from the plants in pots in different hours of the day based on the weather being sunny or rainy and rested them in 8-hidroxyquinoline pretreatment solution for 4 hours and fixated them in acetic alcohol during the studies on the genus *Crocus*.

In reference [19], α-bromonaphthalene is used as the pretreatment solution on the root tips the researcher has collected for the examination of mitosis during the studies on the species *Cucumis melo*. In references [19, 37], researchers have rested the flower sprouts directly in the Carnoy's fixative without using a pretreatment solution during their meiosis examinations they have conducted using pollen mother cells.

In reference [27], cytotaxonomical studies were made on several *Musci* species deployed among the Aegean region of Turkey. The researcher cultured the samples she has brought in the laboratory by ensuring the humidity of the material at 10-15 ^{0}C in petri dishes. As the new suckers develop, they were cut from the plant at an hour close to midnight and were fixated in the Carnoy's fixative at 18-20 ^{0}C for 3 hours.

If acetic alcohol is used as a fixative and the samples are put in this solution after being taken from the pretreatment solution, there is no need to place the samples in another solution or in ethyl alcohol to be able to preserve them for a long period, because, acetic alcohol esterifies and the acid loses its effect in time. Also, since the glacial acetic acid and alcohol mix esterifies in time and since they lose their effect as a fixative in time, this mixture should be prepared right after the root tips are removed from the pretreatment solution. Also, the small bottles in which the samples are to be preserved should be chosen carefully. Bottles with a capacity of 5 cc would be adequate to hold the samples. These small bottles may be used during the period when the root tips collected from the plant for the pretreatment. The time and whether conditions when the root tips are collected for the pretreatment should definitely be noted on the bottle, because this data will provide information about when mitosis divisions occur in general. This information will be helpful in determining on what time and in which weather conditions root tips should be collected in order to observe the chromosomes in the metaphase stage. It would be practical to take the pretreatment solution from the bottle with an injector carefully and this way, it will be ensured that there are not any liquids left in the bottle. Also, before the root tips are taken from the pretreatment solution and put in the fixative, the pretreatment solution drops remaining on the samples should be removed with a blotting paper. If the samples are put in the fixative without paying attention to this step, the purity of the fixative may change and the required effects may not be realized on the chromosomes. If the bottle caps are made of plastic or if the structure of the caps is similar to plastic, it may get fractured in time. Because the bottle includes acid and the corrosive effects of acid are well known. If the caps are fractured, the acetic alcohol inside the bottle will evaporate and the samples will dry. On the other hand, even if the cap is not fractured, the acetic alcohol in the bottle will vaporize, if the sides of the cap allow air to get in; thus the samples will dry and they will become unusable. For this reason, the cap should be covered with a cloth plaster (1 cm wide depending on the size of the bottle) carefully, without leaving any space for air between. If the samples will be preserved for a long time, they should be checked regularly to see if they have dried. If the acetic alcohol level of the bottle has decreased, adding ethyl alcohol on the sample would be sufficient. If the samples are kept in the refrigerator (+4^{0}C), their storage time would increase and it would be ensured that the samples are maintained without decaying. The samples stored in this manner could be examined for years after they were prepared. In order to examine the chromosomes during meiosis, the formation of pollens (microspore) and the ovum (megaspore) of the phanerogams should be assessed. Pollen mother cells (microspore mother cells) produce pollens as a result of meiosis. Ovule mother cells (megaspore mother cells) produce ovums as a result of meiosis. In short, in order to examine the meiosis of the flower, the pollen mother cells, mother cells of the embryo sac and the embryo cells (ovaries) can be used.

In order to examine pollen mother cells, pretreatment should be applied to very young flower blossoms. After the proper procedure is carried out on the fixated samples, the blossom is opened, the pollen mother cells without a fractured callus wall are chosen by disjoining the anthers and meiosis is observed.

3.1. Dying the chromosomes

For the chromosomes of the collected root tips, at different stages of mitosis to be examined clearly, the samples should be dyed. Also, in order to examine the meiosis of the fixated flower primordium pollens, the samples should be dyed thoroughly. Some researchers have examined the root tips by dying them with Feulgen dye [30, 38, 39]. Crystallized basic fuchsine should be used when preparing the Feulgen dye. If basic fuchsine is in powdered form, the Feulgen dye prepared with this will not dye the chromosomes adequately.

Bands are formed when the chromomeres in polythene chromosomes are in juxtaposition. The part between two bands is called an interband. The bands can be dyed with Feulgen dye or with basic dyes, but interbands cannot be dyed.

If mitosis will be examined by using fixated root tip samples, the most convenient material to dye the chromosomes with would be aceto-orcein. If the pollens in the anthers of flower primordiums will be used as samples to examine meiosis, chromosomes should be dyed with aceto-carmine.

In reference [10, 24, 25], aceto-orcein is used to dye the root tips taken from the fixative when working with some *Crocus* taxa. This way, the photos of the available metaphase stages were taken and the karyograms were prepared. In reference [40], they used the same method to examine the karyotypes in their study related to the seed development and DNA structure of *Cynara scolymus* and *Phaseolus coccineus* seeds with Pb and Cu heavy metal stress.

In reference [27], the researcher rested the *Musci* samples at 15-20 ^{0}C for 10 hours in 2% aceto-orcein after fixation. After the dying process, the samples were examined with Feulgen preparation technique, performed the karyotype analysis and prepared ideograms. The researcher has also stated that the fixation period and the dying characteristics of each species they have worked with was different and for this reason, they had to develop different methods.

The dye acceptance of pollens and consequently the adequate dying of the chromosomes is in direct proportion with their vitality. For that matter, it would be appropriate to carry out a pollen vitality test before the karyological study. The dye acceptability of pollens can be tested on alive samples, samples which are fixated with Carnoy's fixative or 80% alcohol and herbarium samples. In cytological studies, pollen infertility is generally regarded as a measure for meiosis irregularity.

In reference [19], the meiosis of the pollen mother cells examined were obtained from the flower buds along with the root tips when conducting a cytological study on some *Cucumis melo* taxa. The researcher dyed the root tips with nigrosin and examined the chromosomes. He also examined some of the root tip samples with pectinase enzyme and aceto-orcein dye. The researcher examined the meiosis divisions with Fuelgen method. He has dyed the pollen mother cells he had obtained from the anthers of flower buds with 2% aceto-carmine.

There are several ways to prepare aceto-orcein and aceto-carmine and the procedures given below have been tested many times and satisfactory results were obtained [10, 19, 37, 41].

3.2. Preparation of aceto-orcein

5 grams of powdered orcein and 250 cc 45% acetic acid are mixed and shaken. They are boiled for 30 minutes by using a Soxhlet apparatus. The apparatus should certainly be held by a stative. The Soxhlet apparatus looks like a glass tube with a spiral back cooler connected to the volumetric flask, it has a tap for water intake below and a place for water outlet. The volumetric flask under the Soxhlet apparatus is placed on the amiant wire on the heater. A boiling chip should be placed inside the volumetric flask. If there are not any boiling chips available, 1-2 cm long glass bars can be used for the same function. Acetic acid dye mix is poured in the volumetric flask and the heating process is started. The aceto-orcein prepared is filtered after it has been cooled down. Aceto-orcein prepared in this manner shall be ready for use.

3.3. Preparation of aceto-carmine

1 gram of powdered carmine and 200 cc 45% acetic acid are mixed and shaken. They are boiled for 5 minutes by using a Soxhlet apparatus. This duration is ideal for Turkey. For example, if the boiling process for dye preparation would take place at a location in the north of Turkey, a country with colder weather, the boiling duration may be 30 minutes. After the boiling process, 1-2 drops of Fe acetate solution saturated with 45% acetic acid is added to the dye.

http://dx.doi.org/10.5772/56081

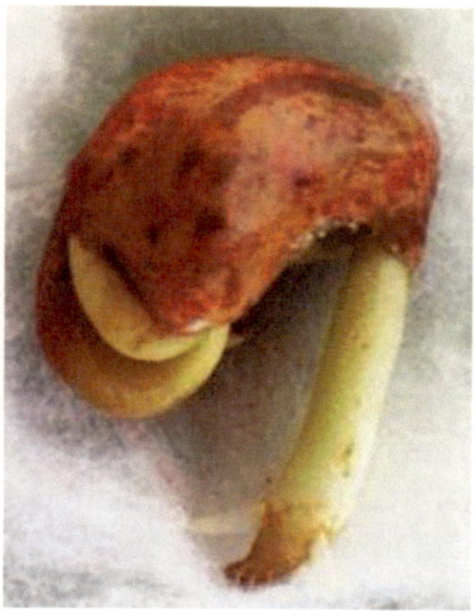

Figure 12. Radicula and primary roots on the germinated *Phaseolus coccineus* seed [40]

Excess Fe acetate settles the carmine. In this case, the dye cannot be used expediently. The aceto-carmine is filtered after being cooled down. Aceto-carmine prepared in this manner shall be ready for use.

3-4 cc of aceto-carmine should be spared before every use. If Fe acetate is not used when preparing aceto-carmine, a nail is placed in the aceto-carmine spared. The iron nail should not remain in the dye for a long time. Because, aceto-carmine with a heightened Fe proportion dyes the cytoplasm in very dark color as well as the chromosomes and it gets extremely difficult to examine the slide. However, if the cytoplasms of the cells are dyed in a dark color, 45% acetic acid can be dropped on the side of the cover slip with the help of a thin pipette. When the acetic acid reaches below the cover slip, it may lighten the color of the cytoplasm. The reason a lighter cytoplasm is required is that, it is preferred when there is a contrast between the cytoplasm and the dyed chromosomes. When there is a contrast between the cytoplasm and the chromosomes, it is easier to examine the chromosomes. Also, the photos of the meiosis phases taken are clearer when there is contrast.

4. The points to take into consideration when taking examination samples

The chromosomes of dicotyle plants are generally examined by using the root tips obtained with the germination of their seeds. The seed embryo is a fertilized mature ovule, which consists of endosperm and testa. When the germination begins, deterioration first takes place in the micropyle area. The radicula starts to grow towards the micropyle. Root hairs emerge on the radicula and primary roots become apparent (Figure 12). Germination varies in accordance with the species.

The testa is a diploid tissue of the sporophyte. The seed coats of beans and groundnuts are thin. It can be thick and rigid as the seed coat of nuts. The variety in the thickness of seed coats may affect the germination of a seed. In addition to this, the seed sizes also differ. For example, the fresh weight of one orchid seed is 0.000002 grams. The seed of *Mora oleifera*, which is 1000 gr, is one of the heaviest seeds known [18]. As it can be seen, if the chromosome examination will be conducted by using the root tips obtained with seed germination, the characteristics of the seed need to be determined clearly and if necessary some pretreatment procedures should be applied before the germination. For example, if the seed coat is thick, it should be sanded or perforated to facilitate the water intake.

The impact of environmental conditions is also important with regard to seed germination. For a successful germination process; the temperature, water and oxygen levels should be adequate. Water is required for the development of the embryo and the enzymatic reactions to start by secreting hormones. Temperature is significant with respect to the functioning of the enzyme. Oxygen is required for the respiration need of the developing seedlings. Although the seeds of some plants germinate in dark, seeds of several plants can only start the germination process after being left under light for a certain amount of time. This pretreatment performed with light can be significant when the seeds absorb water [18, 42].

Therefore, the ecological factors of the environment plant lives in should be determined and a seed germination environment should be prepared accordingly. For this, generally climate cabinets are used. In some instances, even though the conditions required for the seed to be germinated are present, germination does not take place. For example, for the orchid seeds to begin germinating, they should form a mycorrhiza with some fungi types. As it can be seen from the examples, the germination factors of seeds may vary significantly. Thus, more detailed preliminary examinations may be due for the germination of some seeds. In addition to this, if the dicotyle plant examined is endemic, its seeds may be small in quantity or the fertile seeds may be scarce. Also, it is possible for the mature seeds obtained from endemic plants to require more care and time for germination. If the seed of the dicotyle plant is spread around the land as the fruit dries, such as endemic *Linaria corifolia* of the Scrophulariaceae family (Figure 13), it would be appropriate to take the root tips by collecting and germinating these seeds [42]. However, if achene fruits, such as the members of the family Asteraceae; for example endemic *Centaurea zeybekii* or endemic *Jurinea pontica*, are examined (Figure 14, 15), they should directly be subject to germination without attempting to remove the seeds [43-45]. Because, pericarp is fused to the thin seed coat in the grain.

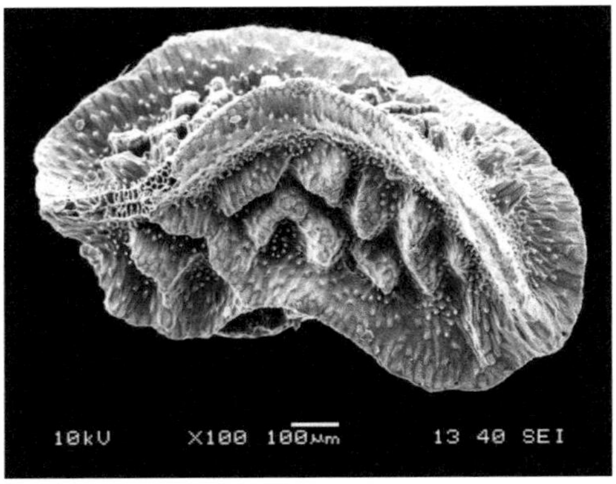

Figure 13. Seed of *Linaria corifolia* (SEM photograph) [43]

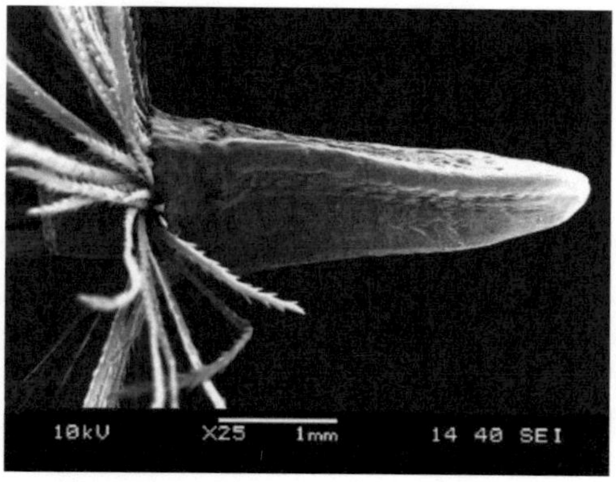

Figure 14. Seed of *Jurinea pontica* (SEM photograph) [43]

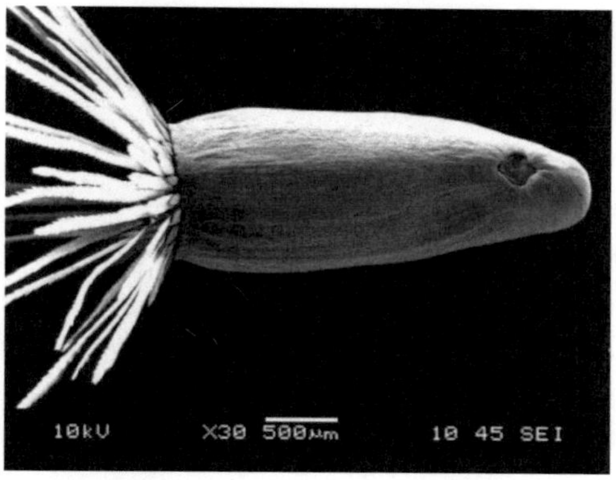

Figure 15. Seed of *Centaurea zeybekii* (SEM photograph) [44, 45]

The germination durations of seeds may vary significantly among plants. Also, the optimum temperature required for the germination of the seed may also vary. Thus, many tests and observations in different places and periods could be needed for the determination of the right germination duration and the optimum temperature for the plant.

Also, sometimes, in order to end the dormancy of the genetic material inside the seeds, germination tests can be made after it is rested in the refrigerator (+4^{0}C) for hours or days. The germination test can be carried out inside a petri dish with a humid blotting paper inside, covered with another petri dish. The point to take into consideration here is this; before placing the blotting paper inside, first a piece of glass in the shape of a square or a rectangle should be put in the petri dish. Later the blotting paper cut in the shape of a circle is placed on the piece of glass. The size of the blotting paper should be smaller than the petri dish. Later, water is poured on the blotting paper, whose center is heightened with the piece of glass. The water should be pure. The water poured on the blotting paper may be 1-2 mm above the surface level. Later, the seeds are placed on the center of the blotting paper which is heightened with the piece of glass. A circular and humid blotting paper of an appropriate size may be placed on the seed as well. This blotting paper can also be placed in the second petri dish after being humidified. This method can work in some instances. For example, if the radicula and the primary roots grow upwards, this humid blotting paper prevents the root tips from getting dry. Because, it is impossible to examine mitosis in dry root tips.

The number of seeds to be placed in the petri dish varies depending on the size and the water absorption capacity of the seed. For example, the swelling capacity of the seeds which belong to Fabaceae family, is high. If a seed with these characteristics is being used, the seeds to be put in the petri dish should be small in number and the water to be poured needs to be plenty. It is important to adjust the amount of water to be poured in the petri dish. If one pours excessive amount of water, it may spill from the sides of the petri dish. If the seeds are observed well during the germination period, water may be added after the level of water in petri dish has decreased and the beginning stages of dryness are observed.

Collecting root tips from a germinated seed in the petri dish relatively easier than collecting the root tips of plants which are grown in fields or on land. The root tip collected from a germinated seed in petri dish is cleaner and there is no risk of tearing the part above the calyptra, where mitosis takes place. Also, the most important point to take into consideration when applying this method is the length of the primary roots shooting from the seed. If the root tip is too long, the part where mitosis takes place can dry. In addition to this, if the root tip is too small, it may get damaged during the dying process and it cannot be examined. It is sufficient for the primary roots to be 1-2 cm long (Figure 16).

Sometimes the seeds placed in a petri dish for germination can be contaminated, they can be molded for example. In this case, they do not shoot root tips. Also, in some instances the seed gets infected after germination. There is a root tip; however, it is impossible to carry out the appropriate chromosome examinations on this root tip, because it is infected. Therefore, the seeds placed in the petri dish should be observed frequently (1-2 times a day).

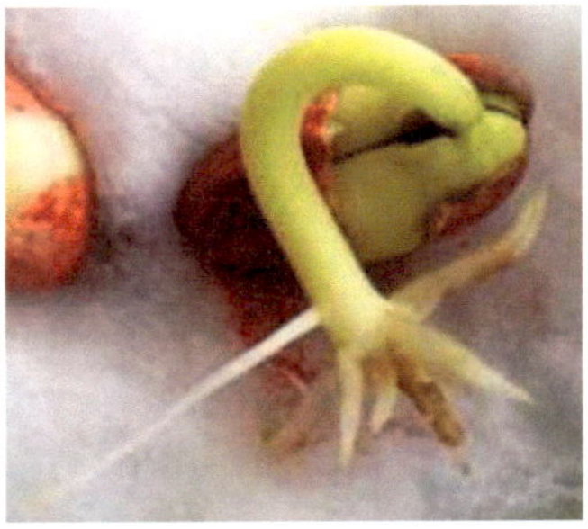

Figure 16. Primary root of the *Phaseolus coccineus* on the left is suitable to collect [40]

It is difficult to collect root tips from dicotyle plants on the land. Especially, if the soil the plant is located on is clayed or stoned, if the plant is on a cliff or on a sloped environment, it is difficult to collect root tips, even though the roots and the lateral roots of the plant do not grow too deep. Also, even if the place the plant is on is flat, if the roots grow deep or if the soil type is not suitable for collecting the root tips, the process of taking root tips will require effort. For

http://dx.doi.org/10.5772/56081

the chromosome examinations of these plants, germinating their seeds would be an easier method which gives useful results.

Perlite can be used for the seeds which are to be germinated. Perlite also is used in greenhouses to grow seedlings from seeds. Torf can also be used for the tests of growing plants in pots. The pots are turned upside down, the torf surrounding the plant is collected carefully and the lateral roots are reached. One should be very careful in order not to damage the root tips.

If the chromosomes to be examined belong to a monocotyle plant and it reproduces with stems or corms like the genus *Crocus* (Figure 17, 18), it should be known that the number of the seeds may be less for these plants. Even if there are plenty of seeds, there is a great probability that many of them are sterile (Figure 19, 20) [10].

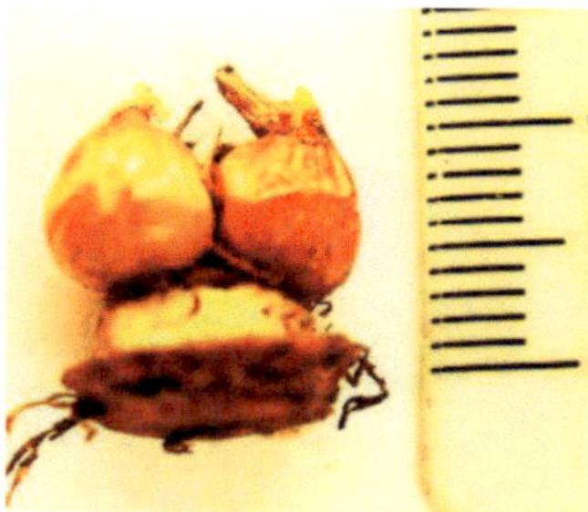

Figure 17. Young corms of *Crocus chrysanthus* [10]

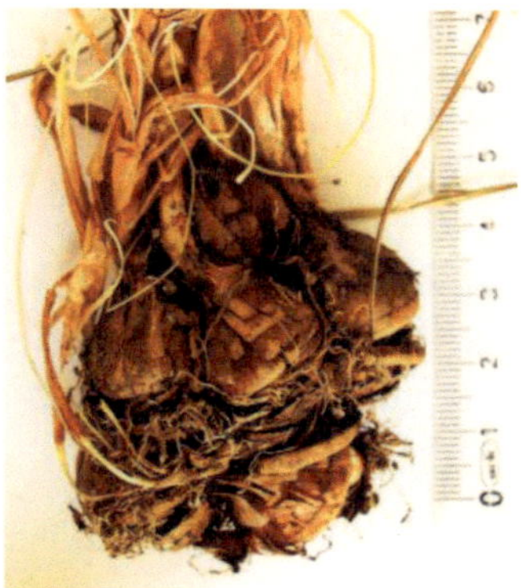

Figure 18. Corms of *Crocus chrysanthus* [10]

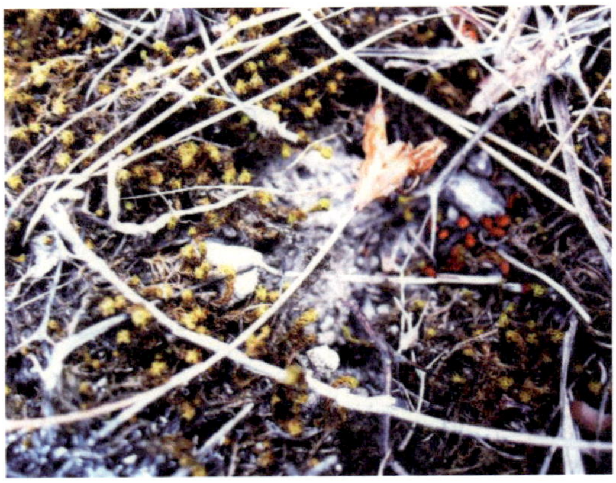

Figure 19. Riped fruit and scattered seeds of *Crocus chrysanthus* [10]

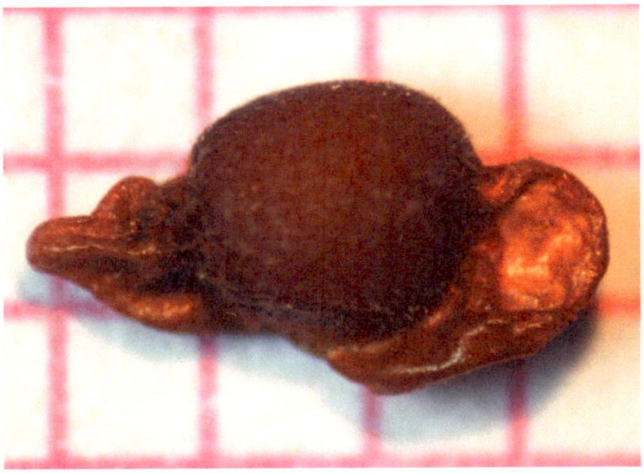

Figure 20. Riped seed of *Crocus flavus* subsp. *flavus* [10]

If the chromosomes of monocotyles (for example Iridaceae or Liliaceae) are to be examined, root tips may be collected on the land. However, the most appropriate and easy method would be to obtain them on the land, sew them on the pot and to try and collect the root tips. If the plants are on a mountain or on highlands, the environment in your house or your garden may not be suitable for the plant to grow. In this case, the plants sown will die. However; if the corms and bulbs are preserved under convenient conditions (in a dry and dark environment), they will give roots the next year. The corms of *Crocus* (Iridaceae) and bulbs of *Colchicum* (Liliaceae) species shoot primary or contractile root tips the following year even if they are not placed under soil or torf.

If root tips are to be collected from monocotyles on land, it should be noted that this process requires extreme attention and patience. The root depth of the plant is examined and a proper garden tool (such as digger, shovel and hoe) needs to be taken to the land. When removing the plant from the land, the distance between the tool and the plant should be maintained. Otherwise, there is a risk of tearing the root or the stem of the plant and rupturing the lateral roots. The plant should be removed with the soil surrounding it and later, the soil and the weed around the plant should be sorted out for the unruptured root tips to be collected. If the soil is clayed, it is difficult to collect root tips since, the soil is sticky. In this case, the corm or the bulb should be taken, the plant should be sown in a pot and the root tips shoot in that environment should be collected. For example, the chromosomes you wish to examine could be of a plant which grows in a mountain, far away from where you live. The region and the climate the plant grows in may not be suitable for you to visit the area often to collect root tips. It is difficult for the researcher to grow this plant, which is adapted to the mountain climate and cold weather, and to collect its root tips. In this case, it may be convenient to sew the samples collected from the land in pots and to take the pot to a mountain near (or another place similar to the original environment of the plant). An area on the mountain or the natural site is surrounded with a wire or a fence, after obtaining the necessary permits from the authorities. The pots are placed in this area. Thus, it may be possible to prevent the pots from getting harmed by some animals.

The root tips of the plants taken from the soil may continue performing mitosis divisions. For this reason, it would be appropriate to use the natural water of the environment in order to prevent the root tips from drying out until they are collected for examinations. For example, if a field study is being conducted on a highland, it would be convenient to use water from the mountain. If the land is snow-covered, it would be best to use melted snow. If the water reserves of the land are scarce, drinking water or pure water may be used to prevent the root tips from drying. However, if the environment is cold, the water used should also be cold. As it is known, temperature affects mitosis.

If the fixated pollens in the anthers of flower primordiums will be used to examine meiosis, samples should be taken during the periods when there are plenty of flower buds. The flower buds should be collected at different times of the day and they should be in different sizes. Because it is extremely difficult to estimate at what time and in which size (necessary maturity) the pollens will be in the appropriate phase to be examined. Thus, it would be beneficial for the study to take many samples while changing the variables.

5. The points to take into consideration when preparing the mitosis or meiosis slides and when performing the examination

If slides are to be prepared by using root tip squash samples, it would be convenient to place the pretreated and fixated root tips 1-2 cm length, collected from the seed or the root in a clean petri dish which includes 70% clean ethyl alcohol. The samples placed in the petri dish should be pre-examined with a stereo microscope. Because, the part of the root to be examined, which is 1-2 mm long and is above the calyptra, may be torn in the sampling process. Also, the samples may be contaminated. These cases are most commonly observed in the root tip collection processes carried out in the fields. If the soil conditions are favorable, the hairy roots may grow and spread in the soil. Sometimes, for example, when the soil is clayed, it will be difficult to collect the root tips. Since the pieces of soil will stick to the roots, the sensitive root tips will be ruptured. Even when the root tip is collected properly from such an environment or a different environment, the soil pieces stuck on the roots should be cleaned before the slides are prepared. There is also a possibility for particles and dirt to remain on the root tips collected from torf or perlite. Thus, before starting the slide preparation process, the samples should be examined in alcohol with a stereo microscope. If the root tips are very dirty, the alcohol in petri dish should be replaced for a couple of times. The cleaning of root tips can be carried out by shaking the samples in alcohol and removing the dirt by using a forceps or a needle.

It would be sufficient for aceto-orcein or aceto-carmine dyes to be filtered for a short time during the preparation process, because, there may be sedimentations in the dyes which are rested for a long period. It may be convenient to transfer small amounts of dye from the total amount stored in dark glass bottles in a dark place to small bottles which can contain 5 cc of liquid. Because, the amount of dye required for an examination is 3-5 cc. The required amount of dye is filtered with a diameter of 2-3 cm prepared blotting or filtering paper. The filtered dye is poured in a middle sized watch-glass. The fixated root tips are placed in here. The watch-glass which contains dye and root tips heated on the burner until it boils. Since there is a small amount of liquid, the boiling process should not take a lot of time. Also, the acetic acid in the dye will evaporate. The samples may dry if the heating process lasts too long, since the acid will be vaporized. In this case, the root tips in the watch-glass will be unusable. The heating process made in a careful way should be repeated three times. After each heating process, the watch-glass is taken aside and another watch-glass larger than the one used is covered on top of it. This should be done very quickly. The purpose here is to prevent the acetic acid in the dye to vaporize. Also, the point to take into consideration is the size of the watch-glass which is used to cover the watch-glass used. If a significantly larger watch-glass is used to cover the heated watch glass, the acetic acid would vaporize and the dye would dry. If the heating process is carried out carefully, it will enable the maceration of the roots as well as allowing for the dye to perforate in the cells and ensuring the dying of the chromosomes; therefore, there will be no need for hydrolysis.

The slide prepared for mitosis examination does not only reflect one phase of the mitosis. When some cells are in interphase, some may be in anaphase, some in telophase and some may be in metaphase (Figure 21). If lengthened cells are observed in the slide, this shows that not only the necessary part of the root tip required to examine mitosis is squashed. The excessive parts squashed are the cells in the stage of elongation. Also, vascular tissue can be seen in the slide. The reason of this observation is similar to the reason for seeing the elongated cells. Even if there are proper metaphase cells in the slide, the existence of elongated cells and vascular tissue could make it difficult for the chromosomes to be examined. For this reason, one should decide very carefully when determining how much of the root piece will be left in the slide when examining the length of the calyptra shot from the root tip.

The root piece on the slide which is 1-2 mm long has become very soft and is ready to be squashed. The dyed root tip is placed on the slide. After the calyptra is cut with a sharp razor blade (a piece almost in the size of a pinhead), 1-2 mm of the remaining piece is cut and this

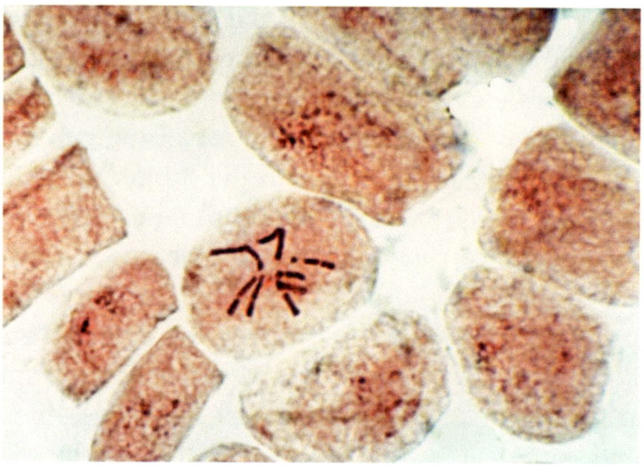

Figure 21. Different phases in a squashed root tip of *Crocus chrysanthus* [15]

piece is placed on the slide. The remaining root piece is thrown away. 1 drop of the aceto-orcein filtered for the study shall be poured on the material. The cover slip is closed on the sample without allowing any air to get in (with an angle equal to 45⁰C). A piece of blotting paper (a little larger than the cover slip) is placed on the cover slip carefully. The blotting paper absorbs the aceto-orcein spilling from the sides of the cover slip. The thumb is placed on the cover slip carefully, without moving the cover slip on the slide. The thumb is not removed, but is moved from side to side for the mitosis cells of the root tip squashed to spread under the cover slip. Thus, the cells which have overlapped and the chromosomes of the cells will be separated from each other and are spread on one plane. As a result, the cells and the chromosomes will be easily examinable.

However, there may be cells in the slide which are not spread on the plane as well as the cells which reflect the chromosomes clearly. In this case, various images of the same cell should be taken using the microscrew (Figure 22). Later, the images are put together and examined. For example, a chromosome observed in one image may not be present in the other. As a result, a karyogram can be prepared with these images.

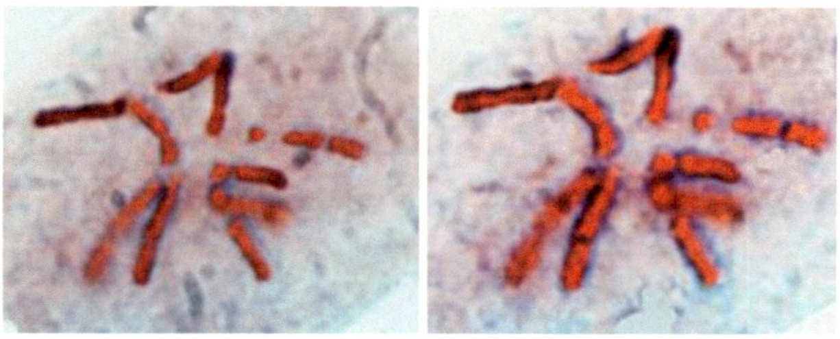

Figure 22. Various images of the same cell of *Crocuschrysanthus* using the microscrew [15]

Sometimes the photographs taken by replacing the microscrew may not be sufficient in providing the chromosome data. In this case, the microscope coordinates of the cell examined are noted in accordance with the objective used. Later, the slide is taken from the microscope flange and is put on a hard surface. A blotting paper is placed on the cover slip once more and the cover slip is pressed with the thumb carefully. This pressure may allow for the chromosomes of the cell, whose coordinates were noted, to be observed individually. If this operation is carried out carefully, there is a great chance that it will be useful. However, even the slightest gliding of the slide may cause the cells to overlap or it may result in the emergence of new cells which have been flattened and cannot be observed clearly. This second squashing process can only work after many practices. As it can be seen, a minor error in the second squashing process may cause the slide to be unusable. Thus, before the second squash and after the coordinates of the examined cell is noted, other photographs of the cells should be taken. So that, when later, the slide is taken from the flange to be squashed once more and the slide ends up being unusable, the negative impact will partially be eliminated.

In some instances, the researcher may need to take a break when observing the phases of mitosis or meiosis. When the slide is being examined as described above, it may only be preserved for 15 minutes, depending on the temperature, because the acetic acid in the aceto-orcein used to dye the chromosomes and the acetic acid in the aceto-carmine used in meiosis examinations will vaporize. Thus, a dried slide is not functional and it cannot be used for examination. In this case, it would be convenient to cover the all sides of the cover slip with paraffin in order to be able to examine it in 1–2 days. For this appliance, the back of the metal spatula should be heated on the burner and it is contacted with the paraffin. The liquid paraffin poured on the metal is applied thinly around the cover slip. The slide prepared in this manner can be maintained for 1-2 days without being dried and it can be used. If the slide is preserved in the refrigerator (+4^{0}C) in a petri dish covered with another petri dish, the life cycle of the slide will increase. Covering of the sides of the cover slip with rubber solution, has the same effect.

It may take a long time to make a careful examination on all the root tip squash under the cover slip with microscope. If the slide is prepared with aceto-orcein (for the examination of mitosis) or with aceto-carmine (for the examination of meiosis), under the sides of the cover slip will begin drying circularly. Since the drying of the slide will prevent us from completing the examination, a small amount of dye shall be added on the side of the cover slip with the help of a needle. It will be observed that the dye steals into the dried parts under the cover slip after a while. The excess dye on the side of the cover slip can be cleaned with a blotting paper. This process will delay the drying process and increase the time allowed for examination.

In some instances Feulgen's dye is used for the chromosomes dying. In this case, 45% acetic acid is dropped on the sample and the slide is covered with the cover slip. The squashing process is carried out carefully. The cover slip may start to dry from the sides when examining the slide, as it does with other dying methods. In order to prevent the drying of the slide, the researcher should drop 45% acetic acid on the side of the cover slip with a needle and should wait for it to steal into the dried parts of the squashed root tip under the cover slip. The excess acetic acid on the side of the cover slip is dried with a blotting paper.

6. Chromosomal abnormalities

Chromosomal abnormalities are observed in plants for various reasons. The existence of a chromosomal abnormality in the cell can also be understood from the morphology of the root or another part of the plant. The chromosomal abnormalities which reflect themselves in the morphological properties can occur with relation to the differentiation and adaptation processes. For example, in reference [10], when examining the problematic species *Crocus chrysanthus*, observed lagging chromosomes (Figure 23) and determined 2n=20+2B as the chromosome number for the plant samples with blackish anthers, which are differentiated and morphologically different suggested as a subspecies in reference 15.

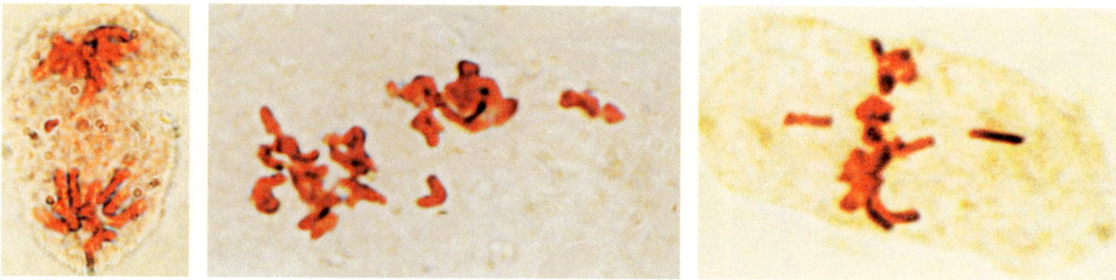

Figure 23. Lagging chromosomes of *Crocus chrysanthus* in different cells [10]

Rapidly increasing world population in recent years brings about an increasing demand for nutrition, which is one of the most important problems for mankind. Various methods have been discussed in order to solve this problem. One of these methods is using chemicals against harmful organisms in plants. The use of pesticides in agricultural areas increases the plant yield; however, some chemical substances may result in pollution in nature and health problems [46].

Modern agriculture and industry depend on a wide variety of synthetically produced chemicals, including insecticides, fungicides, herbicides, and other pesticides. Continual widespread use and release of such synthetics has become an everyday occurrence, resulting in environmental pollution [47]. It was indicated that many cytogenetic studies have been carried out to detect the harmful effect of different pesticides on different plants [48]. These chemicals used at recommended dosage and double the recommended can give rise to abnormal chromosomes and degeneration in meiosis cycle, such as ring shaped chromosomes, linear chromosomes and binding chromosomes [37]. Benomyl, a systemic fungicide, affects germination, mitotic and meiotic activity, and pollen fertility in barley [49]. Besides, the fungicide phosphite reduced polen fertility in *Petunia hybrida, Tradescantia virginiana* and *Vicia faba*, while phosphite, application increased the number of abnormal meiotic cells at all stages in Tradescantia virginiana microspores [50]. Furthermore, some common pesticides (Thiodan, Folithion, Lebaycid, and Kitazin) caused a spectrum of cytogenetic abnormalities such as chromosome fragmentation, lagging of chromosomes, anaphase bridge formation as well as tripolar and tetrapolar spindle formation in barley [51].

The abnormalities occurring in meiosis are very important because they cause sterility in pollens and genetic damage can be transmitted to the offspring via male gametes, leading to congenital abnormalities. It was studied on *Lycopersicon esculentum* that all dosages of the fungicides Agri Fos 400 [80% fosetyl-Al (400 g/l mono- and di-potassium phosphonate)] caused various abnormalities in meiosis when compared with the control (Figure 24-27) [37].

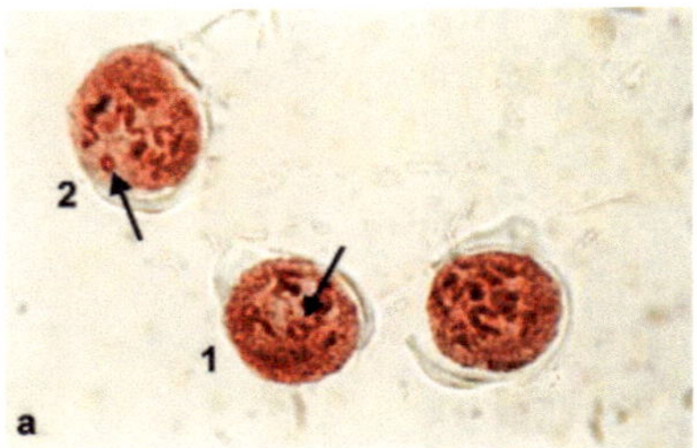

Figure 24. Ring-shaped chromosomes in 400 ml/100 l group a (1, 2) [37]

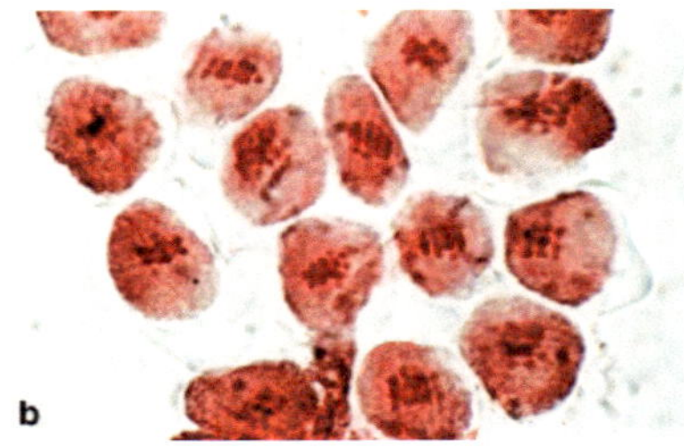

Figure 25. Binding chromosomes in 800 ml/100 l group b [37]

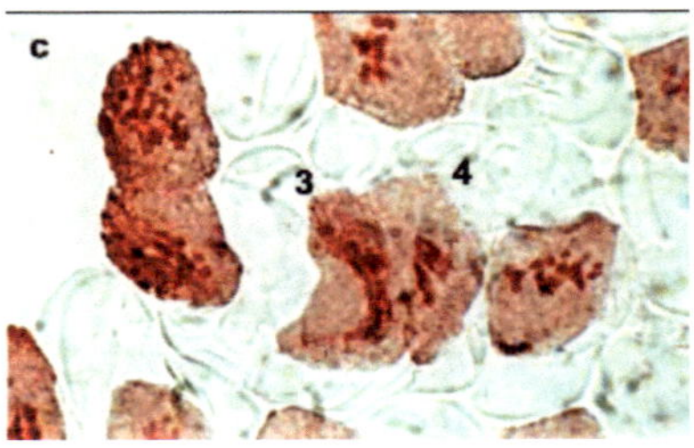

Figure 26. Binding chromosomes and abnormal shape in 800 ml/100 l group c (3, 4) [37]

http://dx.doi.org/10.5772/56081

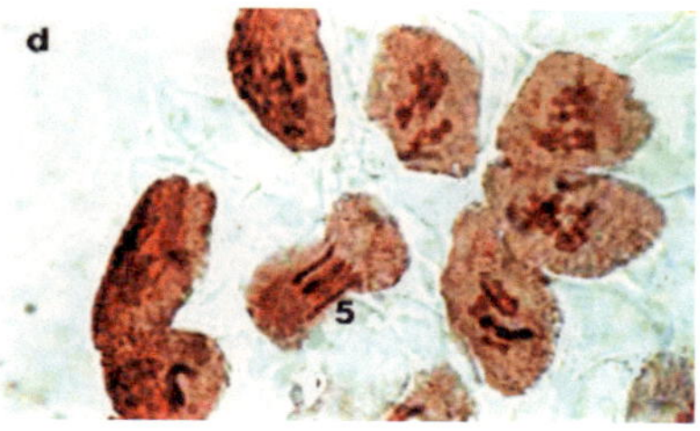

Figure 27. Abnormal shape and linear chromosomes in 800 ml/100 l group d (5) [37]

In another studies, the fungicides Fosetyl-Al (80% Aliette WG 800) and Equation Pro (22.5 % Famoxadone + 30 % Cymoxanil) widely applied on tomato plants (*Lycopersicon esculentum*) grown in greenhouse in Turkey caused various anomalies in polen meiosis such as thread-like, ring shaped, linear and binding chromosomes (Figure 24, 25). This situation could lead to a decreased in the productivity of fruits [52, 53]. In references [54- 56], the effects of fungicide and aplicator application on pollen structure in tomato (*Lycopersicon esculentum*) were investigated. SEM photographs of *Lycopersicon esculentum* as regards control group and non-viable pollen grains in the ACT-2 groups are given below (Figure 28-33).

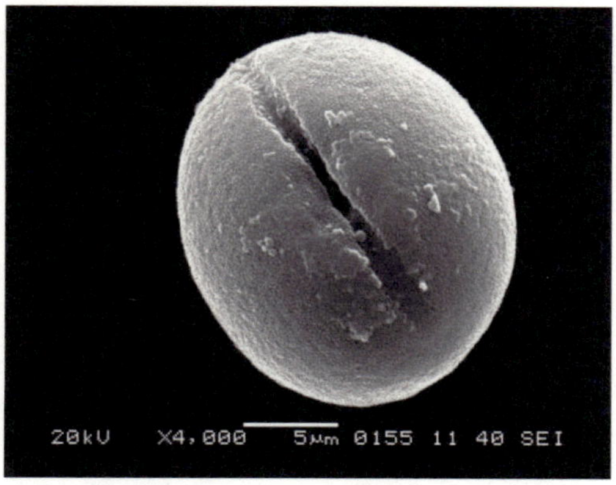

Figure 28. Pollen grain of control group (SEM photograph) [56]

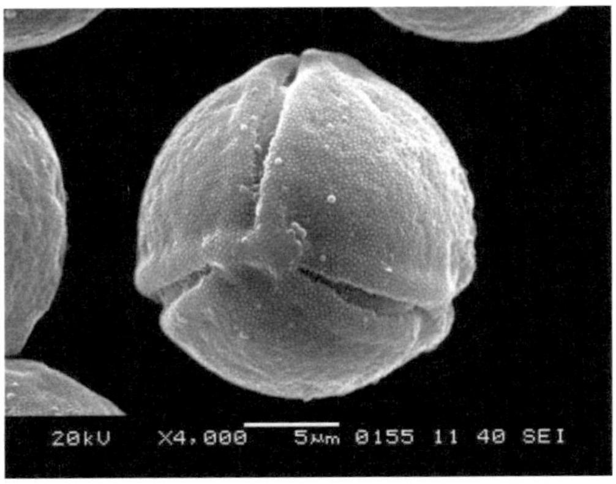

Figure 29. Pollen grain of control group, polar view (SEM photograph) [56]

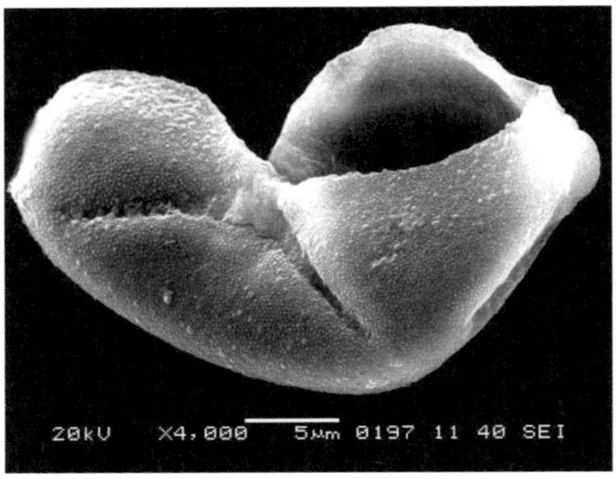

Figure 30. Abnormally shaped pollen grain in 150 cc/100 L. (SEM photograph) [56]

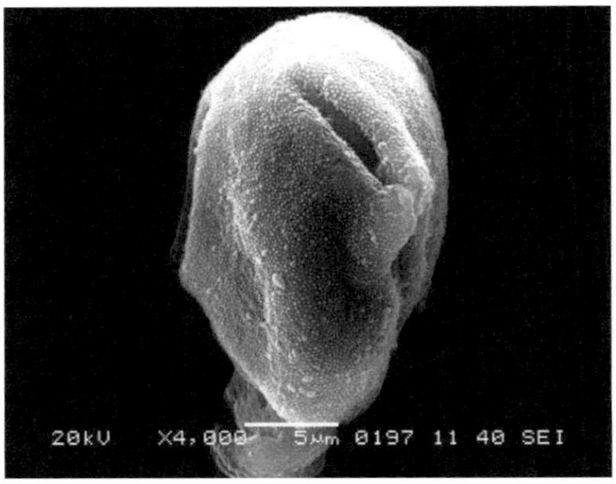

Figure 31. Abnormally shaped pollen grain in 150 cc/100 L. (SEM photograph) [56]

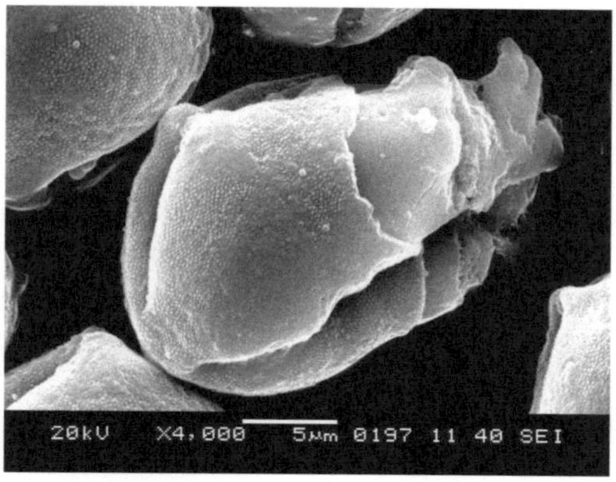

Figure 32. Abnormally shaped pollen grain in 300 cc/100 L. (SEM photograph) [56]

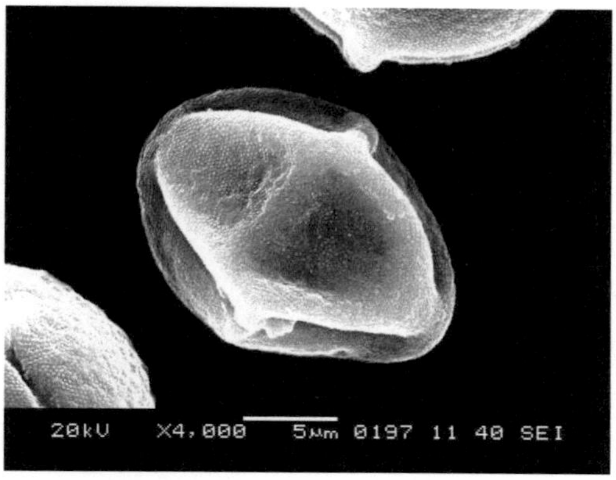

Figure 33. Wrinkled pollen grain in 300 cc/100 L. (SEM photograph) [56]

Agricultural pesticides or hormones commercialized may cause the flowers and pollens of the flowers to have formal differences and abnormalities and it may reduce productivity. The species, *Anemone coronaria* is a flower with corm, which can be grown in greenhouses with no heating between October and May and is very popular in domestic and foreign markets, also, its origin is Mediterranean and it is ecologically advantageous; because of these reasons it has a significant status in export with regard to differentiation. In references [16, 57], it has been pointed out that while there is homogeneity in the pollen sizes of the natural forms of the variety within the species, the pollen sizes, pollen deformations, pollen failure to thrive and vitality of the pollens taken from the members to be traded are significantly different (Figure 34-40). The agricultural pesticides used to enhance and accelerate the growth and blooming can be the reason behind this differentiation. The pollen vitality percentages were determined as a result of the test made with TTC (triphenyltetrazolium chloride) in order to observe the pollen vitality of natural and commercial forms of *Anemone coronaria* taxa. In reference [57], viable pollen ratio of natural *Anemone coronaria* var. *coccinea* is 94%, viable pollen ratio of commercial forms of that taxon is 69%.

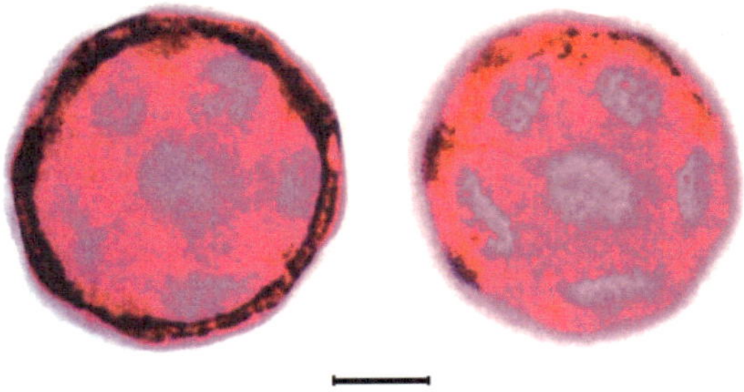

Figure 34. Pollen grains of *Anemonecoronaria* var. *coccinea* as regards control group, scale bar:10 µm (Wodehouse Method used) [16]

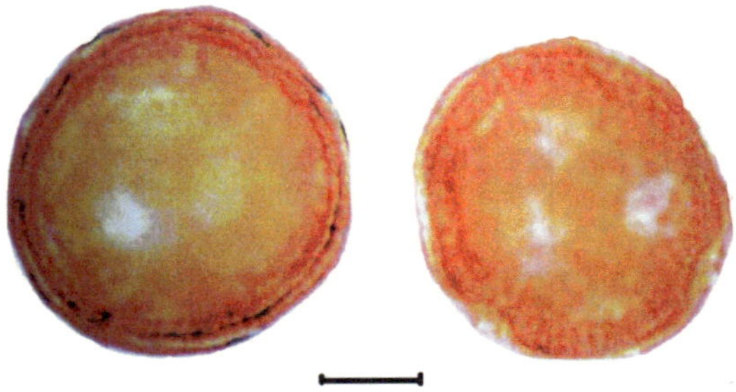

Figure 35. Pollen grains of *Anemone coronaria* var. *coccinea* as regards control group, scale bar:10 µm (Erdtman Method used) [16]

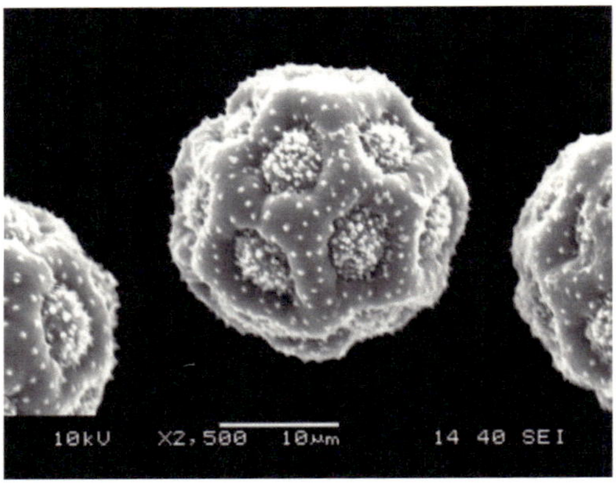

Figure 36. Pollen grain of *Anemone coronaria* subsp. *coccinea* as regards control group (SEM photograph) [57]

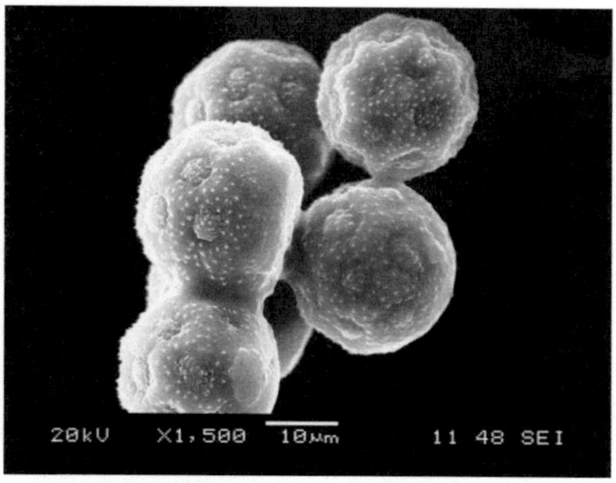

Figure 37. Abnormal shaped pollen grains of *Anemone coronaria* var. *coccinea* as regards commercial group (SEM photograph) [57]

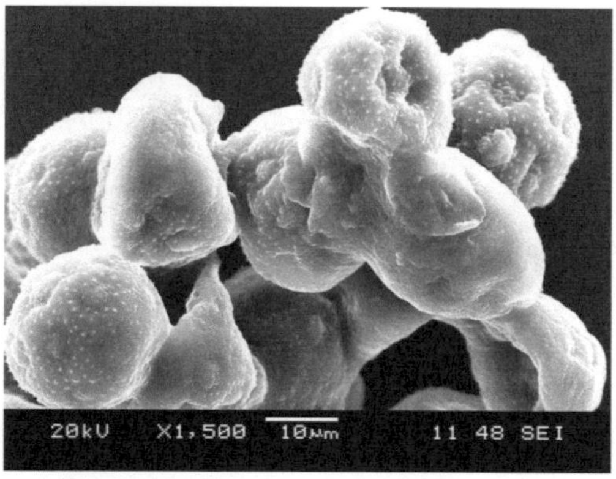

Figure 38. Abnormal shaped pollen grains of *Anemone coronaria* var. *rosea* as regards commercial group (SEM photograph) [57]

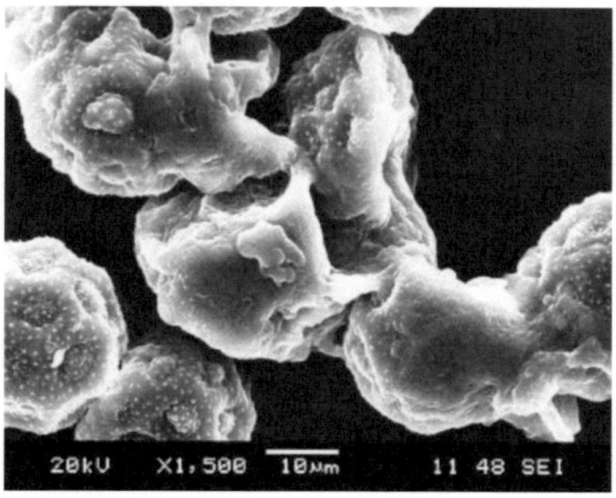

Figure 39. Abnormal shaped pollen grains of *Anemone coronaria* var. *cyanea* as regards commercial group (SEM photograph) [57]

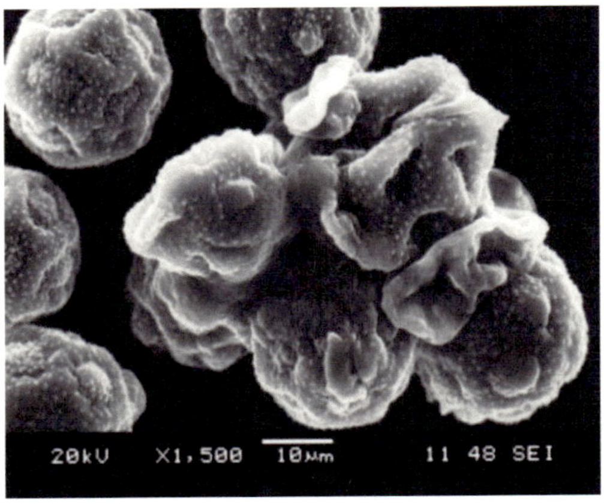

Figure 40. Abnormal shaped pollen grains of *Anemone coronaria* var. *alba* as regards commercial group (SEM photograph) [57]

Also, environmental conditions which are stem from pollution, such as heavy metal stress may cause development disorders and chromosomal abnormalities in plants. For example, in reference [40], they applied different values of Pb stress to artichokes for 5 days and have observed their development. 40, 80, 160, 320, 1280 ppm Pb acetate solution was used. The researchers have also germinated control groups in Hoagland solution. The seeds to which stress are applied, delays in germination were observed and some did not even germinate depending on the stress level (Figure 41). Also, the root tips collected from the seeds have revealed chromosomal abnormalities and deviations.

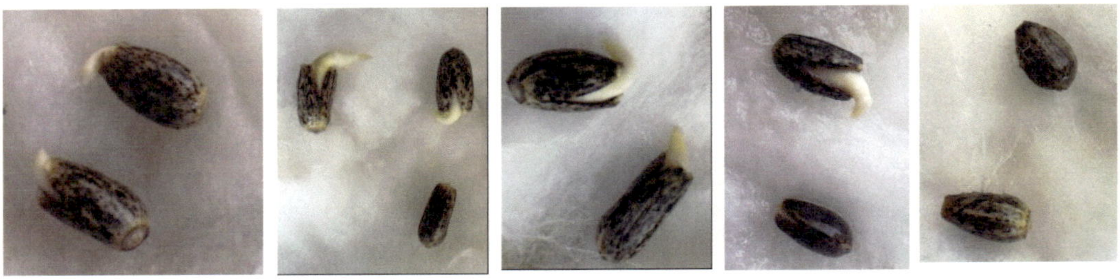

Figure 41. Photographs of germination related *Cynarascolymus* seeds in a row of control group and 40, 80, 160, 320 ppm Pb application [40]

7. Uncontrolled and abnormal cell reproduction of plants

Galls are abnormal growths that occur on leaves, twigs, roots, or flowers of many plants. Most galls are caused by irritation and/or stimulation of plant cells due to feeding or egg-laying by insects such as aphids, midges, wasps, or mites. Some galls are the result of infections by bacteria, fungi, or nematodes and are difficult to tell apart from insect-caused galls. Seeing the insect or its eggs may help you tell an insect gall from a gall caused by other organisms. In general, galls provide a home for the insect, where it can feed, lay eggs, and develop. Each type of gall-producer is specific to a particular kind of plant [58].

The gall structure observed in oak, apple, cherry, nut, walnut and maple trees and grapefruit contain a liquid similar to the gall of the mammals with its green tone and bitter taste. Although many galls do not critically harm the plant, each one of them is a parasite. The parasites causing the gall generation accelerate the uncontrolled cell division of the organism on which they live and as a result cause the number of the cells to increase.

Acknowledgements

Author wants to thank Prof. Dr. Teoman Kesercioğlu for his considerable helpings regarding some chromosomal studies and Dr. İlkay Öztürk Çali for giving the photographs used at figures 24-27. However, author wants to thank her family because of their valuable support in all her life.

Author details

Feyza Candan*

Celal Bayar University, Arts & Science Faculty, Biology Department, MANISA, Turkey

References

[1] Turrill WB. Vistas in Botany. London, New York:Pergamon Press, International series of monographs on pure and applied biology. Division, Botany, 1959-1964.

[2] Tokur S, Zeybek N, Kesercioğlu T. Importance of Cytotaxonomy in Determination of Plants. Anadolu University, Journal of Arts&Science Faculty 1988; 1(1) 17-23.

[3] Graham LE, Graham JM, Wilcox LW. Plant Biology. Prentice Hall, Inc. USA, 1st ed; 2002.

[4] Tsarenko PM. Nomenclatural and taxonomic changes in the classification of "green" algae. International Journal on Algae, 2005; 299-309.

[5] Klug WS, Cummings MR. Spencer CA. Concepts of Genetics. Pearson Education, Inc. Publishing as Prentice Hall, USA, 8th edition; 2006.

[6] Fahn A. Plant Anatomy. Pergamon Press, Oxford; 1982.

[7] Ozyurt S. Plant Anatomy. Erciyes University Publisher, Kayseri, Turkey; 1992.

[8] Sharp LW. Introduction to Cytology. McGraw-Hill Book Company, London; 1934.

[9] Candan F, Kesercioğlu T. Cytaxonomic Investigations on the Species *Crocus chrysanthus* (Herbert) Herbert: proceedings of the International Conference on Environment:Survival and Sustainability, Vol. 2, 19-24 February 2007a, Near East University, Nicosia-Northern Cyprus.

[10] Candan, F. Morphological, anatomical, cytological and palinological investigations on *C. ancyrencis*, *C. sieheanus*, *C. chrysanthus* and *C. flavus* taxa of the genus *Crocus* L. PhD thesis, Science Institute, Celal Bayar University, Manisa, Turkey; 2007b.

[11] Candan F. 7 New Taxa of *Crocus chrysanthus* (Herbert) Herbert from Turkey:proceedings of the Antalya, Turkey:proceedings of the XIth International Symposium on Flower Bulbs and Herbaceous Perennials, 28 Mart-01 Nisan 2012a, Antalya, Turkey.

[12] Candan F. Seed Macromorphological Investigations On 7 New Taxa of *Crocus chrysanthus* (Herbert) Herbert from Turkey:proceedings of the XIth International Symposium on Flower Bulbs and Herbaceous Perennials, 28 Mart-01 Nisan 2012b, Antalya, Turkey.

[13] Candan F. Leaf Anatomical Investigations On 3 New Taxa of *Crocus chrysanthus* (Herbert) Herbert from Turkey:proceedings of the XIth International Symposium on Flower Bulbs and Herbaceous Perennials, 28 Mart-01 Nisan 2012c, Antalya, Turkey.

[14] Candan F. Seed Micromorphological Investigations On 7 New Taxa of *Crocus chrysanthus* (Herbert) Herbert from Turkey:proceedings of the 3rd International Symposium on Sustainable Development. International Burch University, 31 May-01 June 2012d, Sarajevo, Bosnia and Herzegovina.

[15] Candan F, Özhatay N. *Crocus chrysanthus* (Herbert) Herbert s. l. in Turkey, 2012e (article is in press).

[16] Candan F. A Biological investigation on *Anemone coronaria* L. Ms Thesis. Celal Bayar University, Arts&Science Faculty, Biology Department, Manisa, Turkey; 2001.

[17] Heslop-Harrison Y, Shivanna KR. The receptive Surface of the angiosperm Stigma. Annals of Botany, 1977; 41:1233-1258.

[18] Ünal M. Plant Angiosperm Embryology. Nobel Academical Publisher, 5th edition, Turkey; 2011.

[19] Kesercioğlu T. Cytotaxonomical and taxonomical investigations on forms of *Cucumis melo* L. which exist in west Anatolia and which are under culture studies. PhD Thesis, Ege University, Science Faculty, Biology Department, Izmir, Turkey; 1981.

[20] Baboğlu M, Gürel E, Özcan S. Plant Biotechnology Tissue Culture and Applications. Selçuk University Publisher, Konya, Turkey; 2001.

[21] Çapan S. An Investigation on Mitosis Activity and Chromosome Number of *Cucurbita pepo* L. Embryo Cultures. Ms Thesis. Trakya University, Arts&Science Faculty, Biology Department, Edirne, Turkey; 2006.

[22] Collin HA, Edwards HS. Plant Cell Culture. BIOS Scientific Publisher; England, 1998.

[23] Paterson A, Bowers JE, Burow MD, Draye X, Elsik CG, Jiang CX, Katsar CS, Lan TH, Lin YR, Ming R, Wright RJ. Comparative Genomics of Plant Chromosomes. The Plant Cell, 2000; Vol. 12, 1523–1539.

[24] Candan F, Şık L, Kesercioğlu T. Cytotaxonomical studies on some *Crocus* L. taxa in Turkey, African Journal of Biotechnology, 2009; Vol. 8(18), 4374-4377.

[25] Candan F, Kesercioğlu T, Öztürk Çalı İ. A Cytotaxonomical Investigation on 4 Crocus L. Taxa in Anatolia:proceedings in 20. National Biology Congress, 21-25 June 2010, Pamukkale University, Denizli, Turkey.

[26] Inoue S, Iwatsuki Z. A cytotaxonomic study of the genus *Rhizogonium* Brid. (*Musci*). J. Hattori Bot. Lab.1976; 41:389-403.

[27] Aydın Ş. Cytotaxonomical investigations on some *Musci* species which exist in Aegean Region. PhD Thesis, Dokuz Eylül University, Biology Education Department, Izmir, Turkey; 2000.

[28] Mathew B. Crocus: In Davis, P.H. (ed.), The Flora of Turkey and The East Aegean Islands, Edinburgh University, 1984; 8:413-438.

[29] Peurtas MJ, Carmona R. Greater Ability of Pollen Tube Growth in Rye Plants with 2B Chromosomes. Theoretical and Applied Genetics, 1976; 47:41-43.

[30] Elçi Ş. Investigation Methods and Observations of Cytogenetics. 100. Year University Publisher, Van, Turkey; 1994.

[31] Jones RN. B Chromosome Systems in Flowering Plants and Animal Species. International Review of Cytology, 1975; 40:1-100.

[32] Stebbins GL. Chromosomal Evolution In Higher Plants. Addison-Wesley, Reading, MA; 1971.

[33] Gönüz A, Kesercioğlu T, Akı C. Basic Principles of Cytotaxonomy. Çanakkale 18 Mart University Publisher, Çanakkale, Turkey; 2009.

[34] Şık L, Candan F. Ecological properties of some *Crocus* taxa in Turkey. African Journal of Biotechnology, 2009; Vol. 8(9), 1895-1899.

[35] O' Mara JG. Observations on the immediate effects of colchicine. Journal of Heredity, 1939; 30:35-37.

[36] İnce HH. Plant Preperation Techniques. Ege University Publisher; 1989.

[37] Öztürk Çalı İ. Cytogenetic Effects of Fungicide Applications on Meiosis of Tomato (*Lycopersicon esculentum* Mill.). Turkish Journal of Biology, 2009; 33(3): 205-209.

[38] Feulgen R, Rossenbeck H. Mikroskopich-chemischer nachweis einer nucleinsäure von typus der thymonucleinsäure und die darauf beruhende elektive färbung von zellkeren in mikroskopischer präparaten. Hoppe-Seyler's Zeitschrift für Physiologische Chemie, 1924; 135:203-248.

[39] Darlington CD, La Cour LF. The Handling of Chromosomes. Sixth edition, London, George Allen and Unwin Ltd.; 1976.

[40] Candan F, Batır MB, Büyük İ. Determination Of DNA Changes in Seedlings Of Artichoke (*Cynara scolymus* L.) And Runner Bean (*Phaseolus coccineus* L.) Seeds Exposed To Copper (Cu) And Lead (Pb) Heavy Metal Stress, Celal Bayar University Scientific Research Project, 2012 (the project is not finished).

[41] Kesercioğlu T, Öztürk Çalı İ. Effects of pyrimethanil on pollen meiosis of tomato plant (*Lycopersıcon lycopersicum* Mill.). Bangladesh Journal of Botany, 2008; 36(1): 85-88.

[42] Simpkins J, Williams JI. Advenced Biology. Bell&Tlyman LTD. London; 1986.

[43] Öztürk Çalı İ, Candan F. Seed Macromorphological Investigations On Two Endemic Species (*Linaria corifolia* Desf. and *Jurinea pontica* Hausskn. & Freyn ex Hausskn.) From Turkey:proceedings of the International Conference on Climate, Environment and Water Related Matters, BALWOIS, 28 May-2 June 2012f, Ohrid, Republic of Macedonia.

[44] Candan F, Uysal T, Tugay O, Ertuğrul K. Achene Macromorphological Investigations on 21 Endemic Taxa of *Centaurea* Section *Acrolophus* (Asteraceae) From Turkey:proceedings of the International Symposium on Biology of Rare and Endemic Plant Species, BIORARE, 23-27 April 2012g, Fethiye, Turkey.

[45] Candan F, Tugay O, Uysal T, Ertuğrul K. Achene Micromorphological Investigations on *Centaurea* Section *Acrolophus* (Asteraceae) From Turkey:proceedings of the International Symposium on Biology of Rare and Endemic Plant Species, BIORARE, 23-27 April 2012h, Fethiye, Turkey.

[46] Öztürk Çalı, İ. The Effects of Fosetyl-Al Application on morphology and viability of *Lycopersicon esculentum* Mill. pollen. Plant, Soil and Environment, 2008a; 54(8): 336-340.

[47] Martinez-Toledo MV, Salmeron V, Rodelas B. Effects of the fungicide Captan on some functional groups of soil microflora. Applied Soil Ecology, 1998; 7: 245-255.

[48] Marcano l, Carruyo I, Del Campo A. Cytotoxicity and made of action of Maleic hydrazide in root tips of *Allium cepa* L. Environmental Research, 2004; 94: 221-226.

[49] Behera BN, Sahu RK, Sharma CBSR. Cytogenetic hazards from agricultural chemicals 4. Sequential screening in the barley progeny test for cytogenetic activity of some systemic fungicides and a metabolite. Toxicology Letters, 1982; 10(2-3), 195-203.

[50] Fairbanks MM, Hardy GESJ, McComb JA. Mitosis and meiosis in plants are affected by the fungicide phosphite. Australasian Plant Pathology, 2002; 31(3), 281-289.

[51] Grover IS, Tyagi PS. Cytological effects of some common pesticides in barley. Environmental and Experimental Botany, 1980; 20(3): 243-245.

[52] Öztürk Çalı İ. Effects of fungicide on meiosis of tomato (*Lycopersicon esculentum* Mill.). Bangladesh Journal of Botany, 2008b; 37(2): 121-125.

[53] Öztürk Çalı İ, Kesercioğlu T. Effects of Fosetyl-Al, a fungicide on meiosis of *Lycopersicon esculentum* Mill. Bangladesh Journal of Botany, 2010; 39(2): 237-240

[54] Öztürk Çalı İ, Candan F. Effects of a fungucide on the morphology and viability of pollens of tomato (*Lycopersicon esculentum* Mill.). Bangladesh Journal of Botany, 2009; 38 (2):115-118.

[55] Öztürk Çalı İ, Candan F. The effect of fungicide application on pollen structure in tomato (*Lycopersicon esculentum* Mill.) plant. Journal of Applied Biological Sciences, 2009; 3(1): 56-59.

[56] Öztürk Çalı İ, Candan F. The effect of activator application on the anatomy, morphology and viability of *Lycopersicon esculentum* Mill. Pollen. Turkish Journal of Biology, 2010; 34, 281-286.

[57] Candan F, Öztürk Çalı İ. A Palinological Investigation on Natural and Commercial forms of *Anemone coronaria* L. (A. *coronaria* var. *coccinea* (Jord.) Burn, *A. coronaria* var. *rosea* (Hanry) Batt, *A. coronaria* var. *cyanea*, *A. coronaria* var. *alba* Goaty&Pens):proceedings in 10. National Ecology and Environmental Congress, 04-07 October 2011, Çanakkale 18 Mart University, Çanakkale, Turkey.

[58] http://www.mortonarb.org/tree-plant-advice/article/751/plant-galls.html (accesed 10 August 2012).

Chapter 11

The Effects of Different Combinations and Varying Concentrations of Growth Regulators on the Regeneration of Selected Turkish Cultivars of Melon

Dilek Tekdal and Selim Cetiner

Additional information is available at the end of the chapter

http://dx.doi.org/10.5772/55455

1. Introduction

Cucurbits are an economically important family of plants. The majority of the vegetable production in Turkey, for example, derives from the species beloning to the family *Cucurbitaceae.* Despite the importance of cucurbits among vegetable crops worldwide, the development of genomic tools in these species has been rather limited. Although melon production has been improved by conventional plant breeding methods, output is still insufficient. One useful technique in overcoming such problems in melon is functional genomics' studies, and the other one is abiotic stress resistance and improved fruit quality has been gene transfer via *Agrobacterium tumefaciens* mediated transformation. The availability of an optimized plant regeneration system is crucial for genetic transformation techniques as well as obtaining an entire plant. Although Hasanbey and Cinikiz in Turkey, for example, are important commercial melon cultivars used in the breeding programs and molecular biology of fruit ripening and genetic mapping of melons, there is no study to date on the regeneration of these cultivars. The objectives of the present study are thus to develop and optimize an efficient *in vitro* regeneration protocol for *Cucumis melo* L. and investigate the effects of different genotypes and growth regulators on the *in vitro* regeneration of melon. In this paper, we discuss the following topics: general information on the family *Cucurbitaceae,* the importance of melon production both in Turkey and in the world; lastly, the efficiency of *in vitro* culture techniques on melon propagation are presented with data relevant to our laboratory research. We assume that statement of the research findings presented here lead to for further studies on *in vitro* propagation of melon.

1.1. The family cucurbitaceae

The family *Cucurbitaceae* consists of cucumbers and melon as two major commercial vegetable crops and two minor crops, the West Indian Gherkin and the Kiwano, respectively. They are cultivated, economically useful crops [1]. According to the infrageneric classification, the genus *Cucumis* is divided into two subgenera based on the different base chromosome numbers of *Cucumis; Cucumis* subgen. *Cucumis* and. *Cucumis* subgen. *Melo*. Whereas *Cucumis* subgen *Cucumis* has x=7 chromosome numbers, *Cucumis* subgen. *Melo* has x=12 [2]. *Cucumis melo* is the type of the genus *Melo*. As a cucurbit crop, *melon* (*Cucumis melo*) has 552 synonyms and can be divided into three types: cantaloupe melons, musk melons and winter melons [1,3]. Melon is a valuable human food source cultivated in arid and semiarid regions of the world [4]. The family *Cucurbitaceae* is hypothesized to be consisted of the species' open-polination. Due to this open pollination within melon varieties, new melon species have emerged; hence *in vitro* propagation enables *in vitro* conservation of different melon genotypes carrying a variety of desired traits [5].

1.2. The importance of melon production in the world

Melon (*Cucumis melo* L. *2n=2x=24*) is a diploid species with various phenotypic characters due to its adaptation under diverse agroecological conditions from the Mediterranean to Eastern Asia (Figure1).

Melons are grown in both temperate and tropical regions. Due to various morphological variations in its fruit characteristics such as size, colour, shape, taste and texture, melons are hence described an extensive diverse group. In addition, *Cucumis melo* L. can be divided into three groups or types: *Cantaloupensis* (Cantaloup or Musk melon) group, *Inodorous group* (Winter melon or Casaba) and *Reticulatus* (Ananas) group. Genotypes of these three groups can be crossbred [5, 6].

Although Africa is the origin of the melon, the diversification center for this fruit encompasses all Asian countries from Turkey to Japan. China, Turkey, Iran, and USA produce 57% of the melon annual production in the world [3-6].

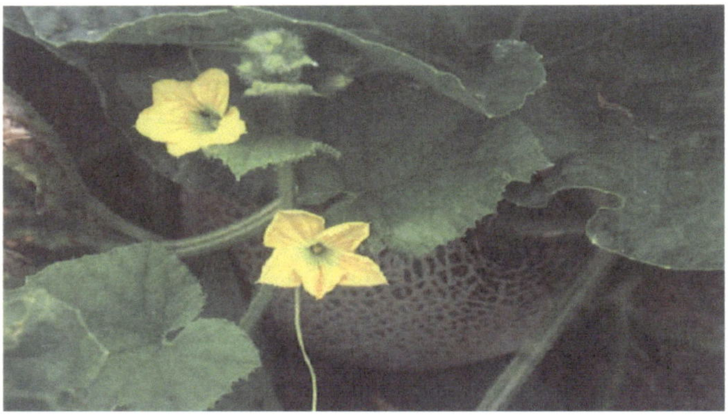

Figure 1. General view of flower and fruit of melon (adapted from [7])

Melon fruits are the valuable food sources with robust vitamin and mineral composition (Table 1) as well as economic values [8].

Composition	*Inodorous Melon Groups*
Overall Compositions	
Water (g)	91.85
Minerals (mg)	218.41
Proteins (g)	1.11
Total Lipid (Fat) (g)	0.10
Carbohydrate (g)	6.58
Fibre, total dietary (g)	0.9
Sugars, total (g)	5.69
Vitamins	
Vitamin K (μg)	2.5
Vitamin C (mg)	21.8
Thiamin (mg)	0.015
Riboflavin (mg)	0.031
Niacin (mg)	0.232
Folate (mcg)	8
Vitamn B6 (mg)	0.163
Vitamin E (mg)	0.05

Table 1. Nutritional compositions of the media used for micropropagation of Hasanbey and Cinikiz melons (value per 100 g of edible portion) *From USDA Nutrient Database, July 2012 [12]

Melons provide several nutrients involving protein (0,6-1,2%/100 g) vitamin E,, vitamin C, and Vitamin K for human metabolic reactions in daily dietary [9, 10]. Melon fruits are used in production of deserts, such as jam, ice cream, yogurt as well as soup (from the juice), pickling and cosmetics [11].

A characteristic skin color and aroma for melons are the primary traits sought by melon breeders. In addition, the development and ripening of melon fruits are very complicated due to the many biochemical and physiological changes comprising cell wall degradation, alteration in pigment biosynthesis, aromatic compounds, and increasing of sugar content. Therefore, performing the ex-situ regeneration of melon is very important for the research focused on improving the agronomic traits of melon *in vitro* conditions.

1.3. The importance of melon production in turkey

Turkey is an important country for cultivation of the economically important plant family *Cucurbitaceae* [13, 14]. Although the nation is not a primary center of melon diversification, it is the second largest producer after China in the world [15]. 38% of vegetable production in Turkey are *Cucurbitaceae* species which are watermelon, melon, cucumber, squash, and pumpkin. Of the 26,7 million tons of melon produced worldwide, 1,749 million tons of production, emerges from Turkey [16, 17] Central Anatolia is the main melon production region in Turkey. Ankara, Balikesir, Diyarbakir, Konya and Manisa are the provinces of highest melon production in Turkey [18]. The main production states are shown in Figure 2 [5,18].

In Turkey, the most popular cultivars are Yuva, Kirkagac, Kislik Sari Kuscular, Hidir, Cumra, Cinikiz and Hasanbey and melons are cultivated on landraces of less than 5 ha in size. Due to climatic conditions, melon harvesting in Turkey can change based on cultivation regions, but generally it is done from June to September [18].

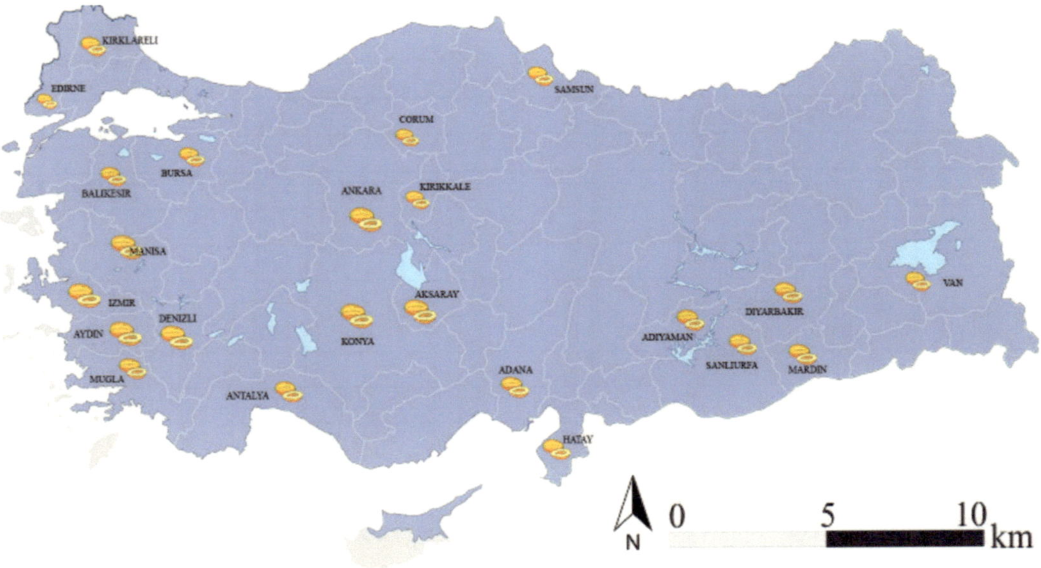

Figure 2. Melon production regions in Turkey

1.4. The importance of in vitro propagation of melon varieties

In vitro propagation provides a great number of clonal plants in a short time. This techique is based on the theory that a new plantlet can be derived from the use of any plant parts (leaf, shoot, root, etc.) on a suitable initial medium [19, 20]. The nutritional composition of a culture medium for optimal growth of a plant tissue is based on plant genotype [20]. Thus, the method established to manipulate plant tissues and cells is not only essential for *in vitro* propagation of valuable plants but also required to regenerate transgenic plants [1, 19]. Due to the fact that most commercial melon varieties have been subjected to viral pathogens, defects in fruit quality and absent yield have resulted in major economic losses [8]. For *in vitro* conservation of melon, *in vitro* propagation among melon varieties, has been implemented to obtain clonally propagated genotypes of melon [21]. In addition, due to the small-sized genome, high polymorphism, and short generation time of the melon, genetic transformation could be possible in the melon [22, 23]. There are several reports of the genetic tranformation of melon with a variety of marker genes, as well as genes for viral resistance, abiotic stress resistance, and fruit quality attributes [13, 24-34] Also some reports suggest that transformation in melon is strictly limited by genotype [26, 28]. This event makes this crop a good target for transformation protocols [35]. It has been shown that genetic transformatin on melon via *Agrobacterium tumefaciens* is limited to a few varieties. Since the difficulty of that melon regeneration is well known [36, 37, 38] the findings of our study on melon regeneration thus hope to constitute a source for further studies on profitable melon breeding.

1.5. Two important turkish melon cultivars: Hasanbey and Cinikiz

The local melon genotypes are the primary production resources of melon production in Turkey [14]. Hasanbey (Figure 3) and Cinikiz melon (Figure 4) varieties are the domestic farmgate *inodorous* melon crops. 85% of melon production in Turkey consists of *Inodorous* (Hasanbey, Cinikiz, Kirkagac, Kuscular, Hirsiz Calmaz and Yuva) and 15% occurs in *Cantaloupensis* (Macdimon, Galia, Polidor and Falez) and *Reticulatus* (Ananas, Topatan, Barada). Moreover, In Turkey Flexuosus melon cultivars and Dudaim type of melons are grown in small quantities [8]. *Cantalupensis* type melons are commonly cultivated in the Mediterranean region of Turkey, whereas the *Inodorous* melons are grown mainly in the Central Anatolia, Aegean and Southeastern Anatolia regions of Turkey. *Inodorous* group has the largest number of cultivars in Turkey [39].

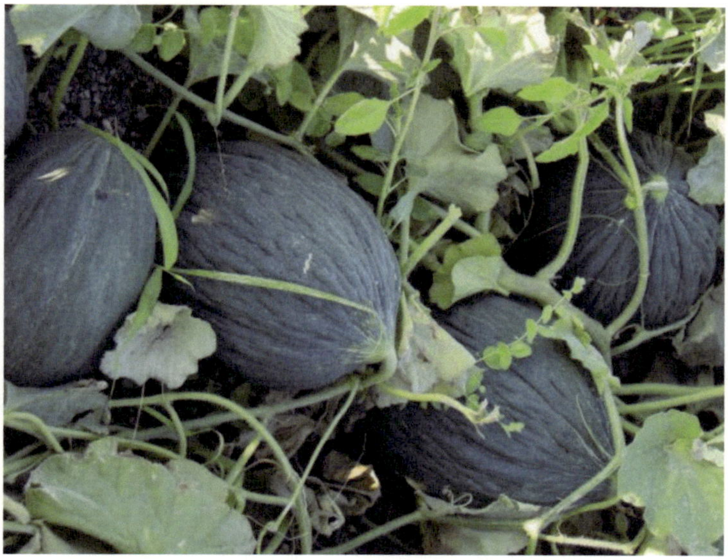

Figure 3. Hasanbey melon fruits(adapted from [40])

Hasanbey melon is commonly grown in Western Anatolia in Turkey. This variety is round and dark green with a long shelf life. The Hasanbey melon cultivar is harvested from August to September due to its late ripening period [4]. Cinikiz melons are grown in the Central Anatolia in Turkey. This melon group has the highest ascorbic acid, sweetness and sugar content. The immature fruits of the Cinikiz melon have a light green skin color with dark green spots; mature fruits, a yellow colored skin [16, 18].

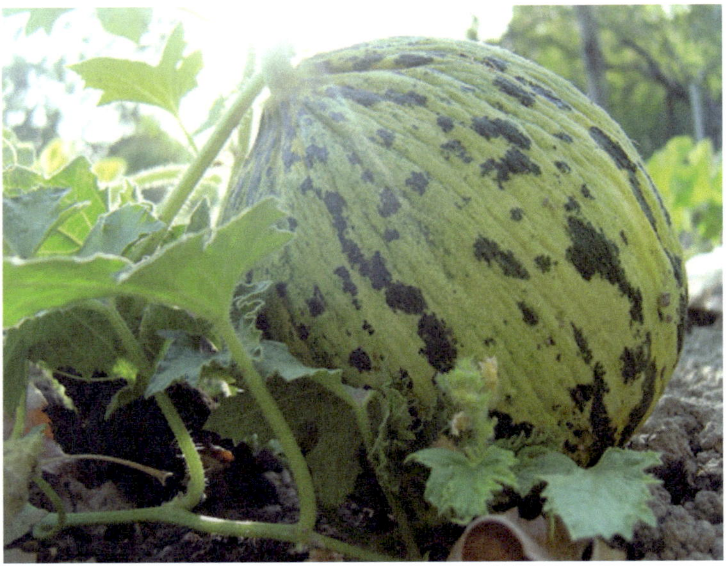

Figure 4. Cinikiz melon fruits (adapted from [41])

Individual plants of the Hasanbey or Cinikiz melon genotypes under *in vitro* conditions develop organs of similar size due to the elimination of environmental conditions and are, genetically controlled. Because of the interspecific and intergeneric incompatibility barriers in melons, some conventional methods such as hybridization and line fixing for improvement of melon cultivars are quite limitied as well as expensive [42, 43]. We assume that the outcomes from the present study may provide good sources for futher transformation studies on the genotypes of Hasanbey and Cinikiz melon groups [10, 44].

In the light of these facts, we hypothesize that an efficient regeneration method of economically important Turkish Cultivars, Cinikiz and Hasanbey, allows comparison of two different melon cultivars in regard to regeneration ability under an identical artificial medium. In the present study, two Turkish melon varieties were tested for *in vitro* regeneration ability cultured on Murashige ans Skoog (MS) media containing different combinations and varying concentrations of growth regulators.

2. Meterials and methods

2.1. Materials

2.1.1. Seed sources

Mature seeds of *Cucumis melo* L. cv. Hasanbey and Cinikiz were used as explants sources. The seeds of Hasanbey and Cinikiz melon varieties were obtained from Laboratory for Plant Biotechnology in Horticulture Department, Agriculture Faculty, Cukurova University, Adana, Turkey.

2.1.2. *Media and culture conditions*

The achievement of *in vitro* tissue culture hinges on the composition of the medium, growth regulators, plant genotypes, explant sources, growth and culture conditions. Culture media used in this study are based on MS salts [20].

After surface sterilization, for the initiation of seed cultures, 10 seeds were placed into 100x15mm petri dishes containing basal MS basal medium with MS vitamins, 3% (w/v) sucrose and 0.75% (w/v) agar for three days. The pH level of the medium was adjusted to 5.7 prior to adding gelling agents. The media were sterilized by autoclaving at 121°C for 20 minutes.

Cultures were incubated in a growth room at 25±2°C at dark for three days. In vitro grown cotyledon pieces of mature seeds were transferred into regeneration medium containing different concentrations of IAA (0.0, 2.5, 5.0 mg L^{-1}), Kin (0.0, 2.5, 5.0 mg L^{-1}) and NAA (0.0, 0.5 mg L^{-1}) for organogenesis. Cotyledon explants were incubated at 25±2°C under 16 h photoperiod provided by cool white fluorescent lamps.

2.2. Methods

2.2.1. *Surface sterilization of seeds*

Melon seed coats were removed and the seeds were dipped into 70% ethanol for ten minutes and kept in 20% sodium hypochlorite with 2 drops of Tween-20 per 100 ml solution with occasional shaking for 10 minutes. The seeds were then rinsed three consecutive times with sterile distilled water and blotted dry in a laminar flow cabinet. After straining the water, the seeds were placed directly on the culture medium under sterile conditions.

2.2.2. *Seed germination*

For seed germination, 10 seeds in each of the 100x15mm petri dishes containing the culture medium containing MS salts [20], MS vitamins and 3% (w/v) sucrose, gelling agent were placed.

Cultures were maintained on a hormone free MS medium for five days in a growth chamber at 25±1°C in darkness.

2.2.3. *Plant regeneration treatments*

In vitro plant regeneration is based on the balance of cytokinin and auxin and the quality of the explant sources during plant development. To evaluate the efficiency of various growth regulators, cotyledon explants were excised from *in vitro* grown seedlings after seed germination and then placed with the abaxial side onto the surface of a solified regeneration medium variants, consisting of MS basal medium supplemented with growth regulators, auxins (NAA and IAA) and cytokinins (Kinetin) in different combinations (see Table 2 for concentrations of growth regulators).

The explants obtained from the part proximal to the apex of the seedling were taken to induction medium. All media were sealed with parafilm and maintained in a growth room at

25±2°C under dark conditions. Every combination of growth regulators was used in the medium for each melon genotype. The experiment was set as a total of 22 treatments for both of the melon genotypes; each treatment was carried out in triplicates containing ten explants in each culture medium.

Concentrations of growth regulators (mg L^{-1}) in the culture media used for propagation		
NAA	**IAA**	**Kinetin**
0	0	0
0	2,5	0
0	2,5	2,5
0	2,5	5,0
0	5,0	0
0	5,0	2,5
0	5,0	5,0
0,5	0	0
0,5	0	2,5
0,5	0	5,0
0,5	5,0	5,0

Table 2. MS media supplemented with different growth regulators for plant regeneration

The regeneration ability of each genotype was then scored weekly for a period of 6 weeks. The data on seed germination and plant regeneration were collected and regenerated plants less than 1 mm in length were not taken into consideration.

3. Results and discussion

3.1. Seed germination

The germination ability of the melon seeds can be affected by both internal and external factors. Since seed size is considered important for better germination [45-47], seeds in similar size were selected for both genotypes. Germination ratio of the Cinikiz melon seeds was found higher (85%) than that of the Hasanbey seeds (78%) under the same culture conditions.

3.2. *In vitro* plant regeneration

In the study presented here, cotyledons from *in vitro* grown seedlings were explant sources. In all experiments, basic MS medium containing MS salts, MS vitamins and sucrose (30 g L^{-1}) was used.

Different concentrations and combinations of IAA (0,0, 2,5, 5,0 mg L^{-1}), Kin (0,0, 2,5, 5,0 mg L^{-1}) and NAA (0.0, 0.5 mg L^{-1}) were investigated to optimize regeneration of two comercially important Turkish melon varieties: Hasanbey and Cinikiz.

There were significant differences between two melon varieties based on the growth regulator concentrations. According to our findings, comparison of the genotypes showed that the Cinikiz melon cultivar has better regeneration abilitythan did the Hasanbey melon. In addition, the maximum shoot regeneration was achieved on MS medium supplemented with 2,5 mg L^{-1} IAA and 2,5 mg L^{-1} Kin was determined the best regeneration medium for both cultivars. Moreover, NAA was foun to be the best growth regulator in the induction of callus of both melon variaties. NAA alone induced direct callus formation, while Kin exhibited synergism with IAA for induction bud formation for both two varieties.

To date propagation of *Cucumis melo* has been reported by different research groups [34, 36, 48, 49, 50, 51]. The main differences between the present study and the earlier ones are the growth regulators used and melon cultivars selected. We used Hasanbey and Cinikiz melon cultivars as explants; while the others used 'Amarillo oro' [48, 51], 'Accent', 'Galia', 'Presto', and 'Viva' [36], 'Revigal' and 'Kirkagac' [34, 50], 'Topmark' [49, 50]. After three weeks on a MS medium free from plant growth regulator, approximately 80% of cotyledon explants gave rise to friable callus (Figure 5). Calli were found from the cut surface of cotyledon explants within 5 days. In a previous study, however, direct shoot formation was obtained from cotyledon explants cultured on MS medium supplemented with 1,0 mg L^{-1} BA [36].

In our study, the media containing 0,5 mg L^{-1} NAA showed that supplying NAA in the medium increased the callus formation, although the IAA and Kin concentration (5 mg L^{-1}) was the identical to that of previous study[36]. The addition of NAA alone in our experiment stimulated formation of the callus. The best callus formation ratios were observed from the media containing 0,5 mg L^{-1} NAA, 5 mg L^{-1} IAA and 5 mg L^{-1} Kin for Cinikiz and Hasanbey melon cultivars 100% and 87%, respectively. The medium containing 0,5 mg L^{-1} NAA, 5 mg L^{-1} IAA and 5 mg L^{-1} Kin stimulated callus growth for Hasanbey melon cultivar. On the contrary, the frequency of callus formation for Cinikiz melon genotype due to NAA concentration was significant. In all medium containing 0,5 mg L^{-1} NAA, high callus formation (100%) from Cinikiz melons' cotyledons was obtained (Table 3).

The calli were white to yellowish; their surface showed structures such as shoot formation and the calli were rarely regenerative. Our result agrees with the reported callus formation from the plants regenerated *in vitro* [50].

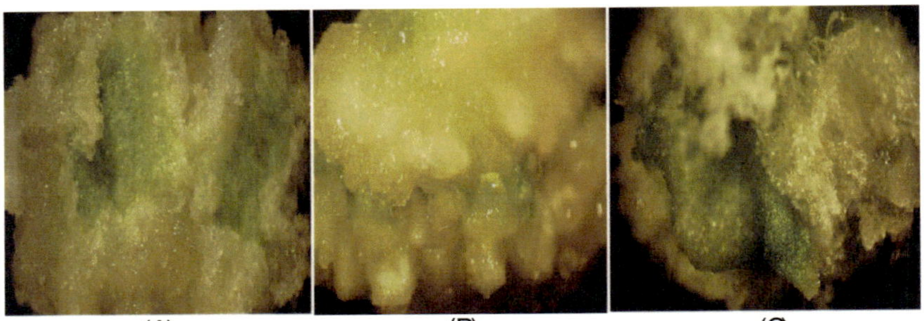

(A) (B) (C)

Figure 5. A) Callus formation from cotyledon explants on the MS hormone free medium, (B) Callus formation from 'Cinikiz' cotyledon explants and (C) 'Hasanbey' cotyledon explants on the MS medium supplemented with 0,5 mg L^{-1} NAA, 5 mg L^{-1} IAA and 5 mg L^{-1} Kin.

In an earlier study on regeneration of melon, shoot buds were obtained at high rates in cotyledon explants [48] and well-developed shoots were observed from calli growing MS media containing 1,5 mg L^{-1} IAA and 6,0 mg L^{-1} Kin.

According to previous study, [48] Kin was essential for shoot formation. *Cucumis melo* L. cv. In our study, Cinikiz gave better shoot production than Hasanbey cultivar. The explants produce fragile and large callus; within 15 days direct shoot organogenesis had occured. The frequencies of bud formation were increased by the combination of 2,5 mg L^{-1} IAA and 2,5 mg L^{-1} Kin compared to 2,5 mg L^{-1} Kin and 0,5 mg L^{-1} NAA. On the other hand, the bud formation of the Hasanbey melon genotype was higher than the Cinikiz melon genotype on the medium including solely 2,5 mg L^{-1} IAA. When the concentration of IAA were increased, the frequency of bud formation for Hasanbey melon variety decreaed. A high frequency of induction of bud for Cinikiz melon genotype occured on the medium supplemented with same concentration of IAA and Kin, but when the concentrations of IAA and NAA were increased with the same level, bud formation for Hasanbey melon was not observed. It was found that IAA and Kin combination at the same concentration (2,5 mg L^{-1}) increased the regeneration ratio. We were able to induce bud formation by culture of the explants on MS medium with 0,5 mg L^{-1} NAA for both melon cultivars. This result is similar to those of early studies on melon regeneration [49, 50] where it was known that the medium containing NAA stimulated callus growth.

Of the growth regulators tested, NAA was the most effective at inducing callus creation from the cotyledons of both two melon genotypes presented here (Table 3).

The media used in the study presented containing IAA alone or in combination with Kin never trigger callus creation. This result is similar to previous studies [43, 48, 49].

Development in regeneration from the melon Hasanbey cotyledon explants on the medium added 2,5 mg L^{-1} IAA and 2,5 mg L^{-1} Kin was found to be slower than with melon Cinikiz.

After 4 weeks in the culture, there was little further development on the explants of Hasanbey melon cultivar compared to that of Cinikiz.

Treatments ($mg\ L^{-1}$)			Variables					
			Callus creation (%)		Bud formation(%)		Shoot regeneration ratio (%)	
			Melon genotypes		Melon genotypes		Melon genotypes	
			Hasanbey	Cinikiz	Hasanbey	Cinikiz	Hasanbey	Cinikiz
IAA	NAA	Kin						
0	0	0	0	0	10	12	0	0
2,5	0	0	0	0	62	50	0	0
2,5	0	2,5	0	0	50	78	50	75
2,5	0	5,0	0	0	37	62	25	12
5,0	0	0	0	0	50	75	0	5
5,0	0	2,5	0	0	50	50	0	0
5,0	0	5,0	0	0	0	62	0	0
0	0,5	0	50	100	25	25	20	15
0	0,5	2,5	50	100	0	12	0	2
0	0,5	5,0	75	100	0	50	12	25
5,0	0,5	5,0	87	100	25	12	0	0

Table 3. Effect of IAA, NAA and Kin concentration on callus creation, bud formation and shoot regeneration percentages of Hasanbey and Cinikiz melon varieties' cotyledons on the medium containing different concentrations of IAA (0,0, 2,5, 5,0 $mg\ L^{-1}$), Kin (0,0, 2,5, 5,0 $mg\ L^{-1}$) and NAA (0,0, 0,5 $mg\ L^{-1}$)

The best results for shoot regeneration were obtained from MS medium supplemented with 2,5 $mg\ L^{-1}$ IAA and 2,5 $mg\ L^{-1}$ Kin for Cinikiz and Hasanbey melon genotypes 75% and 50%, respectively. The results of the regeneration tests are summarized in Table 3.

The regeneration efficiency of Hasanbey and Cinikiz melon using cotyledon explants was evaluated in terms of regenerated plants. Cotyledon organogenesis was induced during incubation and bud formations located along the cut basal edge of the explant were visible on 8 day-old cultures of both of the two melon varieties. On the other hand, the first shoots formed 12 day-old explants of Cinikiz melon. According our results, the Cinikiz melon cultivar gave better results than did the Hasanbey cultivar (Figure 6).

Furthermore, the most important difference was observed in the number of bud induced between the two melons. In the Cinikiz melon young tuberances often clustered in the point of regeneration and shoot meristems developed into leaves(Figure 6-A). In the Hasanbey melon, the first regenerated shoots were observed in 15 day-old cotyledon explants and regenerated shoots were originated from the epidermal layer of the ex-plants (Figure 6-B). These results as those of the previous studies show the clear cut effect of the genotype on regeneration.

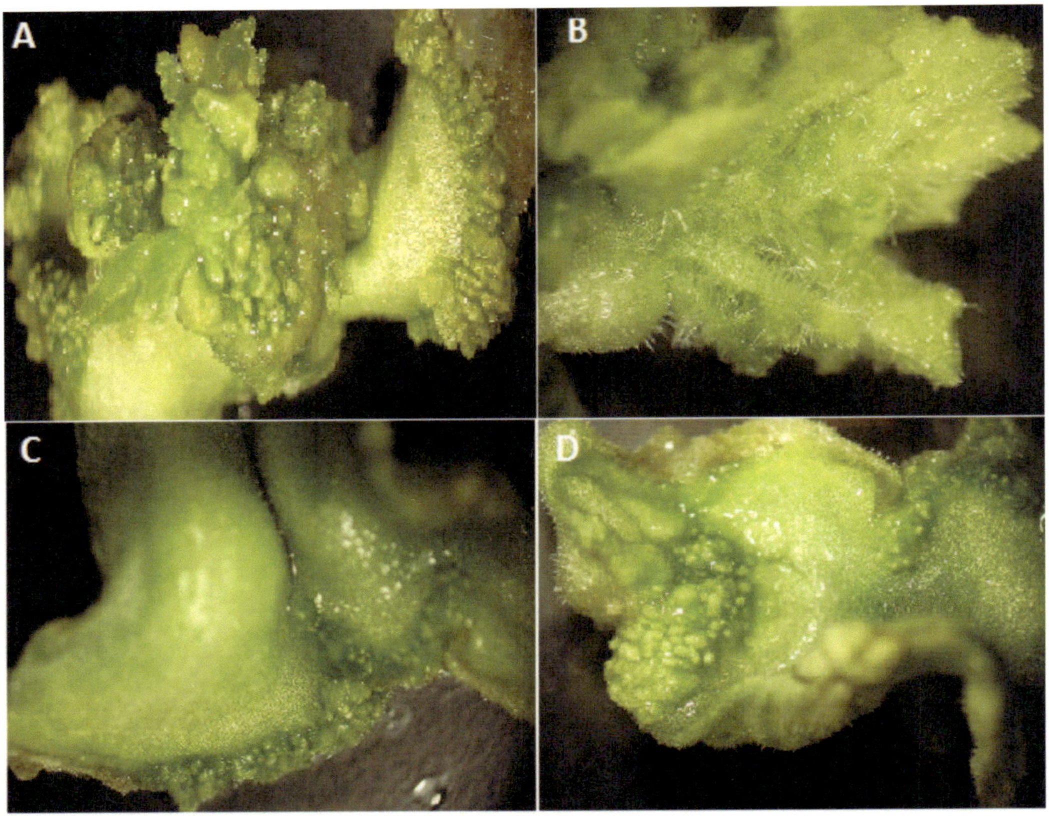

Figure 6. A, B) Shoot formation of Cinikiz melon cultivar on the MS medium added with 5,0 mg L^{-1} IAA and 2,5 mg L^{-1} Kin and (C, D) shoot formation of Hasanbey melon cultivar on the MS medium added 2,5 mg L^{-1} IAA alone

For the Hasanbey genotype, explants which were cultured on the MS medium free from plant growth regulators, showed callus formation with different coloration and appearance after 2 weeks. Most of them were white to yellowish and friable. A mass of small cells initiated the regeneration of the shoot meristems form directly on explants *in vitro*. This result is similar to previous studies [43, 50].

After 3 weeks on the medium, explants developed into buds and about a month on culturing, root formation was observed. As they continued to grow, they became yellow and did not develop into shoots. (Figure 7-A). In addition, some demonstrated necrosis. Shoot formation (50%) for Hasanbey melon genotype was obtained on a MS medium consisting of 2,5 mg L^{-1} IAA and 2,5 mg L^{-1} Kin after 2 weeks. Explants after 3 weeks of culture formed shoot structures, continued to grow, bud formation was not observed at this stage (Figure 7-B).

As a result, it was observed that the melon possessed the ability to regenerate by means of direct organogenesis from cotyledon explants. After 4 weeks in culture the explants enlarged.

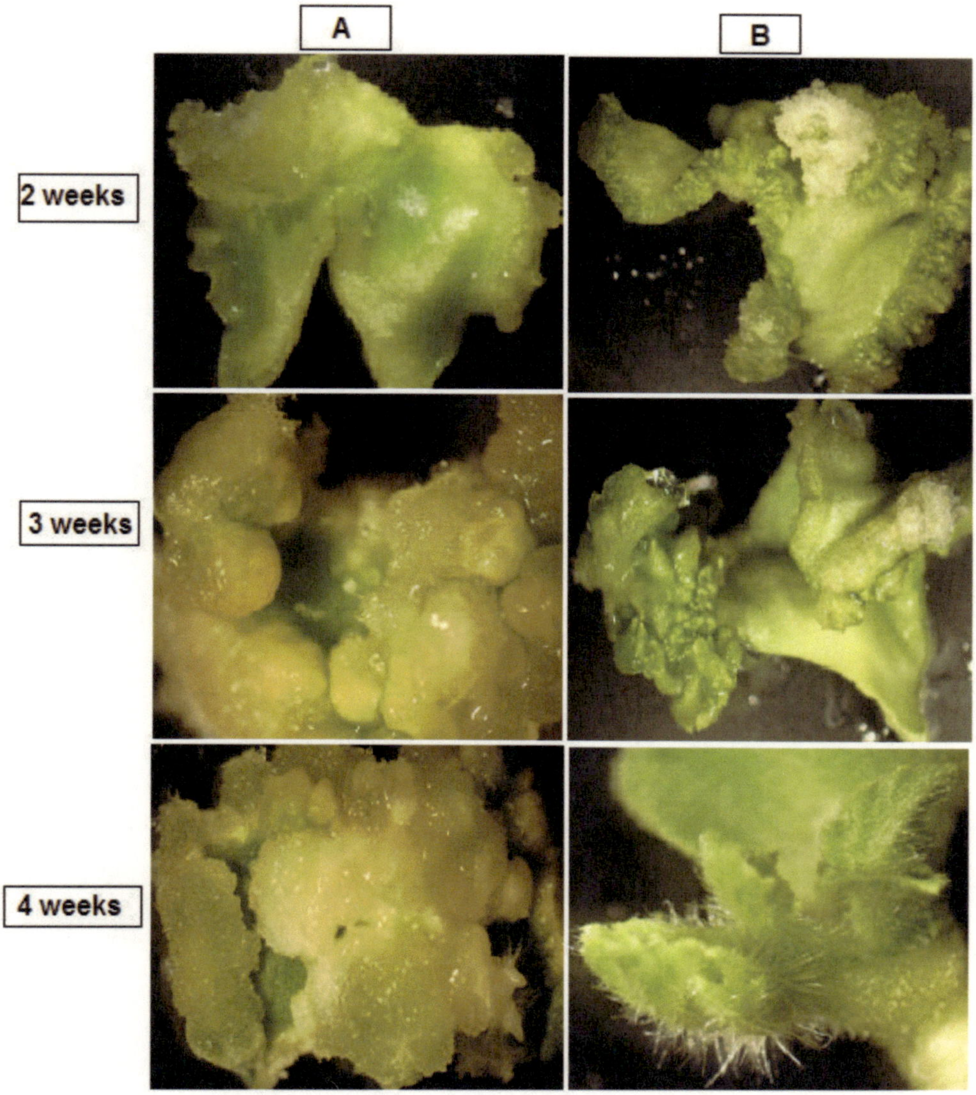

Figure 7. Hasanbey genotypes at different stages of their development. A: Control groups which developed on free plant growth MS medium, B: Explants which developed on MS medium supplemented with 2,5 mg L^{-1} IAA and 2,5 mg L^{-1} Kin

Control groups of Cinikiz melon cultivar developed on the MS medium free from plant growth regulators showed developing callus and roots (Figure 8-A). On the media containing 2,5 mg L^{-1} IAA and 2,5 mg L^{-1} Kin, the highest percentage of shoot regenerants from Cinikiz melon cultivar after 2 weeks was obtained (Figure 8-B).

In contrast by involving the control groups of Cinikiz melon cultivar on the MS medium free from plant growth regulators, shoot formation was observed. After 2 weeks, some young protuberances clustered and developed; after 4 weeks, finger-like structures were observed (Figure 8-B). After 4 weeks, no difference could be determined between protuberances that became leaves from Cinikiz samples.

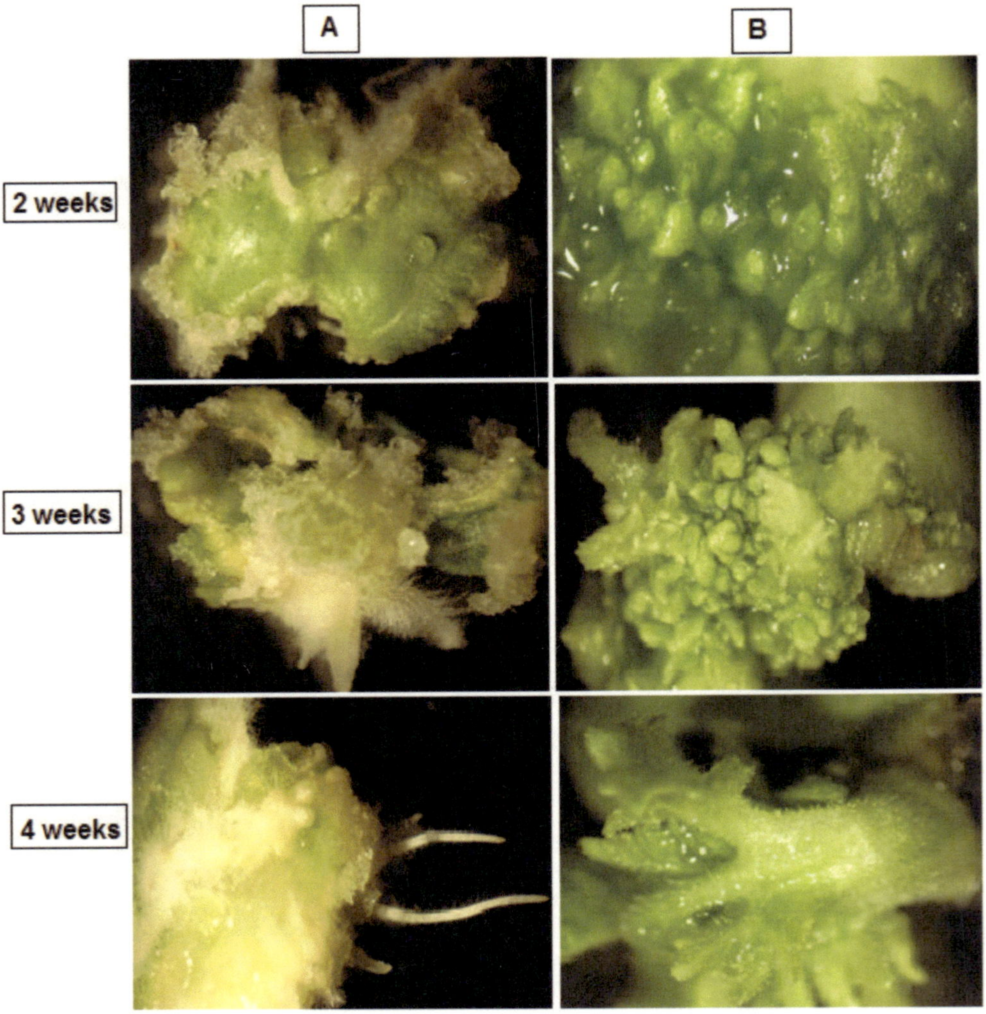

Figure 8. Cinikiz genotypes at different stages of their development. A: Control groups which developed on free plant growth MS medium, B: Explants which developed on MS medium added with 2,5 mg L^{-1} IAA and 2,5 mg L^{-1} Kin

4. Conclusion

Our in vitro propagation results from these two melon varieties, Hasanbey and Cinikiz, were selected as research material for the study presented here due to their importance for the

Turkish agricultural production. Due to open pollination, melon varieties can be more or less stable against environmental factors from one generation to the next. In addition, as can be seen from the results presented here, Hasanbey and Cinikiz melon genotypes can be *in vitro* propagated.

On the other hand, further studies are needed to analyze other Turkish melon varieties and identify the optimum regeneration medium for each genotype. In addition, if the response of the two melon cultivars selected in this study is observed from the point of view of breeder significance, experimental fields should be conducted in future studies. Understanding the role of growth regulators in the development of selected melon cultivars has highly facilitated melon production under controlled environments. Moreover, the resulting information can be also used for research on melon developmental physiology, an intensive continuation of *in vitro* propagation studies is essential, as well.

Acknowledgements

The authors are grateful to Laboratory of Plant Biotechnology in Horticulture Department, Agriculture Faculty, Cukurova University, Adana, Turkey for kindly provided the germplasms used in the study. We also thank Nancy Karabeyoglu for critically reading this manuscript and providing valuable comments for its improvement.

Author details

Dilek Tekdal* and Selim Cetiner

Biological Sciences and Bioengineering Program, Sabancı University, Istanbul TR, Turkey

References

[1] Kirkbride, J. H. Biosystematic Monograph of the Genus *Cucumis* (*Cucurbitaceae*). USA: Parkway Publishers; (1993). http://www.google.com.tr/books?hl=tr&lr=&id=-6rIPLDYg_4C&oi=fnd&pg=PR9&dq=cucurbitaceae&ots=nF-9yr9SF7&sig=wNJUIF-q4QAunk9xZV1_SU-ZXUQ&redir_esc=y#v=onepage&q=cucurbitaceae&f=falseaccessed 11 July 2012).

[2] Achigan-Dako, EG. . Phylogenetic and Genetic Variation Analysis in Cucurbit Species (*Cucurbitaceae*) from West Africa: Definition of Conservation Strategies. Göttingen: Cuvillier Verlag, 2008. http://books.google.com.tr/books?id=HLMNiLc2U4sC&pg=PA102&lpg=PA102&dq=A+review+of+the+cucurbitaceae&source=bl&ots=jn2vB5PN0h&sig=TY7VJ_KI2Io9X_wEFLLc5MlND4&hl=tr&sa=

X&ei=JTYRUOTpKa_O4QSmtYD4Dw&ved=0CEIQ6AEwADgK#v=onepage&q=A%20review%20of%20the%20cucurbitaceae&f=false (accessed 26 July 2012).

[3] Jeffry, C. A Review of The *Cucurbitaceae*. Botanical Journal of The Linnean Society. (1980). , 81, 233-247.

[4] Sivritepe, N, Sivritepe, H. O, & Eris, A. The Effects of NaCl Priming on Salt Tolerance in Melon Seedlings Grown Under Saline Conditions. Scientia Horticulturae. (2003). , 97, 229-237.

[5] Kucuk, A, Abak, K, & Sari, N. Cucurbit Genetic Resources Collections in Turkey. In: Diez MJ, Pico B, Nuez F. Cucurbit Genetic Resources in Europe: proceedings of the First Ad Hoc Meeting on Cucurbit Genetic Resources, 19 January (2002). Adana, Turkey.

[6] Pèrin, C, Hagen, L. S, Conto, V. D, Katzir, N, Danin-poleg, Y, Portnoy, V, Baudracco-arnas, S, Chadoeuf, J, Dogimont, C, & Pitrat, M. A Reference Map of *Cucumis melo* Based on Two Recombinant Inbred Line Populations. Theoretical and Applied Genetics. (2002). , 104, 1017-1034.

[7] Educational Series of Farmers-44http://www.jains.com.tr/uploaded/kavun-karpuz-yetistiriciligipdf1.pdfaccessed 23 July (2012).

[8] Ekbic, E, Fidan, H, Yildiz, M, & Abak, K. Screening of Turkish Melon Accessions for Resistance to ZYMV, WMV and CMV. Notulae Scientia Biologicae. (2010). , 2(1), 55-57.

[9] Lorenz, O. A, & Maynard, D. N. Knott's Handbook for Vegetable Growers. John Wiley & Sons, Inc, USA, (1988). p.

[10] Li, Z, Yao, L, Yang, Y, & Li, A. Transgenic Approach to Improve Quality Traits of Melon Fruits. Scientia Horticulturae. (2006). , 108, 268-277.

[11] Wien, H. C. The Cucurbits: Cucumber, Melon, Squash and Pumpkin (H.C. Wien). The Physiology of Vegetable Crops. CAB International, Wallingford, Oxon. (1997). , 9, 345-386.

[12] [12]Agricultural Researh Service National Agricultural LibraryUSDA. National Nutrient Database For Standard Reference. http://ndb.nal.usda.gov/ndb/foods/show/2373accessed 24 July (2012).

[13] Fang, G. R, & Grumet, R. *Agrobacterium tumefaciens* Mediated Transformation and Regeneration of Musk Melon Plants. Plant Cell Reports. (1990). , 9, 160-164.

[14] Sari, N, Tan, A, Yanmaz, R, Yetisir, H, Balkaya, A, Solmaz, I, & Aykas, L. General Status of Cucurbit Genetic Resources in Turkey: proceedings of the IXth Eucarpia Meeting on Genetics and Breeding of *Cucurbitaceae*, May (2008). INRA, Avignon (France)., 21-24.

[15] Food and Agriculture OrganizationFAO. Value of Agricultural Production. FAOSTAT. http://faostat3.fao.org/home/index.html#SEARCH_DATAaccessed 26 July (2012).

[16] Sensoy, S, Buyukalaca, S, & Abak, K. Evaluation of Genetic Diversity of Turkish Melons (*Cucumis melo* L.) Based on Phenotypic Characters and RAPD Markers. Genetic Resources and Crop Evolution. (2007). , 54, 1351-1365.

[17] Solmaz, I, Sari, N, Mendi, Y. Y, Kacar, Y. A, Kasapoglu, S, Gursoy, I, Suyum, K, Killi, O, Serce, S, & Yildirim, E. Characterization of Some Melon Genotypes Collected from Eastern and Central Anatolia Region of Turkey. Acta Horticulturae. (2010). , 871, 187-196.

[18] Kolayli, S, Kara, M, Tezcan, F, Erim, F. B, Sahin, H, Ulusoy, E, & Aliyazicioglu, R. Comparative Study of Chemical and Biochemical Properties of Different Melon Cultivars: Standard, Hybrid and Grafted Melons. Journal of Agricultural and Food Chemistry. (2010). , 58, 9764-9769.

[19] Bhojwani, S. S, & Razdan, M. K. Plant Tissue Culture: Theory and Practice, a Revised Edition. The Netherlands: Elsevier; (1996).

[20] Murashige, T, & Skoog, F. A Revised Medium for Rapid Growth and Bioassays with Tobacco Tissue Cultures. Physiologia Plantarum. (1962). , 15, 473-497.

[21] Adelberg, J, Rhodes, B, Skorupska, H, & Bridges, W. Explant Origin Affects The Frequency of Tetraploid Plants From Tissue Culture of Melon. HortScience. (1994). , 29, 689-692.

[22] Arumanagathan, K, & Earle, E. D. Nuclear DNA Content of Some Important Plant Species. Plant Molecular Biology Reporter. (1991). , 9, 208-209.

[23] Guis, M, Roustain, J. P, Dogimont, C, Pitrat, M, & Pech, J. C. Melon Biotechnology. Biotechnology and Genetic Engineering Reviews. (1998). , 15, 289-311.

[24] Dong, J. Z, Yang, M. Z, Jia, S. R, & Chua, N. H. Transformation of Melon (*Cucumis melo* L.) and Expression from The Cauliflower Mosaic Virus 35S Promoter in Transgenic Melon Plants. Nature Biotechnology. (1999). , 9, 858-863.

[25] Yoshika, K, Hanada, K, Nakazaki, Y, Minobe, T, & Oosawa, K. Successful Transfer of The Cucumber Mosaic Virus Coat Protein Gene to *Cucumis melo* L. Ikushugaku Zasshi. (1992). , 42, 278-285.

[26] Gonsalves, C, Xue, B, Yepes, M, Fuchs, M, Ling, K, Namba, S, Chee, P, Slingtom, J. L, & Gonsalves, D. Transferring Cucumber Mosaic Virus-White Leaf strain Coat protein Gene into *Cucumis melo* L. and Evaluating Transgenic Plants for Protection Against Infections. Journal of The American Society for Horticultural Science. (1994). , 119(2), 345-355.

[27] Valles, M. P, & Lase, J. M. *Agrobacterium* Mediated Transformation of Commercial Melon, cv 'Amarillo oro'. Plant Cell Reports. (1994). , 13, 145-148.

[28] Gaba, V, & Feldmesser, E. Amit Gal-On H, Antigus Y. Genetic Transformation of a Recalcintrant Melon (*Cucumis melo* L.) Variety. Proc. *Cucurbitaceae*'94: Evaluation and Enhancament of Cucurbit Germplasm, (1995). , 188-190.

[29] Ayub, R, & Guis, M. Ben Amor M, Gillot L, Roustan JP, Latch A, Bouzayen M, Pech JC. Expression of ACC Oxidase Antisense Gene Inhibits Ripening of Cantoloupe Melon Fruits. Nature Biotechnology. (1996). , 14, 862-866.

[30] Curuk, S. Studies on *in vitro* Regeneration and Genetic Transformation in Some Melon (*Cucumis melo* L.) Cultivars. PhD thesis. Cukurova University Adana; (1999).

[31] Bordas, M, Montesinos, C, Dabuza, M, Salvador, A, Roig, A. L, Serrano, R, & Moreno, V. Transfer of The Yeast Salt Tolerence Gene HAL1 *Cucumis melo* L. *in vitro* Evaluation of Salt Tolerence. Transgenic Research. (1997). , 6, 41-45.

[32] Guis, M, Ben-amor, M, Latche, A, Pech, J. C, & Roustain, J. P. A Reliable System for The Transformation of Cantaloupe Charentais Melon (*Cucumis melo* var. cantalupensis) Leading to a Majority of Diploid Rejenerants. Scientia Horticulturae. (2000).

[33] Galperin, M, Patlis, L, Ovadial, A, Wolf, D, Zelce, A, & Kenigsbuch, D. A Melon Genotype with Superior Competence for Regeneration and Transformation. Plant Breeding. (2002). , 122, 66-69.

[34] Yalcin-mendi, Y, Ipek, M, Serbest-kobaner, S, Curuk, S, Aka-kacar, Y, Cetiner, S, Gaba, V, & Grumet, R. *Agrobacterium*-Mediated Transformation of 'Kirkagac 637' A Recalcitrant Melon (*Cucumis melo*) Cultivar with ZYMV Coat Protein Encoding Gene. European Journal of Horticultural Science. (2004). , 69, 258-262.

[35] Abrie, A. L, & Staden, J. V. Development of Regeneration Protocols for Selected Cucurbit Cultivars. Plant Gowth Regulation. (2001). , 35, 263-267.

[36] Dirks, R, & Buggenum, V. M. *In vitro* Plant Regeneration from Leaf and Cotyledon Explants of *Cucumis melo* L. Plant Cell Reports. (1989). , 7, 626-627.

[37] Ray, D. G, Mcolley, D. W, & Michael, E. C. High Frequency Somatic Embryogenesis from Quiescent Seed Cotyledons of *Cucumis melo* Cultivars. Journal of The American Society for Horticultural Science. (1993). , 118, 425-432.

[38] Chovelon, V, Restier, V, Dogimont, C, & Aarrouf, J. Histological Study of Shoot Organogenesis in Melon (*Cucumis melo* L.) After Genetic Transformation. In: Pitrat M, (eds.) Eucarpia2008: IXth Eucarpia Meeting on Genetics and Breeding of *Cucurbitaceae*, EUCARPIAMay (2008). INRA, Avignon, France., 2006, 21-24.

[39] Abak, K. Melons from Turkey: main types and their charactheristics. Proc. 23th Geisenheim Meeting: International Training Course for Quality Inspectors for Fruit, Vegetables and Ware Potatoes. February (2001). Geisenheim, 61-68., 12-14.

[40] IofferA place to Buy, Sell and Trade. Rare Anatolian Hasanbey Melon 30 Seeds. http://www.ioffer.com/i/rare-anatolian-hasanbey-melon-seeds.accessed 24 July (2012).

[41] Organik Production of CorluMelon. http://www.corluorganik.com/Sayfa/Kavunaccessed 24 July (2012).

[42] Rhimi, A, & Fadhel, N. B. Boussaid. Plant Regeneration via Somatic Embryogenesis from *In vitro* Tissue Culture in Two Tunisian *Cucumis melo* cultivars Maazoun and Beji. Plant Cell, Tissue and Organ Culture. (2006). , 84, 239-243.

[43] Gaba, V, Schlarman, E, Elman, C, Sagee, O, Watad, A. A, & Gray, D. J. *In Vitro* Studies on the Anatomy and Morphology of Bud Regeneration in Melon Cotyledons. In Vitro Cellular and Developmental Biology-Plant. (1999). , 35, 1-7.

[44] Lester, G, & Shellie, K. C. Postharvest Sensory and Physichemical Attributes of Honey Dew Melon Fruits. HortScience. (1992). , 27(9), 1012-1014.

[45] Nerson, H. Seed Production and Germinability of Cucurbit Crops. Seed Science and Biotechnology. (2007). , 1(1), 1-10.

[46] Vaughton, G, & Ramsey, M. Relationship Between Seed Mass, Nutrients, and Seedling Growth in *Banksia cuminghamii* (Proteaceae). International Journal of Plant Science. (2001). , 162, 599-606.

[47] Nerson, H. Relationship Between Plant Density and Fruit and Seed Production in Muskmelon. Journal of The American Society for Horticultural Science. (2002). , 127, 855-859.

[48] Moreno, V, Garcia-sogo, M, Granell, I, Garcia-sogo, B, & Roig, L. A. Plant Regeneration from Calli of Melon (*Cucumis melo* L., cv. 'Amarillo Oro'). Plant Cell, Tissue and Organ Culture. (1985). , 5, 139-146.

[49] Chee, P. P. Plant Regeneration from Cotyledons of *Cucumis melo* 'Topmark'. HortScience. (1991). , 26(7), 908-910.

[50] Curuk, S, Ananthakrishnan, G, Singer, S, Xia, X, Elman, C, Nestel, D, Cetiner, S, & Gaba, V. Regeneration *In vitro* from the Hypocotil of *Cucumis* Species Produces Almost Exclusively Diploid Shoots, and Does Not Require Light. HortScience. (2003). , 38(1), 105-109.

[51] Souza, F. V, Garcia-sogo, B, Souza, A. S, San-juan, A. P, & Moreno, V. Morphogenetic Response of Cotyledon and Leaf Explants of Melon (*Cucumis melo* L.) cv. 'Amarillo oro'. Brazilian Archives of Biology and Technology. (2006). , 49, 21-27.

Chapter 12

The Effect of Lead and Zeolite on Hematological and Some Biochemical Parameters in Nile Fish (*Oreochromis niloticus*)

Hikmet Y. Çoğun and Mehmet Şahin

Additional information is available at the end of the chapter

http://dx.doi.org/10.5772/53076

1. Introduction

The elemental lead (Pb) occurs naturally in the environment as well as being produced by mining and manufacturing activities [1]. Lead and its compounds are serious pollutants of the aquatic environment. Moreover, several authors also agree that toxic and non-biodegradable metals such as lead accumulate in many fish species, causing various diseases such as renal [2, 3], hepatic lesions [4], endocrine impairment [5] and effect of cell membrane lipids in cells of the central nervous system.

Zeolites are used in industry, agriculture, environment protection and even in medicine. Zeolites have a relatively high Si/Al compositional ratio which gives it is special ion-exchange selectivity for large monovalent cations. Natural or synthetic zeolites (sodium aluminum silicates) are known to easy adsorb metal ions by exchange reactions [6].

Oreochromis niloticus is a widely used species in aquaculture for food supply and as a bio-indicator of water contamination [7]. Fish hematological parameters are often determined as an index of their health status [8].

Hematological indices such as hematocrit (Hct), hemoglobin (Hb), red blood cells (RBCs), white blood cells (WBCs) and plasma enzyme activities such as AST (aspartate aminotransferase), ALT (alanine aminotransferase), stress hormone cortisol and choline esterase have been used as an indicator of metal pollution in the aquatic environment [9-11].

There is a strong correlation between lead and zeolite that have been found in aquatic organisms and several authors have demonstrated that zeolite protects against lead and also other heavy metals in the experiment [12, 13]. There are numerous biological mechanisms between lead and zeolite. These mechanisms are (I) ion-exchange and (II) adsorb metal ions by exchange reactions [6, 14]. This effects decreases homeostatic mechanisms on fish.

The aim of this study was to determine the effects on hematological and some biochemical parameters on adult *Oreochromis niloticus* exposed to sublethal concentration of lead and zeolite for 10 and 20 days.

2. Materials and methods

Freshwater fish *O. niloticus* were obtained from pools and acclimatized in the laboratory for two months at 25±1°C. After this period the mean body size and body mass of the animals were 15.9±1.87 cm and 56.5±2.15 gr., respectively. We used fish Nile tilapia, *Oreochromis niloticus*, is a teleost widely distributed around the world with economic importance for fisheries [15].

Water quality characteristics in tanks;

- Temperature: 25±1°C
- pH: 8.4±0.8
- Dissolved Oxygen: 7.6±0.5 mg/L
- Total Hardness: 184.5±4.38 $CaCO_3$ mg/L
- Total Alkalinity: 278.2±8.7 $CaCO_3$mg/L

The effects of lead and zeolite were shown as 0.1 mg/L Lead (Pb), 0.1 mg/L Lead+0.1 g/L Zeolite (PbZ1), 0.1 mg/L Lead+0.2 g/L Zeolite (PbZ2) and Control (C). A total of 4 aquariums sized 40x100x40 cm in height were divided into two groups. These were filled with 100 L. aerated class aquarium tanks. Nine fish were put in each aquarium (3 repetition x 3 fish). One aquariums of the first group contained 0.1 mg Pb/L (PbC12, 2 H2O) solutions and two aquariums of the second group contained 0.1 mg/L Lead+0.1 g/L Zeolite and 0.1 mg/L Lead +0.2 g/L Zeolite solutions and one aquarium was used as a control. All fish were fed with Pinar Yem at a concentration of 1 % of their body mass per day.

Fish were anaesthetized with MS-222 blood was collected from each fish by cutting the caudal peduncle. Fish blood was collected for hematological parameters. The blood was centrifuged at 4000 rpm over 10 min at 15 ^{0}C to obtain the serum. Blood samples were sent to Cukurova University (Balcalı Hastahanesi, Merkez laboratory) for hematological analysis. The serum was divided in two portions from the ephandof tubes, first portion for cortisol and cholineesterase, second portion for ALT and for AST, ALT and AST activities. Those analyses were determined using UV test technique [16]. The serum samples were frozen and stored -20^{0}C until required for assays. Cortisol, ALT, AST and cholinesterase were determined by ROCHE Hitachi E-170 and DPP.

Data are presented as mean ± standard error. For the statistical analysis, it was used one-way analysis of variance (ANOVA) followed by Student Newman–Keul's test using SPSS 10.0 statistical software (SPSS Inc., Chicago, IL). Differences were considered significant if $P < 0.05$.

3. Results and discussion

No mortality was observed at concentrations of the lead and its zeolite mixtures studied during the experiments. The statistical analysis was done with "SNK" differences among groups were measured to be significant at $p<0.05$ and showed Table 1 and 2.

	Enzymatic parameters			
Treateds	Cortisol (ug/dL)	ALT (uL)	AST (uL)	Cholinesterase (uL)
C	5.76±0.03 **a**	14.33±1.20 **a**	126.0±2.64 **a**	776.3±5.78 **a**
Pb	6.73±0.08 **a**	18.00±0.01 **b**	121.1±0.57 **b**	649.0±6.11 **b**
PbZ1	4.30±0.13 **b**	9.66±0.66 **c**	98.00±1.00 **c**	313.6±3.17 **c**
PbZ2	3.12±0.30 **c**	8.66±0.65 **a**	88.0±0.57 **b**	214.6±0.66 **c**

Letters a, b,and c show the differences between groups (P < 0.05).

Table 1. Enzymatic changes Mean±SE (N=6) of the fish *O. niloticus* exposed to Pb, PbZ1 and PbZ2 over 10 days

	Enzymatic parameters			
Treateds	Cortisol (ug/dL)	ALT (uL)	AST (uL)	Cholinesterase (uL)
C	5.77±0.03 **a**	15.66±0.88 **a**	126.3±0.88 **a**	790.3±5.17 **a**
Pb	7.28±0.09 **b**	20.33±0.87 **b**	132.6±0.88 **b**	529.0±3.21 **b**
PbZ1	3.81±0.18 **c**	11.66±0.66 **c**	112.6±1.20 **c**	431.3±3.84 **c**
PbZ2	3.26±0.17 **c**	7.33±0.66 **b**	109.0±0.57 **c**	302.0±1.52 **c**

Letters a, b,andc show the differences between groups (P < 0.05).

Table 2. Enzymatic changes Mean±SE (N=6) of the fish *O. niloticus* exposed to Pb, PbZ1 and PbZ2 over 20 days

Zeolite may decrease the toxicity of lead in water and Pb may form a complex with Zeolite. Hb, Hct, RBCc and WBCc levels decreased Pb, PbZ1 and PbZ2 exposed fish at both exposure periods (Fig 1-4). The exposures of Pb, PbZ1 and PbZ2 did not cause any significant changes in RBCc and WBCc levels of fish at 10 days while they caused a decrease in its levels at the end of the exposure period.

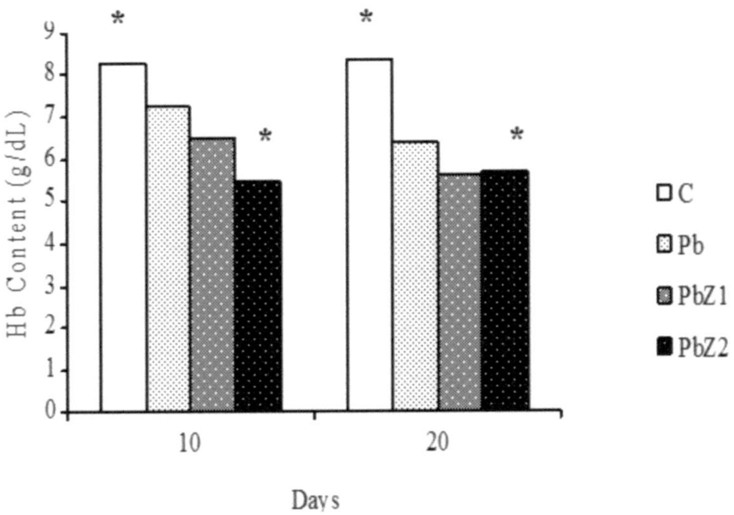

Figure 1. Serum Hemoglobin levels in *O. niloticus* to lead and its zeolite mixtures for 10 and 20 days. Data are expressed as mean ± standard error (N = 6). * shows significant differences between time for the same exposure group ($P < 0.05$).

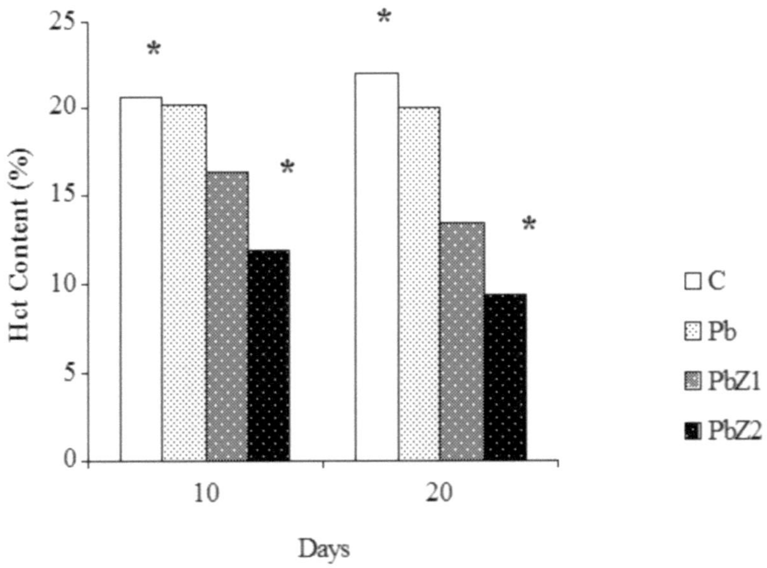

Figure 2. Serum Hemotocrit levels in *O. niloticus* to lead and its zeolite mixtures for 10 and 20 days. Data are expressed as mean ± standard error (N = 6). * shows significant differences between time for the same exposure group ($P < 0.05$).

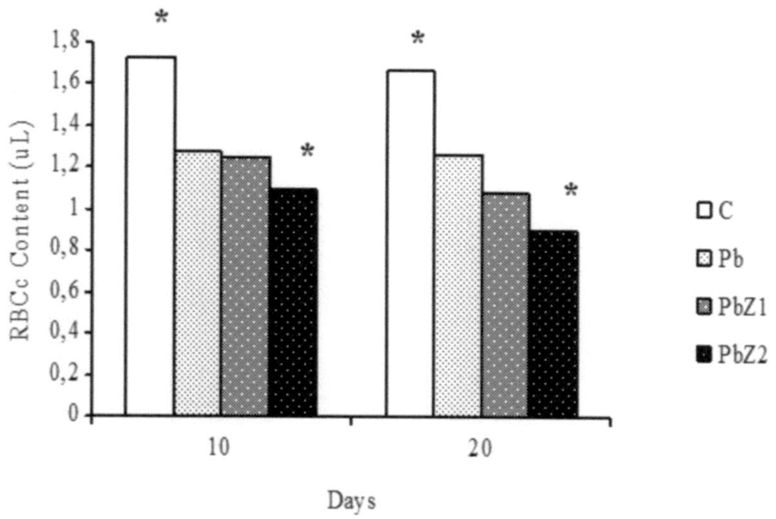

Figure 3. Serum RBCc levels in *O. niloticus* to lead and its zeolite mixtures for 10 and 20 days. Data are expressed as mean ± standard error (N = 6). * shows significant differences between time for the same exposure group ($P < 0.05$).

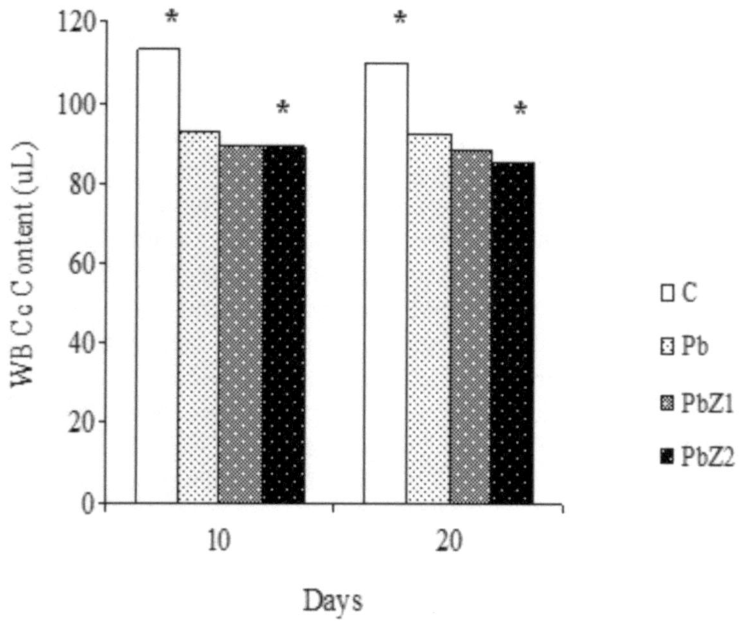

Figure 4. Serum WBCc levels in *O. niloticus* to lead and its zeolite mixtures for 10 and 20 days. Data are expressed as mean ± standard error (N = 6). * shows significant differences between time for the same exposure group ($P < 0.05$).

Serum Cortisol, ALT, AST and Cholinesterase activities of *O. niloticus* decreased in response to Pb, PbZ1 and PbZ2 exposures when compared to control during 10 and 20 days (Table 1 and 2). At the end of the exposure period elevations in Cortisol, ALT and AST enzyme activities of fish exposed to concentrations of Pb, PbZ1 and PbZ2 compared with metal-treated groups. While the cholinesterase activities of *O. niloticus* decreased to Pb, PbZ1 and PbZ2 at both exposure periods, an increase in AST activities 0.1 mg L^{-1} Pb exposure was observed at 10 days (Table 1 and 2).

4. Hematological parameters

Fig. 1-4 show distribution of hematological (Hb, Hct, RBCc and WBCc) parameters Pb and Pb+Ze mixtures exposed to *O. niloticus* over 10 and 20 days. In blood parameters notable declines were observed at all Pb, PbZ1 and PbZ2 exposure periods (Fig. 1-4). The maximum decrease of 41% Hct and 35 % RBCc were observed in Pb+Ze at 10 days and 55% Hct and 41% RBCc at 20 days.

Lead was classified as a toxic substance for fish. Changes in the erythrocyte profile suggest a compensation of oxygen deficit in the body due to gill damage. Hematological indices are commonly used as indicators of metal pollution in fish [17, 18]. This index reflects respiratory status of animals. In addition to these status, infectious and stress have been shown to influence the fish hematology.

Metals in hematological parameters of fish generally occur due to the osmotic changes resulting in hemodilution (an increase in the volume of plasma, resulting in a reduced concentration of red blood cells in blood) or hemoconcentrations (an increase in the concentration of blood cells resulting from the loss of plasma or water from the bloodstream) [19]. Generally, spleen is responsible for this change. Because, spleen, serving as a potent blood storage organ in some teleost, sequestering blood cell under resting conditions and releasing them to circulating blood associated with various stress [20]. In [4] have been reported that histopathological lesions occur in spleen and intestine lead exposure on *Heteropneustes fossilis*. This also leads to changes in hematological parameters of fish. In this study, the effects of lead and zeolite mixtures decreased red blood cell, hemoglobin content and hematocrit values. Significantly depressed in this study blood parameters, an indicator of Pb, PbZ1 and PbZ2 intoxications, were observed in blood (RBCc and WBCc) ($P<0.005$) of fish at exposure time. This change was, however, not found in 0.1 mg L^{-1} Pb group. This may be zeolite is capable of ion exchange [6, 12].

5. Enzyme activity

In this study, at 10 and 20 days, compared with controls, ALT, AST, Cortisol and Cholinesterase were decreased PbZ1 and PbZ2 concentrations while ALT, AST and Cortisol increased only Pb concentrations. However, Cholinesterase decreased at not Pb, but PbZ1 and PbZ2 combinations ($P<0.005$) during 10 and 20 days.

Plasma cortisol level is widely used as a general indicator of stressful conditions in fish [21, 22]. Despite the interest in plasma cortisol measurement as an indicator of stress, few studies have actually measured the kinetics of cortisol in fish. A study [23], reported that during chronic stress, plasma cortisol back to the resting levels on *Salvelinus fontinalis*. In our study, cortisol levels of fish blood, compared with controls, increased both low and high concentration of lead ($P<0.005$). But, these levels were decreased with lead and zeolite combinations during exposure periods (Table 1 and 2). This may be zeolite is capable of ion exchange [6, 12]. The HPI (The hypothalamo-pituitary-interrenal) axis is activated to produce cortisol and other corticosteroid hormones for the maintenance of disturbed homeostasis [24]. The elevation of cortisol, in this study, it was noted that this may be a function of stimulation to the HPI axis in metal stress.

Serum ALT and AST activities used in diagnosis of damage fish tissues (i.e. gill, muscle, liver) [25]. Determinations of transaminases (AST and ALT) have been useful in the diagnosis of liver and kidney diseases in fish [26]. These enzymes of *O. niloticus* increased in response to lead exposures when compared to control during 10 and 20 days (Table 1 and 2). At the end of the exposure period, the activities of these enzymes in fish exposed to lead were higher when compared with PbZ1 and PbZ2 groups. While the ALT and AST activities increased in fish exposed to only lead concentrations at both exposure periods, an decreased in their activities following PbZ1 and PbZ2 exposure was observed at both exposure days (Table 1 and 2). There are numerous study in this serum activity of fish such as *Sparus aurata* [27] and *Cyprinus carpio* [28]. The researchers concluded that necrosis or disease of liver caused to leakage of this enzyme into blood stream might be responsible for increase of this enzyme in blood.

There are multiple forms of esterase in vertebrates' blood plasma [29]. However, acetyl cholinesterase content of fish blood is present in low concentration compared with other vertebrate [30]. One of the biomarkers most frequently used in fish for the diagnosis of exposure to pollutants is the measurement of the inhibition of the enzyme cholinesterase (ChE) [30]. Table 1 and 2 presents ChE activity in plasma of *O. niloticus* exposure lead and its zeolite combinations during 10 and 20 days. ChE activity was decreased significantly after exposure to Pb, PbZ1 and PbZ2 both days ($P<0.05$). Similar findings have been described by in reference [31]. The high levels of ChE activity found in control fish in this present study, as was previously described in [32].

In conclusion, the data from this investigation which is the blood-based enzymatic and hematological parameters responded to relatively Pb and its mixtures concentrations show useful for monitoring on fish [33, 34]. The hematological data, as well as gross observations from sample handing and fish necropsy, suggest that this data may have been related to erythrocyte fragility (erythrocyte easily broken, damaged, or destroyed) and hemorrhaging exposed to metals [20, 35]. It is possible mechanisms that the decrease in blood parameters may be hemolysis and damage to hematopoietic tissues by lead and its zeolite mixtures.

Further, the decrease of serum enzymatic mechanisms may be indicated liver damage [25, 28 and 36] and may be occurring from Pb and Ze mixtures form.

Author details

Hikmet Y. Çoğun and Mehmet Şahin

*Address all correspondence to: hcogun@kilis.edu.tr

Kilis 7 Aralik University, Faculty of Science and Letters, Department of Biology, Kilis, Turkey

References

[1] Health AG (1987) Water pollution and fish physiology. CRC Pres. Florida USA, 24 p.

[2] Lliopoulou-Georgudaki IJ and Kotsanis N (2001) Toxic Effects of cadmium and Mercury in rainbow Trouth (Oncorhynchus mykiss): A Short-term Bioassay. Bull. Environ. Contam. Toxicol. 66: 77-85.

[3] Gordon N, Taylor A, Bennett PN (2002) Lead Poisoning: Case Studies. British Journal of Clinical Pharmacology. 53(5): 451–458.

[4] Bano Y, Hasan M (1990) Histopathological Lesions in the Body organs of cat-fish (Heteropneustes fossilis) following mercury intoxication. Journal of Environmental Science and Health, Part B: Pesticides, Food Contaminants, and Agricultural Wastes. 25(1): 67-85.

[5] Veena KB, Radhakrishnan C K and Chacko J (1997) Heavy Metal Induced Biochemical Effects in an Estuarine teleost. Indian J. Mar. Sci. 26: 74-78.

[6] Jain SK (1999) Protective Role of Zeolite on Short and Long Term Lead Toxicity in the Teleost Fish Heteropneustes fossilis, Chemosphere. 39(2): 247-251.

[7] Almeida JA, Novelli ELB, Dal-Pai Silva M, and Alves-Junior R (2001) Environmental Cadmium Exposure and Metabolic Responses of the Nile Tilapia Oreochromis niloticus. Environ Pollut. 114: 169–175.

[8] Blaxhall PC and Daisley KW (1973) Routine Haematological Methods for use with Fish Blood. J. Fish Biol. 5: 771-781.

[9] Nemcsok JG and Hughes GM (1988) The Effect of Copper Sulphate on Some Biochemical Parameters of Rainbow trout. Environmental Pollution, 49: 77-85.

[10] Pelgrom SMGS, Lock RAC, Balm PHM and Wendelaar Bonga SE (1995) Effects of Combined waterbone Cd and Cu Exposures on Ionic and Plasma Cortisol in Tilapia Oreochromis mossambicus. Comp. Biochem. Physiol. 111C: 227-235.

[11] Shah SL and Altindag A (2004) Hematological Parameters of Tench (Tinca tinca L.) After Acute and Chronic Exposure to Lethal and Sublethal Mercury Treatments, Bull. Environ. Contam. Toxicol. 73: 911-918.

[12] Jain SK, Raizada AK, Jain K (1997) Protective role of zeolite on lead toxicity in freshwater fish. XIII ISEB, Monopoli, Bari, Italy.

[13] Shrivastava S, Mishra M, Jain SK (2001) Remediation of lead toxicity in fish tissues through zeolite with reference to glycogen content. J Natcon, 13 (2): 231-235.

[14] Tepe Y, Akyurt I, Ciminli C, Mutlu E, Çalışkan M (2004) Protective effect of Clinoptilolite on lead toxicity in Common Carp Cyprinus carpio. Fres Environ Bull, 13 (7): 639-642.

[15] Fontaínhas-Fernandes AA (1998) Tilapia production, In: Aquaculture Handbook, ReisHenriques, M.A.(Ed.), pp. 135-150.

[16] Bergmeyer HU, Horder M and Rej R (1985) International Federation of Clinical Chemistry (IFCC) Scientific Committee. J Clin Chem Clin Biochem. 24:481–495.

[17] Shah SL, Hafeez MA and Shaikh SA (1995) Changes in Hematological parameters and Plasma Glucose in the fish Cyprinus watsoni, in the Exposure to Zinc and Copper Treatment. Pakistan J. Zool 27: 50-54.

[18] Drastichova J, Svobodova Z, Luskova V and Machova J (2004) Effect of Cadmium on Hematological Indices of Common Carp (Cyprinus carpio L.). Bull. Environ. Contam. Toxicol. 72: 725-732.

[19] Tort T and Torres P (1988) The Effects of Sublethel Concentrations of Cadmium on Hematological Parameters in the Dogfish, Scyliorhinus canicula. J. Fish Biol. 32: 277-282.

[20] Yamamoto KI (1988) Contraction of Spleen in Exercised Fresh water Teleost. Comp. Biochem. Physiol. 89A: 65-66.

[21] Pickering AD, Pottiger RG and Christie P (1982) Recover of Brown Trout, Salmo trutta L. from Acute Handling Stress: A Time-course Study. J. Fish Biol. 20: 229-244.

[22] Wendelaar Bonga SE (1997) The stress response in fish. Physiol Rev 7:591–625

[23] Vijayan MM and Leatherland JF (1990) High Stocking Density Affects Cortisol Secretion and Tissue Distribution in Brook Charr, Salvelinus fontinalis. J. Endocrinol. 12: 311–318.

[24] Gagnon A, Jumarie C and Hontela A (2006) Effects of Cu on Plasma Cortisol and Cortisol Secretion by adrenocortical cells of Rainbow Trout (Oncorhynchus mykiss). Aquat Toxicol. 78: 59–65.

[25] De La Tore FR, Salibian A, Ferrari L (2000) Biomarkers Assessment in Juvenile Cyprinus carpio Exposed to Waterborne Cadmium. Environ Pollut. 109: 227–278.

[26] Maita M, Shiomitsu K and Ikeda Y (1984) Health Assessment by the Climogram of Hemochemical Constituents in Cultured Yellowtail. Bull. Jap. Soc. Scient. Fish. 51: 205-211.

[27] Vaglio A, Landriscina C (1999) Changes in Liver Enzyme Activity in the Teleost Sparus aurata in Response to Cadmium Intoxication. Ecotoxicol Environ Saf 43B: 111–116.

[28] Karan V, Vitorovic S, Tutundzic V, Poleksic V (1998) Functional enzymes activity and gill histology of carp after copper sulfate exposure and recovery. Ecotoxol Environ Saf 40:49–55

[29] Augustinssonk B (1961) Multiple Forms of Esterase in Vertebrate Blood Plasma. Ann. N.Y. Acad. Sci. 94: 844-860.

[30] Ellman GL, Courtney KD and Andres Jr V (1961) A New and Rapid Colorimetric Determination of Acetylcholinesterase Activity, Biochem. Pharmacol. 7: 88-95.

[31] Sancho E, Ceron JJ and Ferrando MD (2000) Cholinesterase Activity and Hematological Parameters as Biomarkers of Sublethal Molinate Exposure in Anguilla anguilla, Ecotox. Environ. Saf. 46(1): 81-86.

[32] Ceron JJ, Fernandez MJ, Bernal LJ and Gutierrez C (1996) Automated spectrophotometric Medhod Using 2.2-dithiodipyridine Acid for Determination of Cholinesterase in Whole Blood. J. Assoc. Off. Anal. Chem. Int. 79: 757-763.

[33] Dethloff GM, Schlenk D, Khan S and Bailey HC (1999) The Effects of Copper on Blood and Biochemical Parameters of Rainbow Trout (Oncorhynchus mykiss). Arch. Environ. Contam. Toxicol. 36: 415-423.

[34] Chiu SK, Collier CP, Clark AF and Wynn-Edwards KE (2003) Salivary Cortisol on ROCHE Elecsys Immunoassay System: Pilot Biological Variation Studies. Clin Biochem 36: 211–214.

[35] Al-Attar AM (2005) Changes in Hematological Parameters of the Fish, Oreochromis niloticus Treated with Sublethal Concentration of Cadmium. Pakistan J. Biologycal Sci. 8(3): 421-424.

[36] Cogun HY and Şahin M (2012) The Effect of Zeolite on Reduction of Lead Toxicity in Nil Tilapia (Oreochromis niloticus Linnaeus, 1758). Kafkas Univ Vet Fak Derg. 18 (1): 135-140.

Chapter 13

Microorganisms in Biological Pest Control — A Review (Bacterial Toxin Application and Effect of Environmental Factors)

Canan Usta

Additional information is available at the end of the chapter

http://dx.doi.org/10.5772/55786

1. Introduction

In this section, the topic in biological control of pests considered. will take place. There has been an increased interest in biological control agents in last decade. More number of biocontrol agents was screened for their efficacy and environmental impact including mammalian safety. Many organisms have been investigated as potential agents for vector mosquito control, including viruses, fungi, bacteria, protozoa, nematodes, invertebrate predators and fish. However, most of these agents were shown to be of little operational use, largely because of the difficulty in multiplying them in large quantities. Some species of organisms, those that have been introduced from elsewhere may be pest to other organisms as well. They are pests to the extend which efforts must have been made to control them both in terrestrial and aquatic/ freshwater environments [1]. Prior to the advent of chemical pesticides, predators which are natural enemies of those specific pests, were an important subject in biological sciences with respect to agriculture and forest pest control.

Pesticides that include insecticides, herbicides, and fungicides are employed in modern agriculture to control pests and to increase crop yield. In both developed and developing countries, the use of chemical pesticides has increased dramatically during the last few decades. Control of pests with synthetic chemicals results in several problems. The residues ofthese synthetic insecticides cause toxic effects on wild life (e.g.,birds, beneficial insects like honeybees). These chemical insecticides also induce harmful chemical changes on non-target insects/pests on their predators, parasites, etc. They can also be harmful to humans and domestic animals. Other environmental concern is the contamination of ground water [2]

In addition, there have been several recent research on biological control of marine pests [3]. The introduction of marine pests to new habitats is as old as nautical experience. Atlantic shipworms were quite possibly the first for the applicaiton of some new predator, Mytilus gallprovincialis, and the western Atlantic populations of the European green crab have planted themselves so firmly as a neutralized part of the biota. Many other introductions, such as polychaetes, amphipods are cryptic and have been considered species with natural cosmopolitan distributions [4]

Agriculture and forests form an important resource to sustain global economical, environmental and social system. For this reason, the global challenge is to secure high and quality yields and to make agricultural produce environmentally compatible. Chemical means of plant protection occupy the leading place as regards their total volume of application in integrated pest management and diseases of plants. But pesticides cause toxicity to humans and warm-blooded animals.

Despite many years of effective control by conventional agrochemical insecticides, a number of factors are threatening the effectiveness and continued use of these agents. These include the development of insecticide resistance and use-cancellation or de-registration of some insecticides due to human health and environmental concerns. Therefore, an eco-friendly alternative is the need of the hour. Improvement in pest control strategies represents one method to generate higher quality and greater quantity of agricultural products. Therefore, there is a need to develop biopesticides which are effective, biodegradable and do not leave any harmful effect on environment [5].

2. Biological pesticides

The biopesticides are certain types of pesticides derived from such natural materials as animals, plants, bacteria, and certain minerals. For example, canola oil and baking soda have pesticidal applications and are considered biopesticides. Even at the end of 2001, there were approximately 195 registered biopesticide active ingredients and 780 products. Biopesticides are biochemical pesticides that are naturally occurring substances that control pests by nontoxic mechanisms. They are living organisms (natural enemies) or their products (phytochemicals, microbial products) or byproducts (semiochemicals) which can be used for the management of pests that are injurious to crop plants. Biopesticides have an important role in crop protection, although most commonly in combination with other tools including chemical pesticides as part of Bio-intensive Integrated Pest Management.

They are biological pesticides based on pathogenic microorganisms specific to a target pest offer an ecologically sound and effective solution to pest problems. They pose less threat to the environment and to human health. The most commonly used biopesticides are living organisms, which are pathogenic for the pest of interest. These include biofungicides (*Trichoderma*), bioherbicides (*Phytopthora*) and bioinsecticides (*Bacillus thuringiensis, B. sphaericus*). The potential benefits to agriculture and public health programmes through the use of biopesticides are considerable [6].

The advantages of using biopesticides (in place of other chemical ones are based on these factors:

- Ecological benefit; inherently less harmful and less environmental load.
- Target specificity; designed to affect only one specific pest or, in somecases, a few target organisms,
- Environmental beneficiency; often effective in very small quantities and often decompose quickly, thereby resulting in lower exposures and largely avoiding the pollution problems.
- Suitability; when used as a component of an integrated pest management (IPM) programs, biopesticides can contribute greatly.

3. Microbial pesticides

They come from naturally occurring or genetically altered bacteria, fungi,algae, viruses or protozoans. Microbial control agents can be effective and used as alternatives to chemical insecticides. A microbial toxin can be defined as a biological toxin material derived from a microorganism, such as a bacterium or fungus. Pathogenic effect of those microorganisms on the target pests are so species specific. The effect by microbial entomopathogens occurs by invasion through the integument or gut of the insect, followed by multiplication of the pathogen resulting in the death of the host, e.g., insects. Studies have demonstrated that the pathogens produce insecticidal toxin important in pathogenesis. Most of the toxins produced by microbial pathogens which have been identified are peptides, but they vary greatly in terms of structure, toxicity and specificity. [7].

These microbial pesticides offer an alternative to chemical insecticides with increased target specificity and ecological safety so that they are used either uniqly or in combination with other pest management programmes. One definition for integrated pest management (IPM) which is most relevant to this practice comes from Flint and van den Bosch [1981]: "It is a ecologically based pest control strategy that relies heavily on natural mortality factors and seeks out control tactics that disrupt these factors as little as possible. Ideally, an integrated pest management program considers all available pest control actions, including no action, and evaluates the potential interaction among various control tactics, cultural practices, weather, other pests, and the crop to be protected"[8].

These microbials as biocontrol agents present u beneficiancy. They have efficiency and safety for humans and other nontarget organisms. They leave less or no residue in food. They are ecologically safe, so that other natural enemies are free of their threatening, leading to preservation of other natural enemies, and increased biodiversity in managed ecosystem. So, microbial agents are highly specific against target pests so they facilitate the survival of beneficial insects in treated crops. This may be the main reason that microbial insecticides are being developed as biological control agents during the last three decades.

Microorganism e.g., a bacterium, fungus, virus or protozoan as the active ingredient can control many different kinds of pests, although each separate active ingredient is relatively specific for its target pest. For example, there are fungi that control certain weeds, and other fungi that kill specific insects. One bacterial species like *Bacillus thuringiensis* may be more effectiv on *Aedes aegypti* while one another *B. sphaericus* strain can be effective on a different types of mosquito like *Culex quinquefasciatus* [9].

3.1. Advantages of microbial insecticides

Individual products differ in important ways, but the following list of beneficial characteristics applies to microbial insecticides in general.

- The organisms used in microbial insecticides are essentially nontoxic and nonpathogenic to wildlife, humans, and other organisms not closely related to the target pest. The safety offered by microbial insecticides is their greatest strength.
- The toxic action of microbial insecticides is often specific to a single group or species of insects, and this specificity means that most microbial insecticides do not directly affect beneficial insects (including predators or parasites of pests) in treated areas.
- If necessary, most microbial insecticides can be used in conjunction with synthetic chemical insecticides because in most cases the microbial product is not deactivated or damaged by residues of conventional insecticides. (Follow label directions concerning any limitations.)
- Because their residues present no hazards to humans or other animals, microbial insecticides can be applied even when a crop is almost ready for harvest.
- In some cases, the pathogenic microorganisms can become established in a pest population or its habitat and provide control during subsequent pest generations or seasons.
- They also enhance the root and plant growth by way of encouraging the beneficial soil microflora. By this way they take a part in the increase of the crop yield.

3.2. Disadvantages of microbial insecticides

Naturally there are also the limitations which are listed below, but do not prevent the successful use of microbial insecticides. These factors just provide users to choose effective microbial products and take necessary steps to achieve successful results.

- Because a single microbial insecticide is toxic to only a specific species or group of insects, each application may control only a portion of the pests present in a field and garden. If other types of pests are present in the treated area, they will survive and may continue to cause damage. Conventional insecticides are subject to similar limitations because they too are not equally effective against all pests. This is because of selectivity indeed and this negative aspect is often more noticeable for both general predators, chemicals and microbials. On the other hand predators and chemicals may be danger for other beneficial insects in threatened area.
- Heat, desiccation (drying out), or exposure to ultraviolet radiation reduces the effectiveness of several types of microbial insecticides. Consequently, proper timing and application procedures are especially important for some products.

http://dx.doi.org/10.5772/55786

- Special formulation and storage procedures are necessary for some microbial pesticides. Although these procedures may complicate the production and distribution of certain products, storage requirements do not seriously limit the handling of microbial insecticides that are widely available. (Store all pesticides, including microbial insecticides, according to label directions.)

- Because several microbial insecticides are pest-specific, the potential market for these products may be limited. Their development, registration, and production costs cannot be spread over a wide range of pest control sales. Consequently, some products are not widely available or are relatively expensive (several insect viruses, for example).

PATHOGEN	PRODUCT NAME	HOST RANGE	USES AND COMMENTS
BACTERIA			
Bacillus thuringiensis var. *kurstaki* (*Bt*)	Bactur®, Bactospeine®, Bioworm®, Caterpillar Killer®, Dipel®, Futura®, Javelin®, SOK-Bt®, Thuricide®, Topside®, Tribactur®, Worthy Attack®	caterpillars (larvae of moths and butterflies)	Effective for foliage-feeding caterpillars (and Indian meal moth in stored grain). Deactivated rapidly in sunlight; apply in the evening or on overcast days and direct some spray to lower surfaces or leaves. Does not cycle extensively in the environment.
Bacillus thuringiensis var. israelensis (*Bt*)	Aquabee®, Bactimos®, Gnatrol®, LarvX®, Mosquito Attack®, Skeetal®, Teknar®, Vectobac®	larvae of *Aedes* and *Psorophora* mosquitoes, black flies, and fungus gnats	Effective against larvae only. Active only if ingested. *Culex* and *Anopheles* mosquitoes are not controlled at normal application rates.. Does not cycle extensively in the environment.
Bacillus thuringiensis var. *tenebrinos*	Foil® M-One® M-Track®, Novardo® Trident®	larvae of Colorado potato beetle, elm leaf beetle adults	Effective against Colorado potato beetle larvae and the elm leaf beetle. Like other *Bts*, it must be ingested. It is subject to breakdown in ultraviolet light and does not cycle extensively in the environment.
Bacillus thuringiensis var. *aizawai*	Certan®	wax moth caterpillars	Used only for control of was moth infestations in honeybee hives.
Bacillus popilliae and *Bacillus lentimorbus*	Doom¨, Japidemic¨,® Milky Spore Disease, Grub Attack®	larvae (grubs) of Japanese beetle	The main Illinois lawn grub (the annual white grub, *Cyclocephala* sp.) Is NOT susceptible to milky spore disease.
Bacillus sphaericus	Vectolex CG®, Vectolex WDG®	larvae of *Culex, Psorophora,* and *Culiseta* mosquitos, larvae of some *Aedes* spp.	Active only if ingested, for use against *Culex, Psorophora,* and *Culiseta* species; also effective against *Aedes vexans.* Remains effective in stagnant or turbid water
FUNGI			
Beauveria bassiana	Botanigard®, Mycotrol®, Naturalis®	aphids, fungus gnats, mealy bugs, mites, thrips, whiteflies	Effective against several pests. High moisture requirements, lack of storage longevity, and competition with other soil microorganisms are problems that remain to be solved.

PATHOGEN	PRODUCT NAME	HOST RANGE	USES AND COMMENTS
Lagenidium giganteum	Laginex®	larvae of most pest mosquito species	Effective against larvae of most pest mosquito species; remains infective in the environment through dry periods. A main drawback is its inability to survive high summertime temperatures.
PROTOZOA			
Nosema locustae	NOLO Bait®, Grasshopper Attack®	European cornborer caterpillars, grasshoppers and mormon crickets	Useful for rangeland grasshopper control. Active only if ingested. Not recommended for use on a small scale, such as backyard gardens, because the disease is slow acting and grasshoppers are very mobile. Also effective against caterpillars.
VIRUSES			
Gypsy moth nuclear plyhedrosis (NPV)	Gypchek® virus	gypsy moth caterpillars	All of the viral insecticides used for control of forest pests are produced and used exclusively by the U.S. Forest Service.
Tussock moth NPV	TM Biocontrol-1®	tussock moth caterpillars	
Pine sawfly NPV	Neochek-S®	pine sawfly larvae	
Codling moth granulosis virus (GV)	(see comments)	codling moth caterpillars	Commercially produced and marketed briefly, but no longer registered or available. Future re-registration is possible. Subject to rapid breakdown in ultraviolet light.
ENTOMOGENOUS NEMATODES			
Steinernema feltiae (=*Neoaplectana carpocapsae*) *S. riobravis*, *S. carpocapsae* and other *Steinernema* species	Biosafe®, Ecomask®, Scanmask®, also sold generically (wholesale and retail), Vector®	larvae of a wide variety of soil-dwelling and boring insects	*Steinernema riobravis* is the main nematode species marketed retail in the U.S. Because of moisture requirements, it is effective primarily against insects in moist soils or inside plant tissues. Prolonged storage or extreme temperatures before use may kill or debilitate the nematodes.
Heterorhabditis heliothidis	currently available on a wholesale basis for large scale operations	larvae of a wide variety of soil-dwelling and boring insects	Not commonly available by retail in the U.S.; this species is used more extensively in Europe. Available by wholesale or special order for research or large-scale commercial uses.
PATHOGEN			
Steinernema scapterisci	Nematac®S	late nymph and adult stages of mole crickets	*S. scapterisci* is the main nematode species marketed to target the tawny and southern mole cricket. Best applied where irrigation is available. Irrigate after application.

(Agricultural Entomology, University of Illinois at Urbana-Champaign. ENY-275 IN081)

Table 1. Microbial Insecticides: A summary of products and their uses.

3.2.1. *Entomopathogenic fung*

Entomopathogenic fungi are important natural regulators of insect populations and have potential as mycoinsecticide agents against diverse insect pests in agriculture. These fungi infect their hosts by penetrating through the cuticle, gaining access to the hemolymph, producing toxins, and grow by utilizing nutrients present in the haemocoel to avoid insect immune responses [10]. Entomopathogenic fungi may be applied in the form of conidia or mycelium which sporulates after application. The use of fungal entomopathogens as alternative to insecticide or combined application of insecticide with fungal entomopathogens could be very useful for insecticide resistant management [13].

The commercial mycoinsecticide 'Boverin' based on *B. bassiana* with reduced doses of trichlorophon have been used to suppress the second-generation outbreaks of *Cydia pomonella* L. Anderson *et al.* (1989) detected higher insect mortality when *B. bassiana* and sublethal concentrations of insecticides were applied to control Colorado potato beetle (*Leptinotarsa decemlineata*), attributing higher rates of synergism between two agents [14].

The use of the insect-pathogenic fungus *Metarhizium anisopliae* against adult *Aedes aegypti* and *Aedes albopictus* mosquitoes has also been reportedThe life span of fungus-contaminated mosquitoes of both species was significantly reduced compared to uninfected mosquitoes. The results indicated that both mosquito species are highly susceptible to infection with this entomopathogen [15].

3.2.2. *Viral pesticides*

There are more than 1600 different viruses which infect 1100 species of insects and mites. A special group of viruses, called baculovirus, to which about 100 insect species are susceptible, accounts for more than 10 percent of all insect pathogenic viruses. Baculoviruses are rod-shaped particles which contain DNA. Most viruses are enclosed in a protein coat to make up a virus inclusion body. Alkaline condition of insect's midgut dissolves the protein covering and the viral particles are released from the inclusion body. These particles fuse with the midgut epithelial cells, multiply rapidly and eventually kill the host. But, viral pesticides are more expensive than chemical agents. Furthermore, many baculoviruses are host specific. Therefore they cannot be used to control several different pests. The action of baculoviruses on insect larvae is too slow to satisfy farmers. These viral preparations are not stable under the ultraviolet rays of the sun. Efforts are being made to encapsulate baculoviruses with UV protectants to ensure a longer field-life.

First well-documented introduction of baculovirus into the environment which resulted in effective suppression of a pest occurred accidentally before the World War II. Along with a parasitoid imported to Canada to suppress spruce sawfly *Diprion hercyniae*, an NPV specific for spruce sawfly was introduced and since then no control measures have been required against this hymenopteran species. In the past, the application of baculoviruses for the protection of agricultural annual crops, fruit orchards and forests has not matched their potential. The number of registered pesticides based on baculovirus, though slowly, increases steadily. At present, it exceeds fifty virus formulations, some of them being the same baculovirus preparations distributed under different trade names in different countries [16].

NPVs and GVs are used as pesticides but the group based on nucleopolyhedrosis viruses is much larger. The first viral insecticide Elcar™ was introduced by Sandoz Inc. in 1975Elcar™ was a preparation of *Heliothis zea* NPV which is relatively broad range baculovirus and infects many species belonging to genera *Helicoverpa* and *Heliothis*. HzSNPV provided control of not only cotton bollworm, but also of pests belonging to these genera attacking soybean, sorghum, maize, tomato and beans. In 1982 Sandoz decided to discontinue the production. The resistance to many chemical insecticides including pyrethroids revived the interest in HzSNPV and the same virus was registered under the name GemStar™. HzSNPV is a product of choice for biocontrol of *Helicoverpa armigera*]. Countries with large areas of such crops like cotton, pigeonpea, tomato, pepper and maize, e.g. India and China, introduced special programs for the reduction of this pest by biological means. In Central India, *H.armigera* in the past was usually removed by shaking pigeonpea [17].

The well-known success of employing baculovirus as a biopesticide is the case of *Anticarsia gemmatalis* nucleopolyhedrovirus (AgMNPV) used to control the velvetbeen caterpillar in soybean. In the early eighties this program was performed in Brazil. Since then, over 2,000,000 ha of soybean have been treated with the virus annually. Recently, after many new emerging pests in the soybean, this number dropped down. Although the use of this virus in Brazil is the most impressive example of viral bioregulation worldwide, the virus is still obtained by *in vivo* production mainly by infection of larvae in soybean farms. The demand for virus production has increased tremendously for protection of four million hectares of soybean annually. Because large scale *in vivo* production of baculoviruses encounters many difficulties the high demand for AgMNPV require studies dealing with inexpensive *in vitro* production of the virus. The use of AgMNPV in Brazil brought about many economical, ecological and social benefits. On the basis of this spectacular success of a baculovirus pesticide, it is needless to say that the advantages of biopesticides over chemical pesticides are numerous [18].

3.2.3. Protozoa

Protozoan pathogens naturally infect a wide range of insect hosts. Although these pathogens can kill their insect hosts, many are more important for their chronic, debilitating effects. One important and common consequence of protozoan infection is a reduction in the number of offspring produced by infected insects. Although protozoan pathogens play a significant role in the natural limitation of insect populations, few appear to be suited for development as insecticides.

As an other example, the Microsporidia include species promising for biological control. Microsporidian infections in insects are thought to be common and responsible for naturally occurring low to moderate insect mortality. But these are indeed slow acting organisms, taking days or weeks to make harm their host. Frequently they reduce host reproduction or feeding rather than killing the pest outright. Microsporidia often infect a wide range of insects. Some microsporidia are being investigated as microbial insecticides, and at least one is available commercially, but the technology is new and work is needed to perfect the use of these organisms [12]

3.2.4. Microscopic nematods

To be accurate, nematodes are not microbial agents. Instead, they are multicellular roundworms. Nematodes used in insecticidal products are, however, nearly microscopic in size, and they are used much like the truly microbial products discussed previously. Nematodes are simple roundworms. Colorless, unsegmented, and lacking appendages, nematodes may be free-living, predaceous, or parasitic. Many of the parasitic species cause important diseases of plants, animals, and humans. Other species are beneficial in attacking insect pests, mostly sterilizing or otherwise debilitating their hosts. A very few cause insect death but these species tend to be difficult (e.g., tetradomatids) or expensive (e.g. mermithids) to mass produce, have narrow host specificity against pests of minor economic importance, possess modest virulence (e.g., sphaeruliids) or are otherwise poorly suited to exploit for pest control purposes. The only insect-parasitic nematodes possessing an optimal balance of biological control attributes are entomopathogenic or insecticidal nematodes in the genera *Steinernema* and *Heterorhabditis*Nematodes used for insect control infect only insects or related arthropods; they are called entomogenous nematodes [19]

The entomogenous nematodes *Steinernema feltiae* (sometimes identified as *Neoaplectana carpocapsae*), *S. scapteriscae, S. riobravis, S. carpocapsae* and *Heterorhabditis heliothidis* are the species most commonly used in insecticidal preparations. Within each of these species, different strains exhibit differences in their abilities to infect and kill specific insects. In general, however, these nematodes infect a wide range of insects. On a worldwide basis, laboratory or field applications have been effective against over 400 pest species, including numerous beetles, fly larvae, and caterpillars.

The infectious stage of these nematodes is the third juvenile stage often referred to as the J3 stage or the "dauer" larvae. Nematodes in this stage survive without feeding in moist soil and similar habitats, sometimes for extended periods. *Steinernema* species infect host insects by entering through body openings--the mouth, anus, and spiracles (breathing pores). *Heterorhabditis* juveniles also enter host insects through body openings, and in some instances are also able to penetrate an insect's cuticle. If the environment is warm and moist, these nematodes complete their life cycle within the infected insect. Infective juveniles molt to form adults, and these adults produce a new generation withing the same host. As the offspring mature to the J3 stage, they are able to leave the dead insect and seek a new host [20]

Nosema locustae has been used to reduce grasshopper populations in rangeland areas, and adequate control has been achieved when treatments were applied to large areas while hoppers were still young. Although not all grasshoppers in the treated area are killed by *Nosema locustae,* infected hoppers consume less forage and infected females produce fewer viable eggs than do uninfected females. *Nosema locustae* persists on egg pods to provide varying degrees of infection the following season. The effectiveness and utilization of *Nosema locustae* for rangeland grasshopper control are likely to increase as research continues. This single-celled protozoan infects and kills over 90 species of grasshoppers, locusts, and some species of crickets. Nosema Iocustae is non-toxic to humans, livestock, wild animals, birds, fish, and pets. Should be applied early in the season as over-wintering hoppers emerge. Unfortunately, small, one-pound packages of *Nosema locustae* preparations developed for sale to gardeners and homeowners offer much less utility or none. The mobility of grasshoppers, coupled with the fact that infected hoppers are not killed until a few weeks after they ingest the pathogen, means that application of baits containing *Nosema locustae* to individual lawns or gardens is unlikely to reduce grasshopper densities or damage substantially [21].

3.2.5. Bacterial biopesticides

Bacterial biopesticides are the most common and cheaper form of microbial pesticides. As an insecticide they are generally specific to individual species of moths and butterflies, as well as species of beetles, flies and mosquitoes. To be effective they must come into contact with the target pest, and may require ingestion to be effective. Bacteria in biological pesticides survive longer in the open than previously believed. Bacterial pathogens used for insect control are spore-forming, rod-shaped bacteria in the genus *Bacillus*. They occur commonly in soils, and most insecticidal strains have been isolated from soil samples. The *Bacillus* genus encompasses a large genetic biodiversity. *Bacilli* are present in an extremely large area of environments ranging from sea water to soil, and are even found in extreme environments like hot springs [22]. This bacterium could be one of the major sources of potential microbial biopesticides because it retains several valuable traits [23].

First of all, *Bacilli*, like *B. subtilis*, are well-studied organisms. Secondly, the US Food and Drug Administration (USFDA) has granted the "generally regarded as safe" (GRAS) status to *Bacillus subtilis* which is thus recognized non-pathogenic. This is of course essential with respect to its application as a biopesticide. Thirdly, *Bacilli* have the capacity to produce spores which are extremely resistant dormancy forms capable to withstand high temperatures, unfavorable pH, lack of nutrients or water, etc. [24]. They are produced by the bacteria when environmental conditions are unfavorable which probably helps these microorganisms to survive in the phytosphere. The phenomenon can also be exploited in industrial production as sporulation can be induced at the end of cultures. course essential regarding its application as a biopesticide [25].

Bacterial insecticides must be eaten to be effective; they are not contact poisons. Insecticidal products comprised of a single *Bacillus* species may be active against an entire order of insects, or they may be effective against only one or a few species.

3.2.6. Bacillus thuringiensis, BT

Bacillus thuringiensis (Bt) is an aerobic, gram positive, spore forming soil bacterium that shows unusual ability to produce endogenous different kinds of crystals protein inclusions during its sporulation. *B. thuringiensis* (commonly known as 'Bt') is an insecticidal bacterium, marketed worldwide for control of many important plant pests - mainly caterpillars of the Lepidoptera (butterflies and moths) but also mosquito larvae, and simuliid blackflies that vector river blindness in Africa. The commercial Bt products are powders containing a mixture of dried spores and toxin crystals. They are applied to leaves or other environments where the insect larvae feed. The toxin genes have also been genetically engineered into several crop plants. The method of use, mode of action, and host range of this biocontrol agent may differ within other Bacillus insecticidal species [10]

The *Bacillus* species, *Bacillus thuringiensis,* has developed many molecular mechanisms to produce pesticidal toxins; most of toxins are coded for by several *cry* genes. Since its discovery in 1901 as a microbial insecticide, *Bacillus thuringiensis* has been widely used to control insect pests important in agriculture, forestry and medicine. Its principal characteristic is the synthesis of a crystalline inclusion during sporulation, containing proteins known as endotoxins or Cry proteins, which have insecticidal properties [26]. The crystal protein inclusions are composed of one or more crystal (Cry) and cytolytic (Cyt) toxins which are also called δ-endotoxins or insecticidal crystal proteins. Some of these proteins are highly toxic to certain insects but they are harmless to most other organisms including vertebrates and beneficial insect. Since their insecticidal potential has been discovered, it has been produced commercially and accepted as a source of environment friendly biopesticide all over the world.

There are different strains of *B. thuringiensis*. Each strain of this bacterium produces a different mix of proteins, and specifically kills one or a few related species of insect larvae. While some Bt's control moth larvae found on plants, other Bt's are specific for larvae of flies and mosquitoes. The target insect species are determined by whether the particular Bt produces a protein that can bind to a larval gut receptor, thereby causing the insect larvae to starve.The most widely used strains of *B. thuringiensis* have started against three genera of mosquitos; *Culex, Culiseta* and *Aedes*[

Their study has shown that Bt spores can survive both on the ground and in animals. What's more, wind, rain and animals can carry them to neighbouring areas. In the splashing rain drops they can even "hop" from the ground up onto leaves - another means of transport. Bt bacteria are also known to be able to easily transfer their toxicity genes to other bacteria in the application area.

When the bacteria were sprayed on cabbage plants, and they were found to have killed all the cabbage white butterfly larvae. In addition, though, the field study revealed that the bacteria are able to survive for a considerable time. After spraying, by far the majority of the spores were found to be present in the upper two centimetres of the soil, *National Environmental Research Institute of Denmark.* "Their toxic effects disappeared after a few days, but half of the bacteria were still surviving as spores 120 days later, and one fifth were still alive after a year. They existed in a dormant state, however, and did not produce toxins, although the spores are able to germinate later and produce insecticide again," explain microbiologists Bjarne Munk Hansen and Jens Chr. Pedersen of the National Environmental Research Institute. Until now it has generally been believed that the majority of Bt bacteria disappear rapidly after they have been sprayed. "It was thought that when the toxic effect disappeared, the bacteria had also disappeared. What in fact happens, though, is that the bacteria convert to a dormant stage and become spores," continue the two scientists.

In the present era of transgenic technology, insecticidal toxins of *Bacillus thuringiensis* (Bt) assume considerable significance in the production of insect resistant crops such as cotton, maize, potato, rice etc. This review also describes about biology of Bt toxin, recent progress in the development of Bt technology, evolution of resistant insect populations against Bt and management strategy.

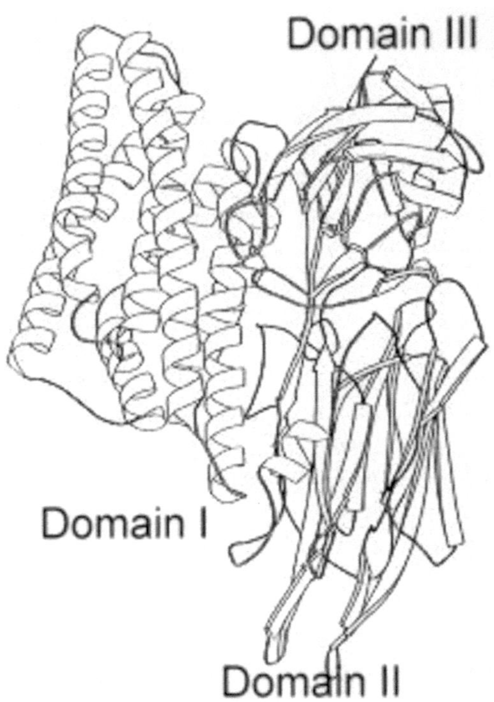

Figure 1. Different domains involved in the toxicity of *B.thuringiensis* toxin in the mid-gut of targeted insect. Source:Sharma et al., 2000. *Bt* bacteria are used by farmers, foresters and gardeners to destroy butterfly larvae, mosquito larvae and beetles. The Danish field study, which was undertaken in 1993 and 1994, is one of the first in the world where plants have been systematically sprayed with *Bacillus thuringiensis* bacteria, and where the research has been ecologically oriented. In contrast, the numerous field studies undertaken by the producers of biological pesticides have been oriented to commercial considerations.

Scientists Per Damgaard and Jørgen Eilenberg at the Royal Agricultural University in Denmark, have also observed examples of spores germinating in living but weakened flies. The flies were already suffering from a severe fungal infection of the lower abdomen, and it was exactly there that the spores germinated. They showed that, the bacterial spores germinate well in dead insects, as the two scientists confirmed by feeding spore and toxin-treated food to larvae of the large cabbage white butterfly.

Under good growth conditions a spore can produce up to a thousand million new spores in a single insect larva.

"There are no previous examples of the spores reproducing in living organisms, although they appear to be able to do so in dead flies. The advantage for the bacterium is that the spores can be spread when the fly moves around," continue Bjarne Munk Hansen and Jens Chr. Pedersen.

Gene	Target pest	References
Cry 1A(b)	Striped stem borer and leaf folder	Fujimoto et al. (1993)
Cry 1A(b)	Yellow stem borer and striped stem borer	Wunn et al. (1996)
Cry 1A(b)	Yellow stem borer and striped stem borer	Ghareyazie et al. (1997)
Cry 1A(b)	Yellow stem borer	Datta et al. (2002)
Cry 1A(b)	Yellow stem borer	Alam et al. (1999)
Cry 1A(b)/ Cry 1A(c)	Leaffolder and yellow stem borer	Tu et al. (2000)
Cry 1A(b)/ Cry 1A(c)	Yellow stem borer	Ramesh et al. (2004)
Cry 1A(c)	Yellow stem borer	Nayak et al. (1997)
Cry 1A(c)	Yellow stem borer	Khanna and Raina (2002)
Cry 1A(c)	Striped stem borer	Liu et al. (2002)
Cry 2A	Leaffolder and yellow stem borer	Maqbool et al. (1998)
Cry 2A/ Cry 1A(c)	Leaffolder and yellow stem borer	Maqbool et al. (2001)
Cry 1Ie	Corn borer	Liu et al., 2004

Table 2. Successful examples to show *B. thuringiensis* genes (originated from *Bacillus thuringiensis*) integration for insect resistance in rice.

Insects can be infected with many species of bacteria but those belonging to the genus Bacillus, as alreadily mentioned, are most widely used as pesticides. *Bacillus thuringiensis* has developed many molecular mechanisms to produce called cry genes [28]. Since its discovery in 1901 over one hundred *B. thuringiensis*-based bioinsecticides have been developed, which are mostly used against lepidopteran, dipteran and coleopteran larvae[29]. In addition, the genes that code for the insecticidal crystal proteins have been successfully transferred into different crops plants by means of transgenic technology which has led to significant economic benefits. Because of their high specificity and their safety in the environment, *B. thuringiensis* and Cry protein toxins are efficient, safe and sustainable alternatives to chemical pesticides for the control of insect pests. The toxicity of the Cry proteins have traditionally been explained by the formation of transmembrane pores or ion channels that lead to osmotic cell lysis [30]. In addition to this, Cry toxin monomers also seem to promote cell death in insect cells through a mechanism involving an adenylyl cyclase/PKA signalling pathway. However, despite this entomopathogenic potential, controversy has arisen regarding the pathogenic lifestyle of *B. thuringiensis*. Recent reports claim that *B. thuringiensis* requires the co-operation of commensal bacteria within the insect gut to be fully pathogenic [31,32].

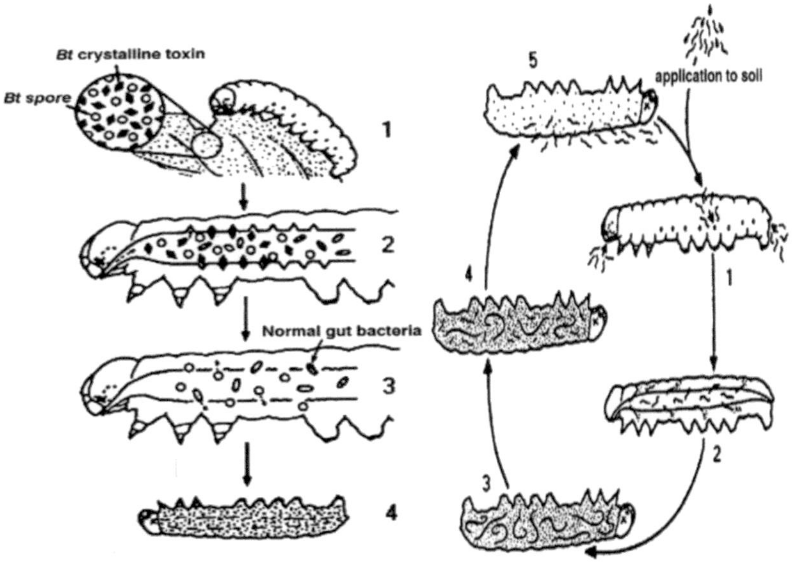

Figure 2. Life cycles of biopesticides, bacteria or nematods, to pest larvas. 1- enter the gut or respiratory system through body openings (mouth, anus, and breathing pores. 2- actively penetrate the gut wall, enter the body cavity, and release bacteria. 3- As it multiplies, host dies of septicemia, Adapted from Woodring,1988

The first developed *Bacillus thuringiensis* insecticidal agent is a mixture of *Bacillus thuringiensis* spores and its toxin. As a pesticide, (BT*)* accounts for over 90 percent of total share of today's bioinsecticide market and has been used as biopesticide for several decades. The discovery of the strain *B. thuringiensis* serovar *israelensis* made possible efficient microbiological control of Diptera Nematocera vectors of diseases, such as mosquitoes (Culicidae) and black flies [33]

In most countries of the world, products are available for control of caterpillars (var. *kurstaki, entomocidus, galleriae* and *aizawai*), mosquito and blackfly larvae (var. *israeliensis*) and beetle larvae (var. *tenebrionis*). Actively growing cells lack the crystalline inclusions and thus are not toxic to insects. The BT preparations remain stable without any disentegration over years even in the presence of UV sun rays. As the insect feeds on the foliage, the crystals too are eaten up. These are hydrolysed in the insect's midgut to produce an active endotoxin. The active toxin binds to receptor sites on gut epithelial cells and creates imbalance in the ionic make-up of the cell. This is seen by swelling and bursting of the cells due to osmotic shock. Subsequent symptoms are paralysis of the insect's mouthparts and gut. So obviously the feeding process is inhibited. [34,35]

Also, a relatively new mechanism of action of Cry toxins have been proposed which involves the activation of Mg2+-dependent signal cascade pathway that is triggered by the interaction of the monomeric 3-domain Cry toxin with the primary receptor, the cadherin protein BT-R1 [26]. The triggering of the Mg2+-dependent pathway has a knock-on effect and initiates a series of cytological events that include membrane blebbing, appearance of nuclear ghosts, and cell swelling followed by cell lysis. The Mg2+-dependent signal cascade pathway activation by Cry

http://dx.doi.org/10.5772/55786

Binding
↓
Conformation change
↓
Insertion
↓
Oligomerization
↓
Pore formation
↓
Cell Lysis

Figure 3. Characterization of the steps require for formation of pores in cell membranes

toxins have been shown to be analogous to similar effect imposed by other pore forming toxins on their host cells when they are applied at subnanomolar concentration [37, 38]

Though the two mechanisms of action seem to differ, with series of downstream events following on from toxin binding to receptors on target cell membranes, there is a degree of commonality in that initially the crystals have to be solubilised in vivo or in vitro, and activated by proteases before and/or after binding to receptors such as cadherin [39, 40]

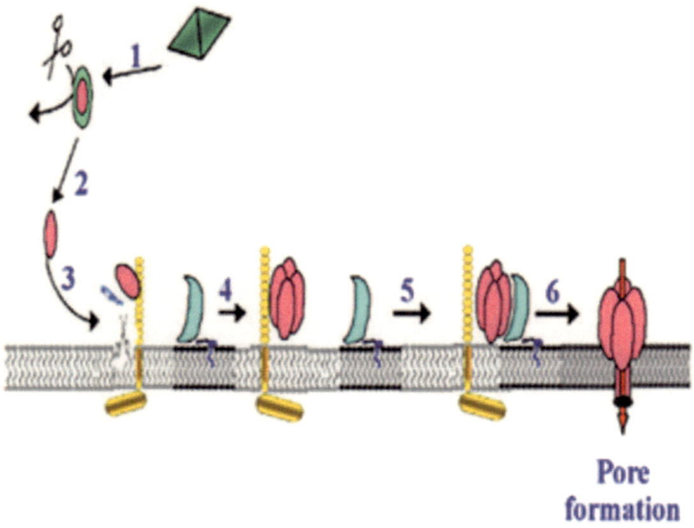

Figure 4. Model of the mode of action of Cry1A toxins. *1* Crystal toxin solubilisation, *2* Initial cleavage by gut proteases, *3* Toxin monomer binding to receptors and second cleavage bymembrane bound protease, *4* Membrane insertion-competent oligomer formation, *5* Binding of oligomeric toxin to receptors, *6* Lytic pore formation

4. Plant-Incorporated-Protectants (PIPs)

One approach, to reduce destruction of crops by phytophagous arthropod pests, is to genetically modify plants to express genes encoding insecticidal toxins. The adoption of genetically modified (GM) crops has increased dramatically in the last 11 years. Genetically modified (GM) plants possess a gene or genes that have been transferred from a different species.

The production of transgenic plants that express insecticidal δ-endotoxins derived from the soil bacterium *Bacillus thuringiensis* (*Bt* plants) were first commercialized in the US in 1996. The expression of these toxins confers protection against insect crop destruction. The lethality of *Bt* endotoxins is highly dependent upon the alkaline environment of the insect gut, a feature that assures these toxins are not active in vertebrates, especially in humans [41]. These proteins have been commercially produced, targeting the major pests of cotton, tobacco, tomato, potato, corn, maize and rice, notably allowing greater coverage by reaching locations on plants which are inaccessible to foliar sprays. There are numerous strains of *Bt*, each with different Cry proteins, and more than 60 Cry proteins have been identified. Most *Bt* maize hybrids express the Cry1Ab protein, and a few express the Cry1Ac or the Cry9C protein, all of which are targeted against the European corn borer (*Ostrinia nubilalis* Hubner) (Lepidoptera), a major pest of maize in North America and Europe. Some recent maize hybrids express the Cry3Bb1 protein, which is targeted against the corn rootworm complex [*Diabrotica spp.* Coleoptera], also a major pest of maize, especially in North America. Cotton expressing the Cry1Ac protein is targeted against the cotton bollworm [*Helicoverpa zea- Lepidoptera*] [42].

Crop target	Gene	Target pest	References
Corn	*Cry 1A(b)*	European corn borer	Koziel et al. (1993)
Soybean	*Cry 1A(c)*	Bollworm and Bud worm	Stewart (1996)
Tobacco	*Cry 2aa2*	Cotton bollworm	De Cosa et al. (2001)
Sugar cane	*Cry 1A(b)*	Stem borer	Arencibia et al. (1997)
Potato	*Cry 5*	*B. thuringiensis* Potato tuber moth	Douches et al. (1998)
Alfalfa	*Cry 1C*	Leaf worm	Strizhov et al. (1996)
Tomato	B. thuringiensis (k)	Tobacco hornworm, tomato pink worm and tomato fruit worm	Dellannay et al. (1989)
Brassica	*Cry 1A(c)*	Pod borer	Stewart (1996)
Cotton	*Cry 1A(b)/(c)*	Lepidoptera	Stewart(2001), Chitkowski et al. (2003)
	Cry 2A	Pink Bollworm	Tabashnik et al. (2002)

Table 3. Development of some other *B. thuringiensis* transgenic crops for insect resistance [35]

5. *Bacillus thuringiensis* applications in agriculture

Bacillus thuringiensis and its products have been formulated into various forms for application as biological control agents. Such formulations could be solid (powdery or granulated) or liquid. Presently there are over 400 of *Bt* based formulations that has been registered in the market and most of them contain insecticidal proteins and viable spores though the spores are inactivated in some products. Formulated *Bt* products are applied directly in the form of sprays). An alternative, and highly successful, method for delivering the toxins to the target insect has been to express the toxin-encoding genes in transgenic plants [43,44]

5.1. *Bacillus sphaericus*, BS

Entomopathogenic bacteria, namely *Bacillus thuringiensis* Bt, have been known from the early 1900's but the control of dipteran species has been establ,shed only since the discovery of *B. thuringiensis* serovar *israelensis* Bti in 1977 and a highly toxic strain of *B. sphaericus* B.s. strain 1593 in [45].

Bacillus sphaericus is the another aerobic bacterium in Bacillus genus that has been used in the biological control of the insects. *Bacillus sphaericus* Bs, like *Bacillus thrungiensis* Bti is a naturally occurring soil bacterium with mosquitoe larvicidal properties from the genus *Bacillus*. It has become an alternative agent for microbial control of mosquitoes since the isolation of highly larvicidal strains of this bacteria. *Psorophora*, and some members of the genus *Aedes*. *Ae. aegypti* and *Ae. albopictus* are insensitive to *B. sphaericus*

The first reported *B. sphaericus* strain (BS) active against mosquito larvae was isolated from Moribund area in Argentina to mosquito larvae of *Culiseta* incidens in 1965 [46]. Strain 2362, isolated from *Simulium* in Nigeria, is not toxic to black flies, but it is regarded as the most promising isolate for field use against mosquitoes. Pasteurization of the soils make the medium selective for *B. sphaericus*. The efficacy of strain 2362 against field populations of mosquitoes from the genera *Culex* has been demonstrated. Since the sixties, when a strain of BS was discovered to have larvicidal activity against mosquito species, a large number of other mosquitocidal Bs strains have been described. The larvicidal activity of this first isolate was so low that its use in mosquito control would not have been considered indeed. But only after isolation in Endonesia from dead mosquito larvae of strain 1593 which exhibited a much higher mosquitocidal activity against *Culex quinquefasciatus* was potential of *Bacillus sphaericus* as a biological control agent for some species of mosquitoes, and used as insecticide in the field as part of vector control programmes [47].

It has terminally located sphearical spores. One of the phenotypic characthers examined was patogenicity of some of them to mosquito larvae. A pro-toxin produced during sporulation as in the case of BT, causes fatal cellular alterations when ingested by larvae of some dipteran species. This bacterium has been used to control *Culex* and *Anopheles* populations in various countries replacing chemical larvicides with certain advantages. They include reduction in cost and selectivity to the target populations. The toxic activity of the *Bacillus sphaericus* strains increased at the time of sporulation, it is logical to look for parasporal inclusions in this bacterium. Since filter sterilized culture supernatants had been shown to be nontoxic, all of the toxin must be retained on or within the cells themselves. In the cells fractioned in the process of sporulation, the cell walls gave more toxic characthere than the cytoplasmic part. On the other hand, the mature spores isolated from the cells were more toxic than the cell wall fraction, thus it appeared that some toxin may be located in several parts of the cell but that the spore contains the highest concentration of the toxin [48,49,50].

Abbott Laboratories has recently formulated a commercial product (Vectolex) of *B. sphaericus* 2362. Generally, *B. sphaericus* strains with high larvicidal activity have been isolated from dead insects and as well as from other sources. However, five isolates of *B. sphaericus* from soil samples in Israel have been reported to belong to phage group three and were found to be as toxic as strain 2362 to *Culex* sp. Larvae. During a screening for entomopathogenic bacteria in soil samples carried out at Cenargen / Embrapa in Brazil, several *B. sphaericus* isolates were obtained [51].

5.2. Systematics of the *Bacillus sphaericus* Neide

According to one the old view *Bacillus sphaericus* is a heterogeneous species of bacteria that contains strains belonging to at least five different DNA homology groups that are sufficiently phenotypically similar without a need to establish each as a new distinct species of which homology group IIA differ from the other genospecies in that it contains strains that are pathogenic for mosquitoe larvae. According to a recent study based on phylogenetic analysis of the 16S rRNA DNA sequences from 58 strains identified as *B. sphaericus*, which were also confirmed by whole-cell fatty acid profiles and other phenotypic determinations, *B. sphaericus*-like strains segregated into seven distinct clusters in a phylogenetic tree and is a genetically and phenotypically a highly heterogeneous taxon. Among these, one cluster represented *B. sphaericus* and another *B. fusiformis*. A third cluster containing all of the pathogenic strains was closely related to or was possibly part of the *B. fusiformis* group. The remaining four groups were distinct and represented unnamed taxa that are more closely related to *B. sphaericus* and *B. fusiformis* than to the psychrophilic, round-spored species, *B. globisporus* and *B. psychrophilus*. The pathogenic strains are members of a distinct group and not of the species *B. sphaericus* sensu stricto. The apparent variability of mosquitoe pathogenicity among *B. sphaericus* strains can partially be explained by this heterogeneity [52].

5.3. Mode of living of *Bacillus* spp. and *Bacillus sphaericus* Neide

The growth of *Bacillus sphaericus* is in four stages depending on the presence of food and water in their environment. These are; (1) lag phase, where active microbial growth is to be commenced, (2) log phase, where there are active bacterial growth and the number of bacteria increases logarithmically, hence the name suggests, and (3) stationary phase, where growth of bacteria ceases due to food limitation and/or some other factors, and (4) death phase, where death of bacteria starts if they are not sporulating. If the bacterium is of a sporulating type like the genus *Bacillus*, then at the late stationary stages sporulation starts and we usually do not speak of death phases for the bacteria in the genus *Bacillus*. *B. sphaericus* starts producing endospores at the last stage of its growth cycle [51,52]

5.4. Endospore formation of *Bacillus sphaericus* Neide

Endospore formation is a trait found in several microorganisms, which can provide positive benefits to agriculture and varying affects in humans as well. Species of *Bacillus, Clostridium, Sporosarcina,* and *Heliobacteria* produce typical endospores. Endospores are formed when a vegetative cell discontinues protein synthesis for proteins needed for normal cell function and instead activates genes specific for sporulation. Endospores are the product of aging cells in environments low in nutients. All of the cell's materials remain inside the protoplast, or core of the endospore, but metabolism is dormant. The endospore is refractile, dehydrated, and surrounded by numerous thick layers of peptidoglycan. The coat, a keratin-like protein, contains diplicolinic acid (DPA) and a high calcium content. These help make the endospore highly heat resistant, boiling, radiation, pressure, dessication and chemical treatment. Endospores also contain large amounts of small acid-soluble spore proteins (SASPs). The function of SASPs is to bind to DNA as a form of protection and to serve as a carbon energy source for when the endospore germinates to form a new vegetative cell [52]

5.5. Growth Cycle of *B. sphaericus* and production extra-cellular enzymes

During their growth cycle, strains of *Bacillus* grow as undifferentiated rod-shaped vegetative cells. Usually when the carbon source (or some other required nutrient) becomes limited, the cell enters a sporulation sequence during which a resistant resting-stage endospore is formed. The process of cellular differentiation leading to spore formation can be divided into three successive phases. Sporulation in *B. subtilis* has been well studied and it includes four stages. The first (stages 0 to II) is the stage of differentiation, and during this there is a single cell type, which eventually contains two completed chromosomes. The phase is completed with the division of this cell into two cells that differ markedly in size, but otherwise appear to be rather similar. In the second phase (stages II to III) the differentiation becomes fixed; the two cells have their own genomes, which presumably functions differently, and by stage III the two cell types differ dramatically. The developing spore at stage III exhibits none of the properties that characterize the mature spore, and the development of these properties takes place in the next phase (stages III to VII). Production of entomopathogenic toxin is a biochemical changes that accompany the morphological changes during sporulation. When fresh medium (or a pulse of a carbon source) is made available, the spore will germinate and produce a vegetative rod-shaped cell [53,54]

Because *B. subtilis,* like other Gram-positive eubacteria, lacks an outer membrane, many of these proteins are directly secreted into the growth medium. In most cases, these secreted proteins are enzymes involved in the hydrolysis of natural polymers such as proteases, lipases, carbohydrases, DNases and RNases. Such degradative enzymes are usually synthesised as part of an adaptive response indeed to changes in the environment. So that the cell to optimally can benefit from available resources.

5.6. Pathogenicity and properties of toxins of *B. Sphaericus*

The bulk of toxicity in Bs comes from the second toxin which is produced at the time of sporulation and it accumulates in the sporangium as a parasporal body, parasporal crystal packed with bacterial spores, in much the same way as that found in *B. thuringiensis.* The crystal of *B. sphaericus* 2362, which becomes visible in the cytoplasm at about stage III of sporulation contains two polypeptides, a 51 kDa protein,P51 and a 42-kDa protein, P42, which together form the binary toxin. The binary toxin consists of two distinct proteins of 51.4 and 41.9 kDa. Both proteins are cleaved by endogenous proteases to form active toxins of 43 and 39 kDa protein subunits that are believed to associate as a hetero-dimer named the binary toxin Bin, in a 1:1 ratio, which form the active hetero-dimer complex [42]. These protein toxins have been sequenced and were found to be unrelated to each other or to the *B. thuringiensis* toxins. The *bin* genes of several highly toxic strains have also been completely sequenced, and their amino-acid sequences have been found to be highly conserved [54].

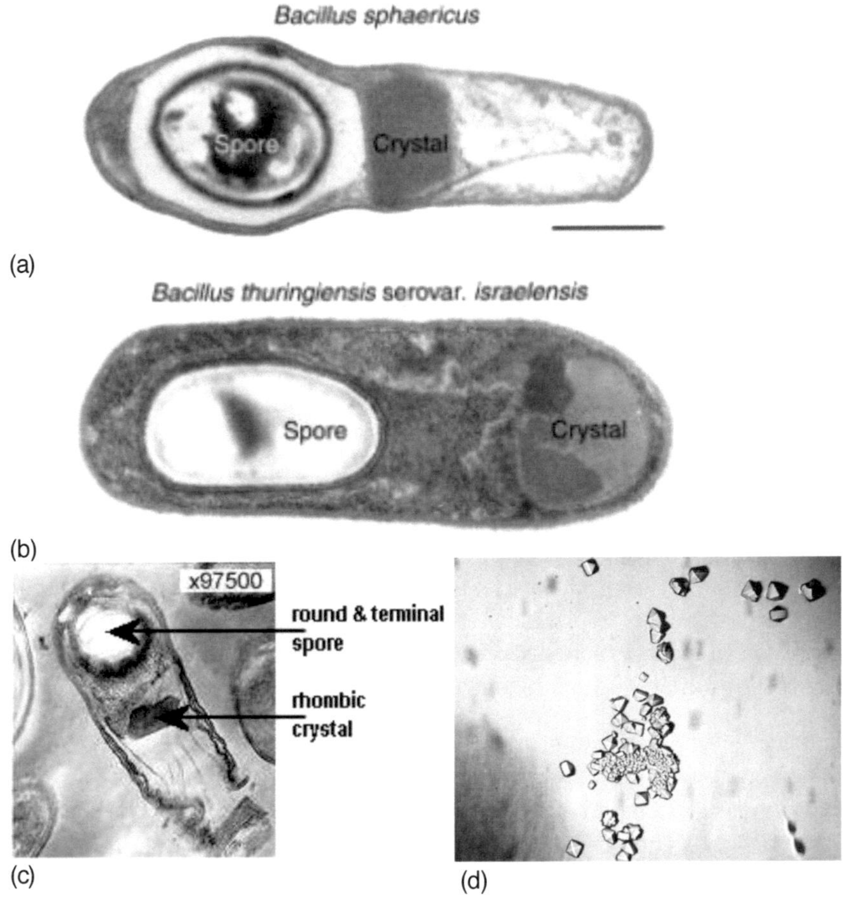

Figure 5. Sporangia of *Bacillus sphaericus* (**a**) and *Bacillus thuringiensis* serovar. *israelensis* (**b**) before the end of the sporulation process as seen by transmission electron microscopy. The parasporal inclusions (crystals), which contain the entomopathogenic toxins, are visible close to the spore. Scale BAR = 0.5 μm (from Regis et al., 2001). A closer view of *B. sphaericus* crystal showing its rhombic shape from the **a** (top) and crystals of the 51 kDa protein of *B. sphaericus* grown using the seeding method. The largest crystals are 0.2 mm in length and have well defined facets consistent with the tetragonal space group. Note that the crystals grow preferentially along the streaking path, which is almost vertical [55]

http://dx.doi.org/10.5772/55786

The two major protein subunits, the 42 and 51 kDa, are both required for full activity and maximum toxicity if they are present in equimolar amounts, suggesting a 'binary toxin' mode of action. Studies on the mode of action of Bin toxin suggested that BinB is responsible for the initial binding to the surface of midgut epithelial cells and that BinA confers toxicity. It was also reported that the BinA compound alone can confer toxicity at high doses These two protein subunits are homologous, with 25% identity and four conserved regions between their sequences. P51 is the primary component of binding to the *Culex* midgut epithelium, while P42 binds efficiently only in the presence of P51 but is responsible for the larvicidal action Upon ingestion by larvae, these proteins are processed to 43 and 39 kDa, respectively. Studies on the mode of action of Bin toxin suggested that BinB is responsible for the initial binding to the surface of midgut epithelial cells and that BinA confers toxicity Neither subunit of the binary toxin is not toxic by itself both BinB and BinA in order to achieve full toxicity and a BinA–BinB or BinA–BinB–receptor complex formation in strains of 1593 and LP1-G of *B. sphaericus* has been proposed to cause larval. In confirmation that both subunits are required for full toxicity in vitro binding studies were performed to show that the N-terminal region of BinB interacts with the larval gut receptor, whereas the C-terminal region interacts with the N-terminal region of BinA, leaving the C-terminal end of BinA to facilitate internalization of the toxin complex. Binding of the binary toxin to midgut epithelium causes swelling of mitochondrial and endoplasmic reticula and enlargement of vacuoles, followed by lyses of epithelial cells, midgut perforation, and the death of larvae. How the Bin toxin causes the death of larvae is not clearly established. There is evidence that a single class of receptor is expressed on the surface of microvilli in the gastric caeca and posterior midgut of susceptible *C. pipiens* and *A. gambiae* and binding of toxin to midgut cells of susceptible mosquitoe larvae is a key step after the initial solubilization and activation of the toxin. A recent report has shown that this binding is specific, and mediated by a receptor with a unique binding site, present at the surface of epithelial cells from *Culex* and *Anopheles*. It was found that BinB alone is involved in receptor binding in *C. pipiens,* whereas both BinA and BinB seem to be involved in receptor binding in *A. Gambiae* [55]

6. Mode of action of the crystal toxin

The mode of action of *Bacillus sphaericus* crystal toxin has only been studied in mosquito larvae. A number of studies have established that the action of the crystal toxin on susceptible larvae involves th efollowing series of steps: (i) ingestion of the crystal- spore- cell complex; (ii) solubilization on th e midgut by the alkaline pH; (iii) processing of the 51- and 42-kDa proteins to 43 and 39-kDa proteins respectively, (iv) binding of toxin proteins to cells of the gastric cecum and posterior midgut; and (v) exertion of a toxic effect by means of a unknown mechanism [56].

6.1. Binding to a specific receptor in the brush- border membrane fractions

After ingestion of the spore-crystal complex by mosquito larvae, the protein crystal matrix quickly dissolves in the lumen of the anterior stomach through the combined action of midgut proteinases and the high pH *Bacillus sphaericus* crystals release the toxin in all species such as *A. aegypti*. Indeed, some studies reported that the differences in susceptibility to Bacillus sphaericus between mosquito species do not result from differences in solubilization and/or activation of the crystal toxin. Physiological effects in midgut start as soon as 15 min. after ingestion of spor crystal complex. Midgut damages may be the same after ingestıon of spore crystals but the semptoms of intoxication produced differ in mosquito species. Large vacuoles or lysosomes appear in *Culex pipiens* midgut cells, whereas large areas of low electron density appear in Anopheles stephensi midgut cells. A generally occuring sypmtom is mitocondrial swelling, described for *C. pipiens* var. *pipiens* and *Aedes stephensi*, as well as for *A. Aegyptin* when intoxicated with a very high dose of spore crystals. The midgut cells are the cells most severely damaged by the toxin, also reported late damage in neural tissue and in skeletal muscel. Ultrastructural effects have been reported in cultured cells, of which swelling of mitochodrial cristae and endoplasmic reticula, followed by enlargement of vacuoles and condensation of mitochondrial matrix [55,56].

6.2. The effectiveness of the toxin

Differences in susceptibility between mosquito species seem to differences at the cellular level.The binding of the crystal proteins, P42 and P51 depend on each other. In addition, the internalization of toxin only seems to occur when both components are present. The hyphothesis that a single receptor is involved in the toxin binding was confirmed by in vitro binding assays using radio-labeled activated crystal toxin and midgut brush-border membrane fractions isolated from susceptible mosquito larva It is assumed that the P42 component is the toxic moiety and the P51 is the binding component, the *B. sphaericus* crystal toxin is more likely to be similar to an A/B toxin than to a binary toxin. The nature of the receptor is still unknown [56].

6.3. Mtx1: Vegetative growth mosquitocidal toxin single protein of 100 kDa

B. sphaericus is also known for the ability of some strains to produce another mosquitocidal toxin. The gene encoding one such toxin, Mtx1 (formerly known as Mtx, Mosquitocidal toxin, Mosquitocidal toxin), was first isolated from the low.

Toxicity *B. sphaericus* strain SSII-1 and has been shown to be widely distributed amongst many, but not all, high and low toxicity isolates of this species [59]. It was later shown that there are other Mtx toxins which are then started to be called Mtx1, Mtx2 and Mtx3 the genes for these toxins have been partially characterized and shown to have an extremely high level of similarity [46]. Unlike the binary toxins Mtx1 is produced as a 100 kDa protein that is processed by trypsin-like proteinases in the mosquitoe gut to yield a product with ADP-ribosyl transferase activity, 27 kDa and a putative receptor binding domain, 70 kDa [56].

In initial experiments, activity of the protoxin was demonstrated against larvae of the mosquitoe, *Culex quinquefasciatus*, and protoxins of *Escherichia coli* cells were shown to be active against *Aedes aegypti* but not the predatory mosquitoe *Toxorhynchites splendens*. In contrast to the Bin toxin, Mtx1 was also found to be highly potent against larvae of *Ae. Aegypti*, on the other hand, Bin toxin shows low or zero toxicity against this insect. This high-level toxicity to

http://dx.doi.org/10.5772/55786

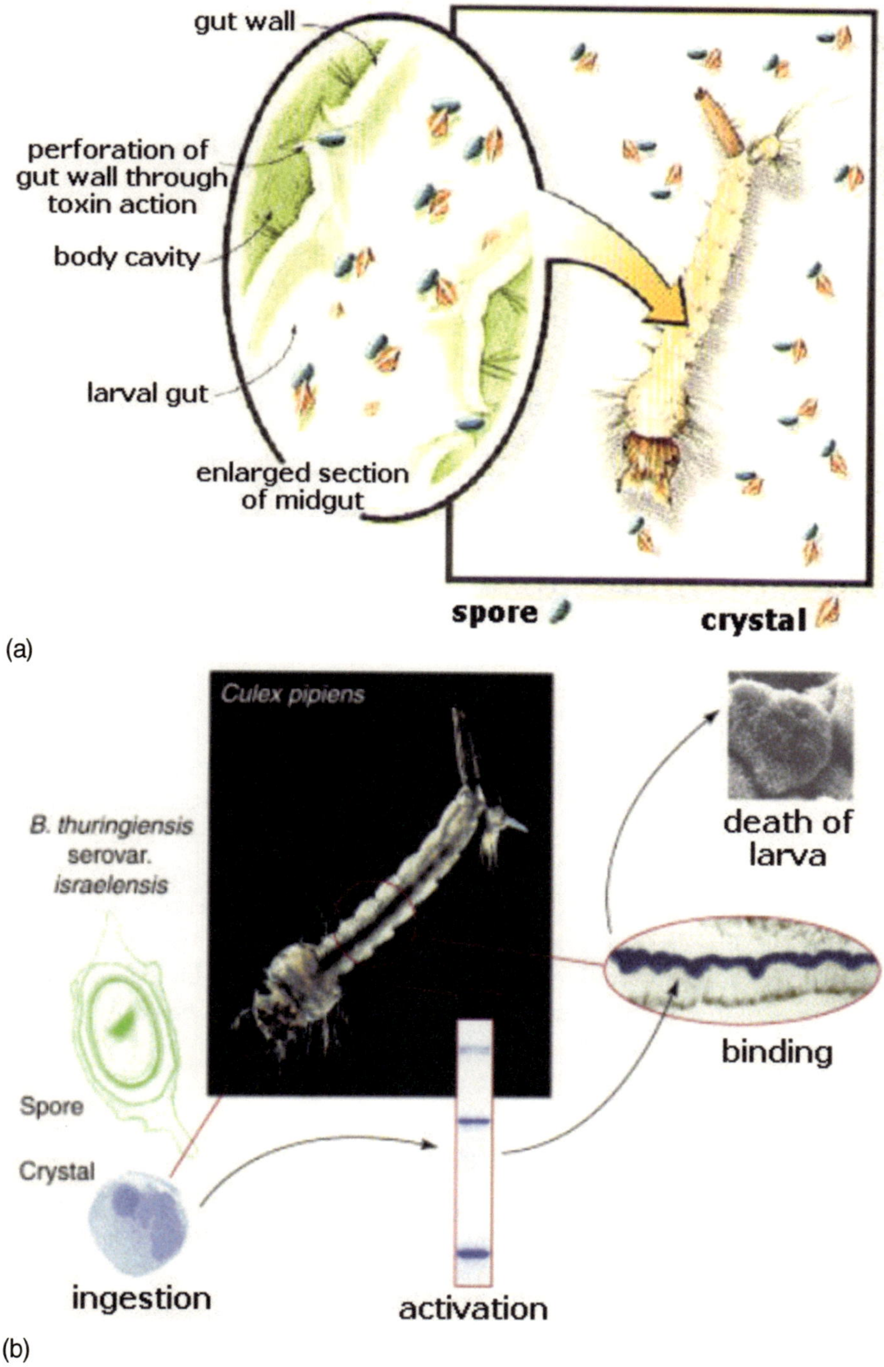

(a)

(b)

Figure 6. Action mechanism of VectoLexBC, a Biological Larvicide of *Bacillus sphaericus* (from Abbott Laboratories, 2003) **a.** top. The mode of action of crystal toxins from an entomopathogenic bacteria *Bacillus thuringiensis* serovar. *israelensis*, in this case **b.** below

Ae. aegypti gives Mtx1 great potential for use, by over-expression, in the strain improvement of *B. sphaericus*. It was proposed that the enhanced toxicity against *Ae. aegypti* would widen the utility of resulting strains whilst the distinct mechanism of action of Mtx1 compared to the Bin toxin would be expected to delay the development of resistance in target *Culex* populations. So far, thus Mtx toxin(s) of *B. sphaericus* may further enhances toxicity of this species both to mosquitoe and non-mosquitoe dipteran species [51].

7. Comparison of The Two Important Insect pathogens of *Bacillius*

Though *B. sphaericus* has a narrower range of host species than the main mosquitoe control agent *B.t.* subsp. *israelensis*, it is able to persist in the environment for a longer time than *B.t.* subsp. *israelensis*, especially in waters polluted with organic materials. However, populations of *Culex* mosquitoes resistant to the binary toxin of *B. sphaericus* have been selected under laboratory conditions. Field resistance, as a consequence of vector control programs based on *B. sphaericus* application, has also been reported in some countries, such as France and Brazil. In spite of massive field usage of *B.t.* subsp. *israelensis* in mosquitoe, chironomid midge, and black fly control, no resistance has been detected in field populations of these dipterans. This event has been explained by the presence of a set of toxic proteins of a different nature that interact synergistically, increasing larvicidal activity of *B.t.* subsp. *israelensis* and suppressing development of resistance [52].

The development of a larvicide for use in public health programmes demands selectivity. It should be active against the target species without affecting humans and other non-target populations. The development of a biological larvicide is a process similar to that of the chemical insecticides in that it aims to identify the ideal concentration and form of administration in the field. Formulation is the process used to convert a technical slurry or powder containing the active ingredient produced by the bacterium into a useful and use larvicide compatible with existing application systems. It should also ensure biological stability of the active ingredient and must have an adequate shelf life. It should be easily produced and administered, conveniently stored, and economic [51,52].

8. Resistance of insects to mosquitoe toxin

It was recently found that the decomposition of organic matter present in aquatic bodies by bacteria lead to the evolution of certain volatile compounds, which attract and/or stimulate gravid female mosquitoes to lay eggs. This finding is a clear indication that bacteria are in great association with mosquito species.

The risk of emergence of resistance should be considered when designing application strategies. *Bacillus sphaericus,* has been shown to recycle in the field conditions and exert larvicidal activity for a long period. Field resistance has been only reported for Bs, while for Bti, it seems more difficult for mosquitoes to develop resistance even under intensive laboratory selection, which may be due to the multiple toxin complex of this bacterium. One mechanism of resistance is the reduced binding of the toxin to the midgut receptor sites. The mechanism of resistance to *B. sphaericus* crystal toxin has been studied extensively in only two *C. pipiens* populations. Bioassays indicated that the resistance level was increased as the treatment increased, and the best way to produce bacterial strains that simultaneaously express different toxins binding to different receptors

One mechanism of resistance is the reduced binding of the toxin to the midgut receptor sites. As genes for production of insecticidal compounds are added to crop plants, developpers devise methods of preventing or managing insecticide resıstance in target pests. The mechanism of resistance to *B. sphaericus* crystal toxin has been studied extensively in only two *C. pipiens* populations. Bioassays indicated that the resistance level was increased as the treatment increased, and the best way to produce bacterial strains that simultaneaously express different toxins binding to different receptors.

Despite the reports of the resistance, the future of *B. sphaericus* in the control of mosquito larvae is promising. Indeed, resistance in the field seems to decline very quickly when treatments are suspended. The best way to prevent resistance has been seemed to produce bacterial strains that simultaneaously express different toxins binding to different receptors. On the other hand, there still exist some resistance or there are some other factors effecting the toxin in the application medium.

Development of mosquitoe larval resistance against the toxin of commercial microbial larvicide *B. sphaericus* has been first studied in cultured mosquito cells and later in *Culex quinquefasciatus* by many authors. It was recently shown that pattern of resistance evolution in mosquitoes depended on continuous selection pressure, and the stronger the selection pressure, the more quickly resistance developed. However repeated exposure of an insect population to *B. thuringiensis* induces the emergence of resistant pests. The number of toxin genes, together with the qualitative and quantitative differences among them and the properties of the resulting toxin, affect the quality of the developed strains [58].

Depending on the formulation and environmental conditions, *B. sphaericus* is generally effective from 1-4 weeks after application. The persistence of toxicity against *Culex quinquefasciatus* larvae, during a considerable period of time, the ability to recyle under certain environmental conditions have been studied.

On the other hand, there still exist some resistance or there are some other factors effecting the toxin in the application medium. The effects of aquatic bacterial proteases have been determined only in one study yet. In that study, about 500 bacterial isolates have been obtained from different aquatic mosquito habitats in Turkiye, and then the B. s. larvacidal toxin proteins have been exposed to these extracellular proteases of these bacterial isolates to establish the preliminary screening of the possible effect of these proteases on the B.s. binary toxin proteins. In this study, it was found that, there are also the effects of the environmental microorganisms specifically bacteria due to their extracellular proteases released in the area naturally, so that the B.s. toxin effectiveness in controlling the mosquitoes, especially *Culex* spp., can be affected by this factor [59,60]. The decrease or variability in the efficiency of the B.s. toxin may be not only due to the genetic capability of the insect organism to develope resistance against the microbial protein, but also due to the environmental microbiological character.

9. Conclusion

The increasing of biological control due to both ecological beneficiancies including the human health as part of world ecology, has been renewed.

The demand for bio-pesticides is rising steadily in all parts of the world. When used in Integrated Pest Management systems, biopesticides' efficacy can be equal to or better than conventional products, especially for crops like fruits, vegetables, nuts and flowers. By combining performance and safety, biopesticides perform efficaciously while providing the flexibility of minimum application restrictions, superior residue and resistance management potential, and human and environmental safety benefits.

In the study in which the sensitivity of the Bs crystal binary toxin to extracellular proteaese of the aquatic microorganisms were detected, it was shown that there are also the effects of the environmental microorganisms due to their extracellular proteases released in the toxin application area naturally. So that, the Bs toxin effectiveness in the controlling the mosquitoes, especially *Culex* spp.can be affected by this factor. The resistance against the microbial entamopathogens by the target organisms, has been usually thought to be genetic capability of the insects, specifically mosquito species. In this study it is found that, the decrease or variability in the efficency of the Bs toxin may be not only due to the genetic capability of the insect organism to develope resistance against the microbial protein, but also may as well be due to the environmental microbiological character [61].

In the future other studies can be done as well to detect the type and charactheristics of the effective proteases released into the Bs toxin application areas, so that the preventive manıp-ulatıons of the Bs toxin protein or some other genetic derivations of the toxin protein may well b eestablished, so that the specific proteaeses would not be able to effct the toxin, while the toxin still can kill the mosquito spp. It is very likely that in future their role will be more significant in agriculture and forestry. Biopesticides clearly have a potential role to play in development of future integrated pest management strategies Hopefully, more rational approach will be gradually adopted towards biopesticides in the near future and short-term profits from chemical pesticides will not determine the fate of biopesticides [62].

Author details

Canan Usta

Gaziosmanpasa University, Natural Sciences and Art Faculty Department of Biology, Turkey

References

[1] Papendick RI, Elliott LF, and Dahlgren RB (1986), Environmental consequences of modern production agriculture: How can alternative agriculture address these issues and concerns? *American Journal of Alternative Agriculture*, Volume 1, Issue 1, Pgs 3-10. Retrieved on 2007-10-10

[2] Lacey, L.A. and Siegel, J.P. 2000. "Safety and Ecotoxicology of Entomopathogenic Bacteria", in *Entomopatgenic Bacteria: From Laboratory to Field Application*

[3] Armand M. Kuris, Lafferty, K. D. 2000. Biological Control of Marine Pests, Ecology, Vol 77 (7) pp. 1989-2000

[4] Chapman, J. W. 1988. Invasion of the Northeast Pacific by Asian and Atlantic Gammaridean Amphipod Crustaceans, Including a New Species of Corophium. J. Of crustacean Biology 8: 364-382

[5] G.M. Nicholson, (2007). Fighting the global pest problem: Preface to the special Toxicon issue on insecticidal toxins and their potential for insect pest control, Toxicon, 2007, vol.49, pp.413–422.

[6] S. Gupta and A.K. Dikshit, Biopesticides: An ecofriendly approach for pest control. Journal of Biopesticides, 2010, vol. 3(1), 186 – 188.

[7] Burges, H.D. 1981. Safety, Safety Testing and Quality Control of Microbial Pesticides. Microbial control of pests and plant diseases. London, Academic Press Inc. 738-768.

[8] Flint, M. L. and R. Van den Bosch. 1981. Introduction to integrated pest management. Plenum Press, New York, 240 pp.

[9] Lacey, L.A., Frutos, R., Kaya, H.K. and Vail, P. 2001. Insect pathogens as biological control agents: Do they have a future? Biological Control 21: 230-248

[10] Meadows, M.P. (1993). *Bacillus thuringiensis* in the environment - ecology and risk assessment. In: Entwistle, P.F.; Cory, J.S.; Bailey, M.J. and Higgs, S. eds. *Bacillus thuringiensis*: an environmental biopesticide; theory and practice. Chichester, John Wiley, USA. pp.193-220.

[11] M.A. Hoy, Myths, models and mitigation of resistance to pesticides. *In:* Insecticide Resistance: From Mechanisms to Management (Denholm, I., Pickett, J.A. and Devonshire, A.L., eds.), New York, CABI Publishing, 1999, pp.111-119

[12] Hoffmann, M.P. and Frodsham, A.C. (1993) Natural Enemies of Vegetable Insect Pests. Cooperative Extension, Cornell University, Ithaca, NY. 63 pp.

[13] A.E. Hajeck and St. Leger, Interactions between fungal pathogens and insect hosts, Annual Review of Entomology, 1994, vol.39, pp.293 - 322.

[14] P. Ferron, Modification of the development of *Beauveria tenella* mycosis in *Melolontha melolontha* larvae by means of reduced doses of organophosphorus insecticides, Entomologia Experimentalis et Applicata, 1971,vol. 14, pp.457 – 466

[15] W.B. Shia and M.G. Feng, Lethal effect of *Beauveria bassiana, Metarhizium anisopliae,* and *Paecilomyces fumosoroseus* on the eggs of *Tetranychus cinnabarinus* (Acari: Tetranychidae) with a description of a mite egg bioassay system, Biological Control, 2004, vol.30, pp.165–173.

[16] C.M. Ignoffo and T.L. Couch, (1981). The nucleopolyhedrosis virus of *Heliothis* species as a microbial pesticide. In: Microbial Control of Pests and Plant Diseases. (Burges,H.D. Ed.), Academic Press. London, 1981, pp.329 - 362.

[17] J. James. Germida, 1984,Persistence of *Nosema locustae* Spores in Soil as Determined by Fluorescence Microscopy, Appl Environ Microbiol. February; 47(2): 313–318

[18] A. Mettenmeyer, Viral insecticides hold promise for bio-control, Farming Ahead, 2002, vol.124, pp.50 – 51.

[19] F. Moscardi, Assessment of the application of baculoviruses for control of Lepidoptera, Annual Review of Entomology, 1999, vol.44, pp.257 –289.

[20] Ma, Juan, Chen, Shulong Li, Xiuhua, Han, Richou, Khatri-Chhetri, Hari Bahadur, De Clercq, Patrick,Moens, Maurice, A new entomopathogenic nematode, *Steinernema tielingense* n. sp. (Rhabditida: Steinernematidae), from north China, 2012, Nematology, Vol: 14- 3, pp. 321-338

[21] Hoch, J., Sonenshein, A., Losick. A (Eds). (1993). *Bacillus subtilis* and other Gram-positive bacteria : biochemistry, physiology and molecular genetics. American Society for Microbiology, Washington, DC.

[22] Harwood, C.R., Wipat, A. (1996). Sequencing and functional analysis of the genome of *Bacillus subtilis* strain 168. *FEBS Letters,* Vol. 389, No. pp. 84-87.

[23] Ongena, M., Jacques, P. (2008). *Bacillus* lipopeptides: versatile weapons for plant disease biocontrol. *Trends in Microbiology,* Vol. 16, No. 3, pp. 115-125.

[24] Piggot, P., Hilbert, D. (2004). Sporulation of *Bacillus subtilis. Current Opinion in Microbiology,* Vol. 7, No. 6, pp. 579-586.

[25] Monteiro, S., Clemente, J., Henriques, A.O., Gomes, R., Carrondo, M., Cunha, A. (2005). A procedure for high-yield spore production by *Bacillus subtilis. Biotechnology Progress* Vol. 21, No. pp. 1026-1031.

[26] E. Schnepf, N. Crickmore, J. Van Rie, D. Lereclus, J. Baum, J. Feitelson, D.R. Zeigler and D.H. Dean, *Bacillus thuringiensis* and its pesticidal crystal proteins, Microbiology and Molecular Biology Reviews, 1998, vol.62, pp.775–806.

[27] Deltcluse A, Barloy F, Thitry I. 1995. Mosquitocidal toxins from various *Bacillus thuringiensis* and *Clostridium bifementans* In *Bacillus thuringiensis*. Biotechnology and Environmental Benefits, ed. HS Yuan, pp. 99-114.

[28] E. Schnepf, N. Crickmore, J. Van Rie, D. Lereclus, J. Baum, J. Feitelson, D.R. Zeigler and D.H. Dean, *Bacillus thuringiensis* and its pesticidal crystal proteins, Microbiology and Molecular Biology Reviews, 1998, vol.62, pp.775–806.

[29] J.Y. Roh, J.Y. Choi, M.S. Li, B.R. Jin and Y.H. Je, *Bacillus thuringiensis* as a specific, safe, and effective tool for insect pest control, J Microbiol Biotechnol, 2007, vol.17, pp. 547-559.

[30] X. Zhang, M. Candas, N.B. Griko, R. Taussig and L.A.Jr. Bulla, A mechanism of cell death involving an adenylyl cyclase/PKA signaling pathway is induced by the Cry1Ab toxin of *Bacillus thuringiensis*, Proc Natl Acad Sci USA, 2006, vol.103, pp. 9897-9902.

[31] N.A. Broderick, C.J. Robinson, M.D. McMahon, J. Holt, J. Handelsman and K.F. Raffa, Contributions of gut bacteria to *Bacillus thuringiensis*-induced mortality vary across a range of Lepidoptera, BMC Biol, 2009, vol.7, pp.11.

[32] Baum JA, Malvar T. Regulation of insecticidal crystal protein production in *Bacillus thuringiensis*. Mol Microbiol. 1995 Oct;18(1):1-12.

[33] E.A Buss and S.G. Park-Brown, Natural Products for Insect Pest Management. ENY-350 (http://edis.ifas.ufl.edu/IN197), 2002.

[34] Milner RJ (1994) History of *Bacillus thuringiensis*. Agric Ecosyst Environ 49(1):9–13

[35] Lambert B, Hofte H, Annys K, Jansens S, Soetaert P, Peferoen M (1992) Novel *Bacillus thuringiensis* insecticidal crystal protein with a silent activity against coleopteran larvae. Appl EnvironMicrobiol 58(8):2536–2542

[36] Zhang X, Candas M, Griko NB, Rose-Young L, Bulla LA (2005) Cytotoxicity of *Bacillus thuringiensis* Cry1Ab toxin depends on specific binding of the toxin to the cadherin receptor BT-R-1expressed in insect cells. Cell Death Differ 12(11):1407–1416

[37] Porta H, Cancino-Rodezno A, Soberón M, Bravo A (2011) Role of MAPK p38 in the cellular responses to pore-forming toxins. Peptides 32(3):601–606

[38] Nelson KL, Brodsky RA, Buckley JT (1999), Channels formed by subnanomolar concentrations ofthe toxin aerolysin trigger apoptosis of T lymphomas. Cell Microbiol 1(1):69–74

[39] Aronson AI, Han ES, McGaughey W, Johnson D (1991) The solubility of inclusion proteins from *Bacillus thuringiensis* is dependent upon protoxin composition and is a factor in toxicity to insects. Appl Environ Microbiol 57(4):981–986

[40] Soberón M, Pardo-López L, López I, Gómez I, Tabashnik BE, Bravo A (2007), Engineering modified Bt toxins to counter insect resistance. Science 318(5856):1640–1642

[41] Zhang XB, Candas M, Griko NB, Taussig R, Bulla LA (2006) A mechanism of cell death involvingan adenylyl cyclase/PKA signaling pathway is induced by the Cry1Ab toxin of *Bacillusthuringiensis*. Proc Natl Acad Sci U S A 103(26):9897–9902

[42] Gómez I, Sánchez J, Miranda R, Bravo A, Soberón M (2002) Cadherin-like receptor bindingfacilitates proteolytic cleavage of helix α-1 in domain I and oligomer pre-pore formation of *Bacillus thuringiensis* Cry1Ab toxin. FEBS Lett 513(2–3):242–246

[43] Jogen Ch. Kalita, The use of biopesticides in insect pest management, 2011, 1 (7), pp169-177

[44] Ali S, Zafar Y, Ali GM, Nazir F (2010) *Bacillus thuringiensis* and its application in agriculture. AfrJ Biotechnol 9(14):2022–2031

[45] George Z., N. Crickmore Department of Biochemistry, School of Life Sciences, University of Sussex, Falmer,BN1

[46] Myers, P. S., and A. A. Yousten. (1980). Localization of a mosquitoe-larval toxin of *Bacillus sphaericus* 1593. Appl. Environ. Microbiol. 39:1205-1211.

[47] Kellen WR, Clark TB, Lindegren JE, Ho BC, Rogoff MH, Singer S 1965. *Bacillus sphaericus* Neide as a pathogen of mosquitoes. *J Invertebr Pathol 7*: 442-448

[48] Charles, J.-F., S. Hamon, and P. (1993). Baumann. Inclusion bodies and crystals of *Bacillus sphaericus* mosquitocidal proteins expressed in various bacterial hosts. Res. Microbiol. 144:411-416

[49] Brownbridge, M. and J. Margalit. (1987). Mosquitoe active strains of *Bacillus sphaericus* isolated from soil and mud samples collected in Israel. J Invertebr Pathol 50: 106-112.

[50] Klein, D., I. Uspensky and S. Braun. (2002). Tightly Bound Binary Toxin in the Cell Wall of *Bacillus sphaericus*. Appl Environ Microbiol. July; 68 (7): 3300–3307.

[51] Charles, J-F and C. Nielsen-LeRoux. (2000). Mosquitocidal Bacterial Toxins: Diversity, Mode of Action and Resistance Phenomena. Mem Inst Oswaldo Cruz, Rio de Janeiro, Vol. 95, Suppl. I: 201-206

[52] Porter, A., E. Davidson, J.-W. Liu. (1993) Mosquitocidal toxins of Bacilli and their genetic manipulation for effective biological control of mosquitoes. Microbiol. Rev. 57: 838-861.

[53] Chiou, C.-K., E. W. Davidson, T. Thanabalu, A. G. Porter and J. P. Allen. (1999). Crystallization and preliminary X-ray diffractionstudies of the 51 kDa protein of the mosquitoe-larvicidal binary toxin from *Bacillus sphaericus*. Acta Cryst. D55, 1083-1085.

[54] Thanabalu, T., C. Berry and J. Hindley. (1993). Cytotoxicity and ADP-ribosylating activity of the mosquitocidal toxin from *Bacillus sphaericus* SSII-1: Possible roles of the 27- and 70-kDa peptides. *J. Bacteriol.* 175, pp. 2314–2320.

[55] Regis L, Oliveira CMF, Silva-Filha MH, Silva SB, Maciel A, Furtado AF 2001. Bacteriological larvicides of diptera disease vectors. *Trends Parasitol 17*: 377-380

[56] Priest FG, Ebdrup L, Zahner V, 1997, Distribution and characterization of mosquitocidal toxin genes in some strains of *Bacillus sphaericus*.J. Appl. Environ., 63(4):1195-8.

[57] Liu, J. W., A. G. Porter, B. Y. Wee, and T. Thanabalu. (1996). New gene from nine *Bacillus sphaericus* strains encoding highly conserved 35.8-kilodalton mosquitocidal toxins. Appl. Environ. Microbiol. 62: 2174-2176.

[58] Nielsen-LeRoux, C., F. Pasquier, J.-F. Charles, G. Sinègre, B. Gaven and N. Pasteur. (1997). Resistance to *Bacillus sphaericus* involves different mechanisms in *Culex pipiens* (Diptera: Culicidae) larvae. J. Med. Entomol. 34:321-327. Abstarct.

[59] Georgihou, G. P., J. I. Malik, M. Wirth, K. Sainato. (1992). Characterization of resistance of Culex to the insecticidal toxins of Bacillus sphaericus 2362. In Univ. Calif., Mosq. Cont. Res. Annu. Repp. pp. 34-35.

[60] Usta, C. Cokmus, Investigation of aquatic bacteria on the effect of *Bacillus sphaericus* binary toxins, 2004. PhD thesis, Aibu. Turkiye

[61] Klein, D., I. Uspensky and S. Braun. (2002). Tightly Bound Binary Toxin in the Cell Wall of *Bacillus sphaericus.* Appl Environ Microbiol. July; 68 (7): 3300–3307.

[62] Charles, J.-F., C. Nielsen-LeRoux, and A. Dele´cluse. 1996. *Bacillus sphaericus* toxins:molecular biology and mode of action. Annu. Rev. Entomol.41:451–472

Chapter 14

Callose in Plant Sexual Reproduction

Meral Ünal, Filiz Vardar and Özlem Aytürk

Additional information is available at the end of the chapter

http://dx.doi.org/10.5772/53001

1. Introduction

The typical plant cell wall is composed of cellulose, hemicellulose, pectin and protein. Cellulose is a polymer of 1,4- β- glucan and found as microfibrils in the cell wall. Callose, a specialized polysaccharide, is also one of the cell wall components in plants, and it appears in some cells or in some cases. It is a 1,3- β- glucan polymer with some 1,6 branches, and it differs from cellulose. Callose and cellulose are synthesized by callose synthase and cellulose synthase located on the plasma membrane, respectively. Callose synthase locates vectorially in the plasma membrane with substrate being supplied from the cytoplasmic side, and the products are deposited on the cell surface [1].

Callose was initially identified by Mangin [2] more than 100 years ago. Afterwards, it is defined by Frey-Wyssling and Muhlethaler [3] as a component of cell walls in higher plants. Although it is not as common as cellulose, its role is very significant. It generally exists in small quantities in structurally different plant tissues, and it has individual properties: (1) High impermeability, (2) Rapid synthesis and easy degradation [4-6]. Callose can be identified with aniline blue by fluorescence microscope or resorsine blue (lacmoid) by light microscope. Aniline blue technique based on the emittance of secondary fluorescence was standardized by Eschrich and Currier [7] and it has been extensively used to identify callose deposition.Callose is deposited between plasma membrane and cellulosic cell wall, and it appears electron-lucent in transmission electron micrographs [8].

Callose plays important roles in many processes during plant development (Table 1). It plays a significant role in the reproductive biology of angiosperms, particularly. Callose wall surrounds the sporocytes while meiosis occurs. Because of its structure, it may provide an isolation barrier sealing off one meiotic cell (pollen mother cell or megaspore mother cell) from another [9]. Waterkeyn [10] suggested that callose plays an important biological role: It acts as a temporary wall to prevent the products of meiosis from cohesion and fusion, and its dissolution results in the release of free spores. It has been proposed that the callose wall functions as a molecular filter isolating the developing microspores from the influence of the surrounding diploid tissue or sister spores [11]. The molecular filter also transmits only signals that are indispensable for meiosis into the meiocytes [12-13]. The temporary isolation of the sporocyte (male as well as female) may be connected with the process of differentiation of the sporocyte. Callose accumulates in the walls of incompatible pollen grains and tubes, and in certain cases, in papillae of stigma following rejection [14].

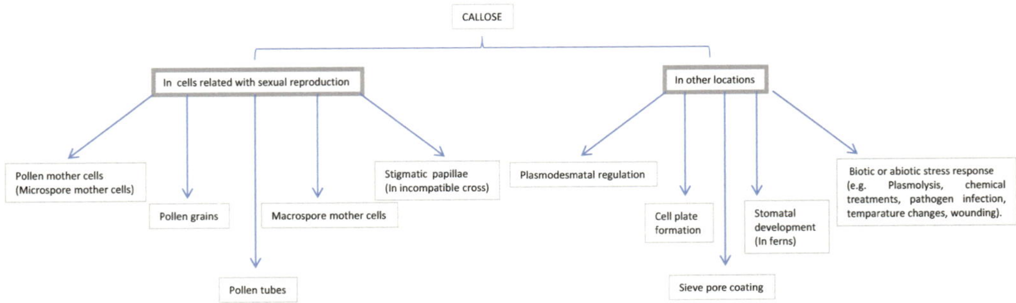

Table 1. Schematic summary of callose deposition in the plant cells.

The synthesis of callose can also be induced by wounding, pathogen infection and physiological stresses [15-16]. Callose is not only a component of the normal sporophytic cell wall when produced in response to wounding [17], but also participates in the formation of a physical barrier against pathogen invasion. It is formed at the penetration sites of fungal hyphae [8] and around lesions in virus-infected plants where it may help to prevent spreading of the virus [18]. Callose localizes at other locations as well, including the cell plate, plasmodesmata, and in sieve plates of phloem [19].

All the events mentioned above point that callose existence is a well organized process. It seems that it provides an isolation period to the cells in normal development and under stress conditions. Although the synthesis and deposition of callose have been studied for many years, the understanding of synthesis mechanism is still incomplete. Over the last several years, however, significant progress has been made, in particular using the model plant *Arabidopsis thaliana* [20]. In the model plant *Arabidopsis thaliana* two independent research groups identified twelve genes encoding putative callose synthase [21-24]. The group of Desh Verma [21] uses the CalS (callose synthase) system to name the twelve genes: *AtCalS1-AtCalS12*. Each of these genes may be tissue-specific and/or regulated under different physiological conditions responding to biotic and abiotic stresses.The callose synthase complex exists in at least two distinct forms in different tissues and interacts with phragmoplastin, UDP-glucose transferase, Rop1 and, possibly, annexin. The Somerville group [24] also refers to the twelve *Arabidopsis* genes as GSL (glucan synthase-like) genes, and has designated them as *AtGSL1* to *AtGSL12* [16]. Phylogenetic analysis of the *AtGSL* family suggests that the *GSL* family can be classified into four main subfamilies according to the phlogenetic analysis based on aligning deduced

GSL amino acid sequences. The first subfamily contains *AtGSL1, AtGSL5, AtGSL8* and *AtGSL10*, the second subfamily contains *AtGSL2, AtGSL3, AtGSL6* and *AtGSL12*, the third subfamily contains *AtGSL7* and *AtGSL11*, and the last subfamily includes *AtGSL4*. A single *GSL* gene can also have diverse functions; for instance, *GSL5* is responsible for the synthesis of wound- and pathogen-inducible callose in leaf tissue, and it also plays an important role in exine formation and pollen wall patterning [16, 25-27].

Although this review will cover the role of callose in the course of sexual reproduction, our purpose is also to draw attention to the formation and importance of callose during normal development and response to biotic and abiotic stresses.

2. Callose in the cells related with sexual reproduction

2.1. Callose in microsporogenesis

Pollen grains in flowering plants are produced as an outcome of meiotic division in pollen mother cells (PMCs). In preleptoten stage, PMCs look alike somatic meristematic cells those are surrounded by a typical cellulose wall. They are connected by plasmodesmata in 200–280 A° diameters. Plasmodesmatal connections also exist between PMCs and tapetal cells, innermost layer of anther wall, at that stage. With the initiation of meiosis, callose deposition starts between plasma membrane and cell wall of microsporocytes, and cytoplasmic connections between tapetum and PMCs are broken. At the prophase I, the PMCs are interconnected by wider cytoplasmic channels which provide cytoplasmic continuity in all microsporocytes of an anther locule. Thus, all PMCs of a pollen sac form a single cytoplasmic entity, the meiocytic syncytium. Although the importance of syncytium is not clear, the cytoplasmic continuities impose a mutual influence of one cell over the other. This probably helps maintaining a close synchrony in meiotic prophase I [28], and with the blockage of cytoplasmic channels, usually at end of prophase I, synchrony is gradually lost. Callose deposition continues through meiosis so that each of the products of meiosis, the tetrad of microspores, is also surrounded by a dense callose (Figure 1a-d). After the completion of meiosis, the callose wall is broken down by callase enzyme activity that is secreted by tapetum releasing free microspores into the pollen sac [29-31].

The development of callose and its degradation a little after the completion of meiosis suggests that callose layer performs some special functions. The callose wall isolates not only the sporogenous tissue from the somatic tissue but also the individual microspores. It gives mechanical isolation to the developing microspores, thereby preventing cell coherence, and by their rapid and total dissolution, sets the microspores free. This layer also functions as a kind of chemical isolation, establishing a selective barrier between genetically different haploid cells that must pass through their developmental stages unexposed to the influence of their sister spore, or of adjoining spores and somatic tissue [28, 32, 33]. Heslop-Harrison and Mackenzie [11] used labelled thymidine in the anthers of *Lilium henryi* and suggest that callose not only acts as a barrier or "molecular filter" to the exchange of at least some macromolecules, but also provides genetic autonomy to each developing sporocyte.

It has also been suggested that callose wall protects the developing sporocytes from harmful hormonal and nutritional influence of the adjoining somatic cells [34, 35]. According to Shivanna [36], isolation is necessary for the PMCs for transition, from the sporophytic phase to the gametophytic phase, and gametophytic genome expression without interference either from other spores or parent sporophytic tissue.

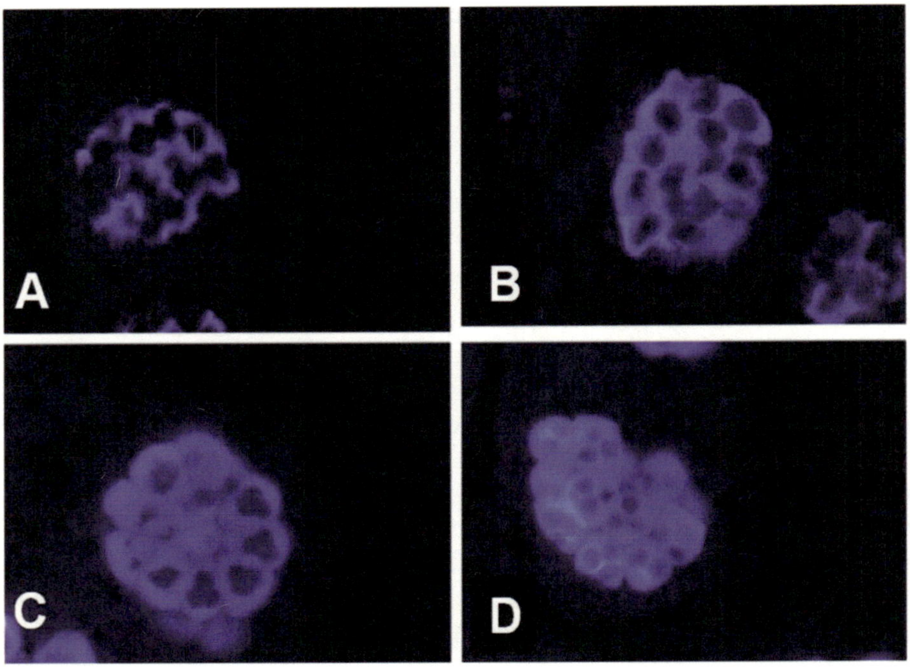

Figure 1. Callose accumulation in the anthers of *Lathyrus undulatus* during microsporogenesis stained with aniline blue. A, B. Prophase I. C. Telophase II. D.Tetrad [129].

Barskaya and Balina [37] studied in Sax beans in order to enlighten the role of callose in the anthers, and examined the effect of atmospheric drought on microsporogenesis. They pointed that moderate drought inflicts considerable damage on sporogenous cells from dehydration, and cells surrounded by callose are not harmed by drought for a certain period of time. The effect of callose is achieved by its ability of water absorption. Undoubtedly, the callose protection is not unlimited. It depends on both the intensity and duration of the drought and the plant's resistance to the drought. When the drought is long and intensive, callose's water source is consumed rapidly, and the anther dies. Similarly Li *et al.* [38] stated that the callose wall isolates meiocytes from other sporophytic tissues and, concurrently, prevents them from dehydration in water stress conditions.

According to Barskaya and Balina [37], callose is a source of carbohydrates for the developing microspores. Following its breakdown, the soluble carbohydrate can be used in their metabolism during their development. Despite the fact that this idea is quite interesting, we think that it seems to have more work.

Irregularities in the deposition of callose around the PMCs and its prematurely breakdown seem to be responsible for male sterility. It has been shown that the PMCs of male sterile lines of *Petunia hybrida* are not enclosed by callose wall after prophase I [39]. It is thought that this abnormality is due to the mistiming of callase in both male sterile *Petunia* [39] and male sterile sorghum lines [40]. In fertile plants, callase enzyme appears only at microspore tetrad stages while in sterile plants strong callase activity is detected during prophase I. It could be concluded that earlier activation of callase enzyme is responsible for cytoplasmic male sterility in *Petunia*. However, it is not known whether this is the only factor that contributes to male sterility. The male sterile plants, therefore, provide only circumstantial evidence that the callose wall has a vital function in microsporogenesis. There is a positive relationship betweeen pH, callase activity and dissolution of callose. Activation of callase in both sterile and fertile anthers is associated with a drop in pH in the anther locule from over pH 7 to around pH 6 that is optimal for callase activity. It is suggested that the time of activation of callase is controlled by regulation of pH in the anther locule [39].

Winiarczyk *et al.* [41] examined callase activity in anthers of sterile *Allium sativum* (garlic) and fertile *Allium atropurpureum*. In *A. sativum*, the extracted callase from the thick walls of microspore tetrads exhibited maximum activity at pH 4.8. Once microspores were released, *in vitro* callase activity reflected the presence of three callase isoforms peaked at three distinct pH values. One isoform, which was previously identified in the tetrad stage displayed maximum activity at pH 4.8. The remaining two novel isoforms were most active at pH 6.0 and 7.3. In contrast to *A. atropurpureum*, three callase isoforms, active at pH 4.8–5.2, 6.1, and 7.3, were identified in the microsporangia that had released their microspores. The callose wall persists around meiotic cells of *A. sativum*, whereas only one callase isoform, with an optimum activity of pH 4.8, is active in the acidic environment of the microsporangium. However, this isoform is degraded when the pH rises to 6.0 and two other callase isoforms, maximally active at pH 6.0 and 7.3, appear. Thus, the researchers concluded that factors that alter the pH of the microsporangium may indirectly affect the male gametophyte development by modulating the activity of callase, and thereby regulating the degradation of the callose wall. They also indicated that a reduction or inhibition of enzyme activity may be caused by the presence of some inhibitors. A number of such inhibitors have been isolated and characterized from legume seeds, cereals, and tubers [42, 43].

Several studies performed on *Arabidopsis* demonstrated that multiple *GSL* genes are involved in pollen development. Enns *et al.* [27] reported that *GSL1* and *GSL5* are necessary in pollen development, and they are responsible for the formation of the callose wall that separates the microspores of the tetrads. They also indicated that these genes also play a gametophytic role later in pollen grain germination.

Callose wall also plays an effective role in the orderly formation of exine. It provides the compounds of cellulosic primexine [44]. Waterkeyn and Beinfait [45] suggested that the callose wall acts like a template or mold for the formation of the species-specific exine sculpturing patterns seen on mature pollen grains. This hypothesis is also supported by the studies in Epacridaceae [46].

It has been reported that there is no callose wall formation during microsporogenesis in *Pergularia daemia* and the exine wall is thin, fragmentary, and it lacks ornamentation [47]. Some hydrophylic plants such as *Amphibolis antartica* [48] and *Halophila stipulaceae* [49] exhibit no detectable callose around microspore tetrads, and pollen grains show no ornamented exine either. Similarly, *Arabidopsis* mutants that produce no callose wall show no ornamented exine either [50]. These results suggest the essential role of callose in the formation of outer wall of pollen grains.

Albert *et al.* [51] investigated the relationship between intersporal wall formation, tetrad shape and pollen aperture pattern ontogeny in *Epilobium roseum* (Onograceae) and *Parranomus reflexus* (Proteaceae). Comparison of apertures within tetrads indicates that the position of apertures is correlated to the last point of callose deposition.

2.2. Callose stage of generative cell in a pollen grain

The mitotic division of a pollen grain results into two unequal cells; a larger vegetative cell and a smaller generative cell. Initially, they are separated by two plasma membranes. The wall of the generative cell is soon formed in between the two plasma membranes [52]. Callose first appears in the region of the wall between the two cells in the pollen grain, and then progresses around the generative cell, completely enveloping it. Gorska-Brylass [53] was the first researcher who pointed that callose exists in the area where the generative cell is separated from the vegetative cell. Later studies have shown that the callose alone, or along with cellulose, is a component of the early formed wall around the generative cell of pollen grains of certain other plants [53-57]. The general rule in researched species is that the callose disappears just before the generative cell moves to the centre of vegetative cell. Generally, the time period where the callose wall appears is short. The isolation period with the callose, comes before the DNA synthesis. Because of that reason, the callose stage of the generative cell is a period where structural and physiological differentiation takes place, and considering the fact that there is no isolation stage in male gamete formation in higher plants, it becomes more significant. Callose provides an adequate isolation barrier for the differentiation of cells related with sexual reproduction. As a result of the isolation, the generative cell confronts a different differentiation period than the vegetative cell has. The callose that becomes visible for a period of time in the border between the two cells in the closed system of the pollen grain has a significant role in both vegetative and generative cell differentiation. It is a well-known fact that isolation is necessary for the expression of gametophytic genome without interference from neighbors [36].

2.3. Callose in pollen tubes

After pollen hydration, a pollen tube emerges at the germination pore. If many germination pores are present, their outgrowth is generally blocked by deposition of callose [58]. When a pollen tube grows out of a pollen grain, the entire cytoplasm that contains the germ units flows continuously towards the tube apex [59]. The pollen tube is surrounded by an outer pectocellulosic wall and an inner homogeneous callose wall [60-61]. Besides as a wall substance, callose occurs as a plug in pollen tubes (Figure 2). A few authors [6, 62, 63] assumpted that inner tube

http://dx.doi.org/10.5772/53001

wall layer and the plug consist exclusively of callose, and concluded that the inner tube wall layer and the plugs contain, in addition to callose, pectin and cellulose. Kroh and Knuimann [64] reported that, in the inner pollen tube wall, and plugs contained microfibrils of cellulose in addition to callose, and "non-cellulosic" microfibrils that had "pectin-like" properties.

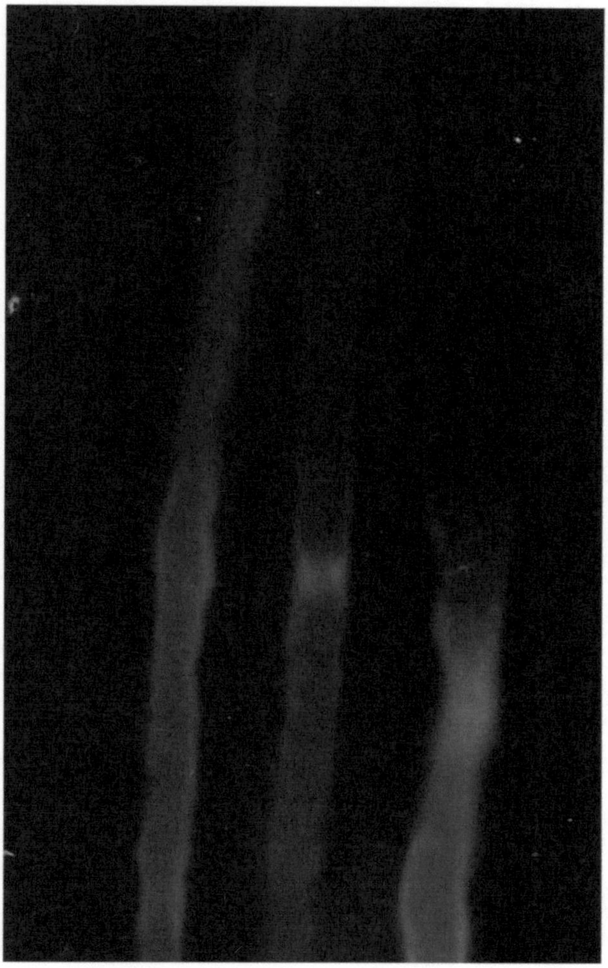

Figure 2. Fluorescence of callose in the compatible pollen tubes of *Petunia hybrida* [78].

As the pollen tubes grow down of the style, depending on the length of pollen tube and the rhythmic growth, a series of callose plugs (Figure 3a,b) sealing off the pollen tube are formed transversely at a regular distance behind the tip [65]. As a result, a fully grown pollen tube is divided into many compartments by callose plugs. The tip of the pollen tube contains only pectin, hemicellulose and cellulose [64, 66]. Closely behind the tip zone an additional cell wall layer is deposited, containing callose. Callose is not deposited on the tip of growing pollen tube.

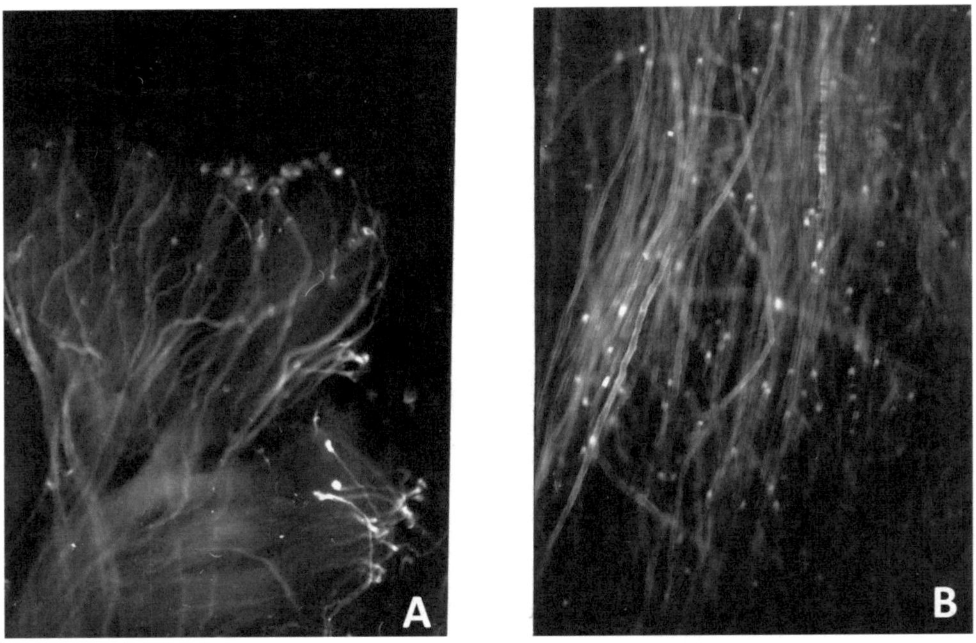

Figure 3. Fluorescent micrographs of compatible pollen tubes of *Petunia hybrida*. A. In stigma B. In style [78].

Generally, callose plugs are believed as mechanical barriers those prevent the plasma at the apex to flow backwards. According to Jensen and Fischer [67], plugs prevent the tubes to shrink. According to Müller-Stoll and Lerch [62], callose is a significant product of the pollen tube metabolism. It arises as a result of a mechanical stimulation of the cytoplasm movement, and this stimulation activates the callose synthesizing enzyme. According to Tsinger and Petrovskaya–Baranova [63], plugs are formed to support the pollen tube wall from the factors such as pressure, dehiscence and mechanical tensions. The callose in the pollen tube wall takes also a role in maintanence of osmotic balance in pollen tubes [65]. As a wall material, however, there must be another reason for the callose deposition. According to the Rubinstein et al. [68] the callose sheath of pollen tube in maize is the target of accumulation of a maize pollen-specific gene, PEX-1, with an extensin-like domain. It might be expected that proteins like extensin would ultimately be involved in supporting the growth of the pollen tube or in facilitating cell to cell signalling between the pollen tube and the style [68]. Much more work is needed before we can truly assess generality and significance of extensin and callose sheat of pollen tube. Giampiero *et al.* [69] examined the distribution of callose synthase and cellulose synthase in tobacco pollen tubes in relation to the dynamics of cytoskeleton and the endomembrane system. Both enzymes are associated with the plasma membrane, but cellulose synthase is present along the entire length of pollen tubes (with a higher concentration at the apex) while callose synthase is located in distal regions. Actin filaments and endomembrane dynamics are critical for the distribution of callose synthase and cellulose synthase.

There is a close relation between incompatibility and callose deposition on pollen tubes. Sexual incompatibility in plants may be interspecific or intraspecific. The latter is also called self-incompatibility and it is of two types: gametophytic self-incompatibility (GSI) and sporophytic self-incompatibility (SSI). An important manifestation of gametophytic incompatibility systems includes abnormal behavior of pollen tube and heavy deposition of callose in it. Linskens and Esser [70] are the first investigators to point the relationship between the incompatibility and the callose amount in pollen tubes. In GSI systems, the rejection reaction take place in the style and the growth of the pollen tube after growing to various extents, about one-third of the transmitting tissue of style ceases. In GSI systems inhibition of pollen tube is generally associated with extensive deposition of callose in the pollen tube [71-76]. Callose deposition increase in the walls and in the plugs of incompatible pollen tubes. In others, callose is deposited even inside the pollen grain, beginning at what appears to be the site of pollen tube emergence [77].

In incompatible pollen tubes of *Petunia hybrida,* the amount of callose is greater than in compatible ones [78]. According to the results of the study on *P. hybrida,* incompatible tubes are characterized by an abnormally increased deposition of callose in the wall. Often, a callose plug is located at the tip to prevent the sperm cells to reach the tip (Figure 4). Furthermore, the callose plugs in these tubes are much longer and greater in number compared to those in compatible tubes (Figure 5a,b). The incompatibility of pollen tubes is also marked by swelling of tips until they burst to death within the style. While some of the incompatible pollen tubes carrying sperm cells in transmitting tissue may burst. Eventually, incompatible tubes stop growing and die. These events have not been found in compatible tubes. The first callose plug formation in incompatible tubes of *P. hybrida* was observed 4 hours after self-pollination, but 8-10 hours after cross pollination in compatible ones. This fact indicates that the formation of callose plugs in incompatible tubes is earlier than the one in compatible ones [78]. According to Tupy's [71] experiments in apple and tobacco, the callose amount in incompatible tubes is twice that of in compatible tubes. The reason of more callose in incompatible tubes of apple and tobacco is longer plugs and intensive callose, respectively.

Although the most common self-incompatibility system is of the gametopytic type, amazingly, little is known about the location of pollen recognition factors in this group plants. After incompatible pollination, when the pollen grains also come in contact with the stigmatic papillae, a callose plug develops at the tip between the cell wall and the plasma membrane [79-80]. There is no plug formation after compatible pollination. The formation of the callose plug in the papillae is very rapid and often visible within 10 minutes after pollination (Figure 6a,b) [81]. The stigmatic papillae react with the production of callose in the papillate cells near the pollen or pollen tube in order to prevent the penetration of pollen tube into stigma and the style. The deposition of callose in *Raphanus* is possibly related to the perforation of the cuticle by the pollen tube, and it can be compared with a wounding effect [82].

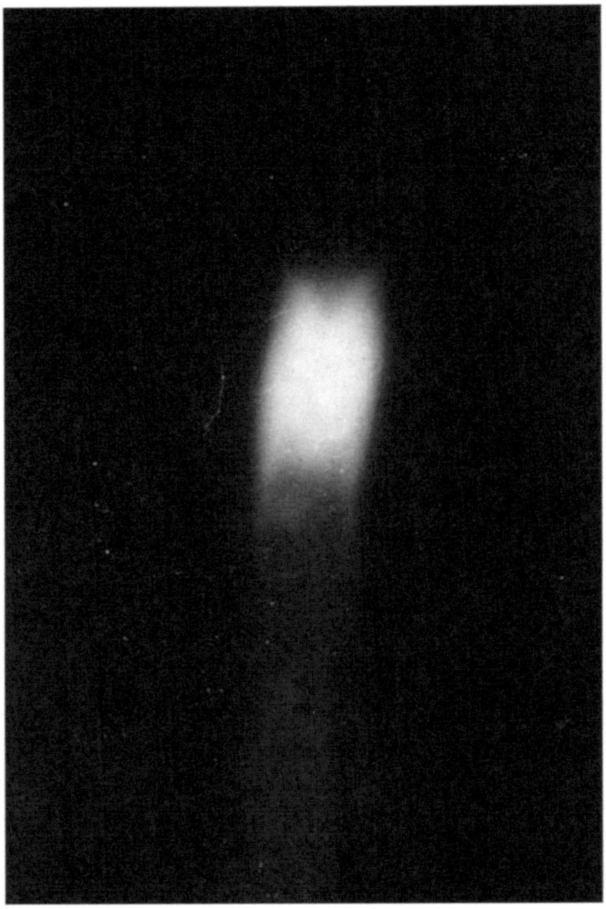

Figure 4. Terminal callose plug in the incompatible pollen tube of *Petunia hybrida* [78].

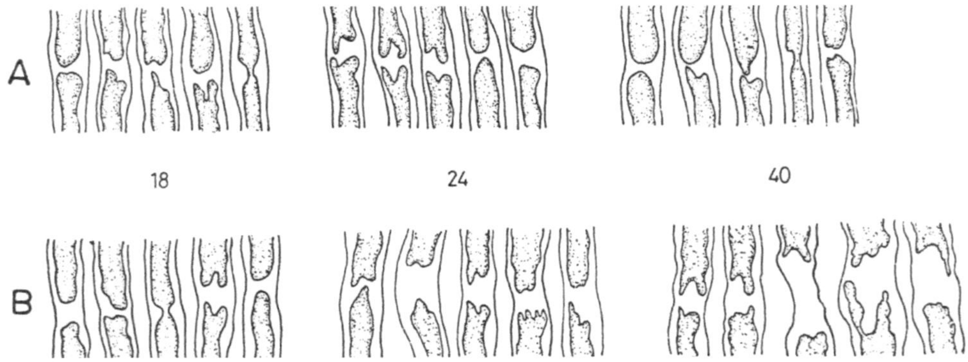

Figure 5. Callose plugs after 18, 24 ,40 hours compatibly pollinated (A) and incompatibly pollinated pistil (B) of *Petunia hybrida* [78].

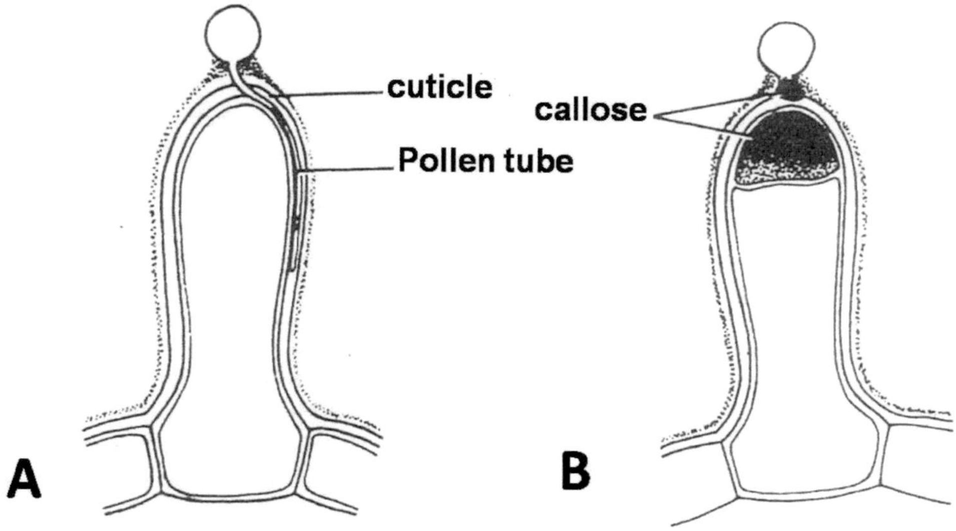

Figure 6. Stigmatic papilla in cross-pollination (A) and self-pollination (B). Note deposition of callose at the tip of pollen tube and in the papilla in self-pollinated stigma [36].

Callose deposition appears to be a Ca^{+2} –dependent process in self-pollinated *Brassica oleracea* since it is abolished by deprivation of Ca^{+2} [83]. Callose formation in the stigma is not a requirement for the demise of self-pollen or incompatibility functions [84].

2.4. Callose in megasporogenesis

Despite there is a similarity on the deposition of callose during megasporogenesis and microsporogenesis, there are evident differences. These differences basically depend on the strong polarization of megaspore mother cell (MMC) and megaspore tetrad. In the course of meiosis of PMCs and microspore tetrads, such polarization does not exist. The polarization in the megasporocyte and megaspore tetrad is very obvious, resulting in the formation of an active megaspore. The unusual accumulation of callose in megasporogenesis is clearly connected with the strong polarization of the cells. The starting of callose deposition in the wall of megasporocyte and its disapperance corresponds with the localization of the active spore in the tetrad [85].

Callose always appears in the early meiotic prophase I. In the *Polygonum* type of embryo sac development callose first deposited at the chalazal pole of the meiocyte in the early prophase I, and the entire meiocyte is usually surrounded by a callose wall at metaphase I. Subsequently, it surrounds the entire cell. Callose deposition continues through meiosis so that each of the products of meiosis, the tetrad of megaspores, is also surrounded by callose. The callose deposites on the cross walls separating individual megaspores, as well. After completion of megasporogenesis, the callose disappears from the wall of the functional megaspore, whereas it frequently remains present in the walls of megaspores which will degenerate. The temporary isolation of the megasporocyte may be connected with the process of differentiation of the sporocyte for basically a new type of development [85].

In such cases, the cell organelles and starch grains are more intensively located in the side of megasporocyte of the active spore in the tetrad. Additionally, cell division occurs in unequally resulting in a larger functional megaspore and smaller non-functional megaspores which will degenerate. Invariably, the active functional megaspore has a callose free wall to allow the passage for the movement substances into it [85]. On the other hand, the non-functional megaspores are surrounded by callose wall for a long time and eventually undergo programmed cell death and degenerate [86].

In the meiotic division of MMC, callose formation was first demonstrated in orchids by Rodkiewicz and Gorska–Brylass [87]. Subsequently, Rodkiewicz [88] identified the callose existence in 43 species from 14 families in angiosperms (Figure 7a-e). We have, now, an impressive list of plants in which callose formation during megasporogenesis has been demonstrated [89-96]. In the course of megasporogenesis, callose exists transiently in the cell walls of plants with mono- or bisporic type of embryo sac development, but it is not detected in the species with a tetrasporic type [88]. It is assumed that the callose wall plays a significant role in the type of embryo sac development, forming a molecular filter that decreases the permeability of the cell wall. In this way, MMC becomes temporarily isolated from the surrounding sporophytic tissue. This isolation enables the cells to undergo an independent course of differentiation, accompanied by the shift from sporophytic to gametophytic gene expression.

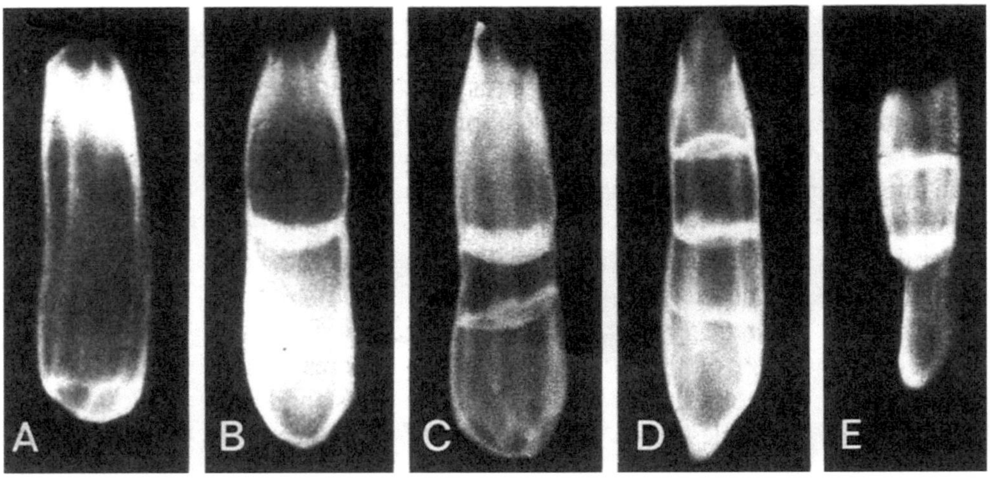

Figure 7. (A-E) Fluorescence of callose in the walls of megasporocytes in *Fuchsia hybrida* [88].

Moreover, callose has alternative roles in sexual reproduction. In *Catananche betacea, Nicotiana tabacum* and *Petunia hybrida*, the two sperm are connected together by a transverse wall as is in *Plumbago zylenica* [97]. However, in *N. tabacum*, the wall appears to be further specialized by the presence of fibrils, small tubules, and callose [98].

http://dx.doi.org/10.5772/53001

It has been known that the pollen tube enters to embryo sac through the filiform apparatus, and after growing, it arrives in the synergid cytoplasm. The content of the pollen tube is discharged in the synergid. In cotton, the content is discharged through a subterminal pore which is invariably on the side facing the chalaza [99]. The end of the discharge is signaled by the formation of a callose plug over the pore, effectively preventing any cytoplasmic flow between the pollen tube and the synergid [100].

Soon after syngamy, the zygote undergoes some changes. Before fertilization, the cell wall that is restricted to the micopylar part of the egg cell, is now complete around the zygote. In several species of *Rhododendron* and in *Ledum groenlandicum* (Ericaceae), a callose wall is laid off around the zygote during the first two days after fertilization [101]. The fact that the wall essentially insulates the newly formed zygote from the influence of cells of a different genotype in the immediate neighborhood probably has some significance in the subsequent induction of the sporophytic divisions [97]. Zygote becomes an isolated cell in the sence that the plasmodesmatal connections with the surrounding cells are blocked.

In apomictic species, the nucellar cells which start an embryonic pathway also show isolation from surrounding nucellar cells with a callose wall [102]. This event is an excellent example of the mystery of callose existence in the cells related with reproduction. It suggests that if a cell takes a role in reproduction, it needs to be isolated for a period by a callose wall.

3. Several other locations of callose and its deposition in response to stress

As we mentioned above, callose plays important roles during sexual reproduction in plants. Besides, callose also appears in several other locations such as plasmodesmata regulation, cell plate formation and responses to multiple biotic and abiotic stresses (including plasmolysis, high and low temperature, many harmful chemical compounds including heavy metals, ultrasounds, pathogen infection and wounding). After stimulation callose synthesis occurs rapidly, and it is deposited as plugs and drops [103, 104].

Callose has been localised particularly to plasmodesmata [105-106]. It has been known that plasmodesmata are the intercellular connections between plant cells that allow cell-to-cell transport of sugars, amino acids, inorganic ions, proteins, and nucleic acids [107]. The accurate function of plasmodesmata depends on what plants require to respond to developmental and/or environmental signals [108]. Thus, callose is deposited at plasmodesmata to regulate the cell to cell movement of molecules by controlling the size of them. Callose can also be deposited at plasmodesmata in response to abiotic and/or biotic stresses [16].

In higher plants during cell division, the first visible evidence of the new cell wall is deposition of the cell plate in an equatorial plane between daughter nuclei. Samuels *et al.* [109] indicated that the callose is the main luminal component of forming cell plate and it forms a coat-like structure on the membrane surface. Callose deposition is followed by the deposition and organization of cellulose and other cell wall components; at the same time, cell plate callose is degraded by β-1,3-glucanase.

In ferns, callose performs multiple roles during stomatal development and function. Callose, in cooperation with the cytoskeleton, is involved in stomatal pore formation, in the mechanism of pore opening and closure and wall thickenings of guard cells [110].

It is now generally recognized that the sieve plate of phloem is one of the several sporophytic locations of callose in higher plants (1). Barratt *et al.* [111] suggest that the callose coating of sieve plates pores is essential for normal phloem transport because it confers favorable flow characteristics on the pores. Callose is synthesized in functioning sieve elements in response to damage and other stresses, such as mechanical situmulation and high temperatures. The wound callose is deposited in the sieve elements of surrounding intact tissue. As the sieve elements recover from damage, the callose disappears from these pores. Callose is also found in sieve elements under cases other than wounding, although its function always seems to be sealing. Definitive callose is deposited in dying cells or sieve elements undergoing elimination due to the formation of secondary tissues. Callose associated with dormancy is found in many perennial plants which have become dormant in the winter. Such dormancy callose is redissolved in the spring in preperation for resumption of transport and growth [112].

Biotic and abiotic stresses induce K^+ efflux and Ca^{2+} influx into the cell. Plasma membrane depolarization may result because of changes in ion fluxes. It has been reported that salicylic acid activates callose synthesis due to the induction of calcium influx into the cell which increases its concentration in the cortical cytoplasm layer [113-115]. In *Arabidopsis,* two hours treatment with salicylic acid increased the content of *AtGSL5* gene that encodes a protein homologous to the catalytic subunit of β-1,3-glucan synthase [116].

Although the mechanisms behind the rapid callose synthesis are not well understood, it has been proposed that callose synthase may be activated by perturbed conditions, leading to some loss of membrane permeability [114, 117]. The membrane perturbation results in membrane leakage and the apoplastic Ca^{2+} leaks into the cytosol. The increment of the local Ca^{2+}concentration activates callose synthase. It is reported that several annexin-type molecules that are known to respond to Ca^{2+} levels interact with callose synthase [118]; Callose synthase may be activated by annexin interaction. After wounding, the membrane lipids may change and affect the activity of callose synthase [119].

Wounding or pathogen invasion can induce reversible callose synthesis in plants. This may ameliorate the results of wounding or stop the pathogen from spreading to other cells or tissues. Synthesis of callose within the sieve pores can help to seal off damage or prepare the cells for developmental changes [69]. Iglesias *et al.* [120] indicated that a silencing mutant of β-1,3-glucanase decrease the plant sensitivity to viruses, after the invasion, the plasmodesmata are found to be smaller than in wild-type plants, because of the accumulation of callose in the plasmodesmata, which is degraded in the wild-type plants.

During the fungal infections, callose is deposited to form beneath infection sites and thought to provide a physical barrier to penetration. However there is little knowledge about the signaling pathway leading to callose synthesis during plant-microbe interaction. Although the induction mechanism is not known, it has been reported that callose is induced in carrot (*Daucus carota* L.) cell suspensions treated with a spirostanol saponin from *Yucca* [121].

Furthermore over-expression of the tomato disease resistance gene *PTO* induces callose deposition [122]. Kohler and Blatt [123] reported that *Arabidopsis* plants treated with the synthetic acquired resistance (SAR) inducer benzothiadiazole (BTH) also increase callose deposition, as well as the expression of resistance genes.

After the powdery mildew *Erysiphe cichoracearum* penetration, callose is deposited along the whole cell margin determined by an intense aniline blue fluorochrome staining in wild-type plants, whereas cells in *CalS12* mutants showed only a punctuate callose staining pattern at the cell periphery. It has been suggested that the punctuate staining pattern in *CalS12* plants may be plasmadesmata callose, because callose is typically deposited in the cell wall area immediately surrounding the orifice of a plasmadesmata, particularly during wounding or aldehyde fixation [25, 124, 125].

Luna *et al.* [126] examined the robustness of callose deposition under different growth conditions and in response to two different pathogen-associated molecular patterns, the flagellin epitope Flg22 and the polysaccharide chitosan on *Arabidopsis*. Based on a commonly used hydroponic culture system, the resarchers found that variations in growth conditions have a major impact on the plant's overall capacity to deposit callose.

The constitutive capacity to quickly synthesize callose on wounding provides cells with the ability to generate a new physical barrier, that seals the injured plant tissue. The physiological machinery involved in the induction and maintenance of callose deposition can be triggered also by metal toxicity, without conferring any apparent protection against metal toxicity. Aluminum-induced callose formation has been studied in detail and used for the secreening of plant genotypes for Al sensitivity, because it is a sensitive and reliable indicator and measure of the level of stress perceived by the plant tissue provided the dynamics of callose turnover, and constitutive synthesis capacity are taken into account [112]. For instance, Vardar *et al.* [127] reported time and dose dependent callose accumulation after Al treatment in the root tips of *Zea mays* (Figure 8).

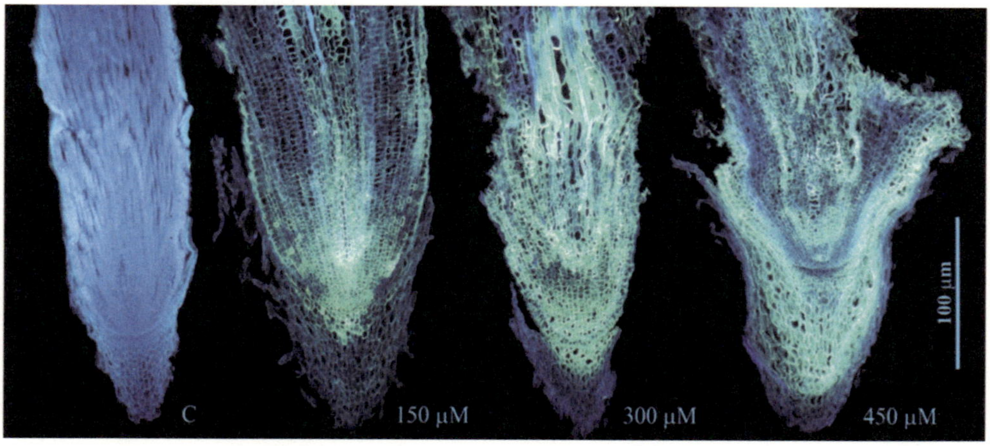

Figure 8. Aluminum-induced root callose deposition (yellowish-green) in maize roots. The seedlings were exposed to aluminum concentrations of 150, 300 and 450 µM AlCl3 (pH 4.5) for 96 h [127].

Among other metals inducing callose formation, only Mn has been studied in some detail [128]. The potential of metal toxicity-induced callose formation to increase understanding of the dynamics and spatial perception of stress within plant tissues has not yet been exploited [112].

4. Conclusion

Callose, which is a 1,3- β- glucan polymer with some 1,6 branches, is involved in diverse biological processes associated with plant development, biotic and abiotic stress responses. Callose plays important roles in the reproductive biology of angiosperms. It appears around microsporocytes and megasporocytes during meiosis. It can be suggested possible that callose is involved in some aspects of meiosis in higher plants. Furthermore it is also involved in plasmodesmata regulation, cell plate formation, in response to multiple biotic and abiotic stresses. Although remarkable progress has been performed, there are still some unexplained cases, such as the biochemical pathway of callose synthesis, functional components of callose synthase complex and signal pathway of callose synthesis. The future perspectives in biochemistry, cell biology, genetics and molecular biology will be helpful improving our knowledge

Author details

Meral Ünal, Filiz Vardar and Özlem Aytürk

Departmant of Biology, Faculty of Art and Sciences, Marmara University, İstanbul, Turkey

References

[1] Taiz, L, & Zeiger, E. Plant Physiology. Redwood City: Benjamin/Cummings Publishing; (1991).

[2] Mangin, L. Observations Sur la Membrane du Grain de Pollen Miur. Bulletin Societatis Botanicorum France (1889). , 36, 274-284.

[3] Frey-wyssling, A, & Muhlethaler, K. Ultrastructural Plant Cytology. New York: Elsevier Publishing Co; (1965).

[4] Eschrich, W. Unteruchungen über den Ab- und Aufbau der Callose. Zeitung Botanik (1961). , 49, 153-218.

[5] Eschrich, W, & Eschrich, B. Das Verhalten Isolierter Callose Gegenüber Wabrigen Lösungen. Berichte der Deutschen Botanischen Gesellschaft (1964). , 77, 329-331.

[6] Waterkeyn, L. Callose Microsporocytaire et Callose Pollinique. In: Linskens HF (ed.) Pollen Physiology and Fertilization. Amsterdam:North- Holland Publishers; (1964). , 52-58.

[7] Eschrich, W, & Currier, H. B. Identification of Callose by its Diachrome and Fluochrome Reactions. Stain Technology (1964). , 39, 303-307.

[8] Stone, B. A, & Clarke, A. E. Chemistry and Biology of (l-3)-β- Glucans. Victoria: La Trobe University Press; (1992).

[9] Knox, R. B, & Heslop-harrison, J. Direct Demonstration of the Low Permeability of the Angiosperm Meiotic Tetrad Using a Fluorogenic Ester. Zeitung Pflanzer Züchter (1970). , 62, 451-459.

[10] Waterkeyn, L. Les Parois Microsporocytaires de Nature Callosique chez *Helleborus* et *Tradescantia.* Cellule (1962). , 62, 223-255.

[11] Heslop-harrison, J, & Mckenzie, A. Autoradiography of Soluble (2-C^{14}) Thymidine Derivatives during Meiosis and Microsporogenesis in *Lilium* Anthers. Journal of Cell Science (1967). , 2, 387-400.

[12] Dong, X, Hong, Z, Sivaramakrishnan, M, & Mahfouz, M. Verma DPS. Callose Synthase (*CalS5*) is Required for Exine Formation during Microgametogenesis and for Pollen Viability in *Arabidopsis*. Plant Journal, (2005). , 42, 315-328.

[13] Rodriguez-garcia, M. I, & Majewska-sawka, A. Is the Special Callose Wall of Microsporocytes an Impermeable Barrier? Journal of Experimental Botany, (2011). , 12, 1659-1663.

[14] Dumas, C, & Knox, R. B. Callose and Determination of Pistil Viability and Incompatibility. Theorotical and Applied Genetics (1983). , 67, 1-10.

[15] Kauss, H. Callose synthesis. In: Smallwood MJ, Knox P, Bowles DJ (eds). Membranes: Specialized Functions in Plants. Oxford: Bios Scientific; (1996). , 77-92.

[16] Chen, X. Y, & Kim, J. Y. Callose Synthesis in Higher Plants. Plant Signaling and Behavior (2009). , 4, 489-492.

[17] Goodman, N, Kiraly, Z, & Wood, K. R. The Biochemistry and Physiology of Plant Disease. Columbia: University of Missouri Press; (1986). , 352-365.

[18] Shimoura, T, & Dijkstra, J. The Occunence of Callose during the Process of Local Lesion Formation. Netherlands Journal of Plant Pathology (1975). , 81, 107-121.

[19] Xie, B, & Hong, Z. Unplugging the Callose Plug from Sieve Pores. Plant Signaling & Behavior (2011). , 6, 491-493.

[20] Nishikawa, S, Zinkl, G. M, Swanson, R. J, Maruyama, D, Preuss, D, & Callose, b. glucan) is Essential for *Arabidopsis* Pollen Wall Patterning, but not Tube Growth. BMC Plant Biology (2005).

[21] Verma DPSHong Z. Plant Callose Synthase Complexes. Plant Molecular Biology (2001). , 47, 693-701.

[22] Brownfield, L, Ford, K, Doblin, M. S, Newbigin, E, Read, S, & Bacic, A. Proteomic and Biochemical Evidence Links the Callose Synthase in *Nicotiana alata* Pollen Tubes to the Product of the *NaGSL1* Gene. Plant Journal (2007). , 52, 147-156.

[23] Brownfield, D. L, Todd, C. D, & Deyholos, M. K. Analysis of *Arabidopsis* Arginase Gene Transcription Patterns Indicates Specific Biological Functions for Recently Diverged Paralogs. Plant Molecular Biology (2008). , 67, 429-440.

[24] Richmond, T. A, & Somerville, C. R. The Cellulose Synthase Superfamily. Plant Physiology (2000). , 124, 495-498.

[25] Jacobs, A. K, Lipka, V, Burton, R. A, Panstruga, R, Strizhov, N, Schulze-lefert, P, & Fincher, G. B. An *Arabidopsis* Callose Synthase *GSL5* is Required for Wound and Papillary Callose Formation. Plant Cell (2003). , 15, 2503-2513.

[26] Nishimura, M. T, Stein, M, Hou, B H, Vogel, J. P, Edwards, H, & Somerville, S. C. Loss of a Callose Synthase Results in Salicylic Acid-Dependent Disease Resistance. Science (2003). , 301, 969-972.

[27] Enns, L. C, Kanaoka, M. M, Torii, K. U, Comai, L, Okada, K, & Cleland, R. E. Two Callose Synthases, GSL1 and GSL5, Play an Essential and Redundant Role in Plant and Pollen Development and Infertility. Plant Molecular Biology (2005). , 58, 333-49.

[28] Heslop-harrison, J. Cell walls, Cell Membranes and Protoplasmic Connections during Meiosis and Pollen Development. In: Linskens HF (ed.). Pollen, Physiology and Fertilization. Amsterdam: North Holland Publishers; (1964). , 39-47.

[29] Steiglitz, H. Role of S Glucanase in Postmeiotic Microspore Release. Developmental Biology (1977). , 1.

[30] Xie, B, Wang, X, & Hong, Z. Precocious Pollen Germination in *Arabidopsis* Plants with Altered Callose Deposition during Microsporogenesis. Planta (2010). , 231, 809-823.

[31] Wan, L, Zha, W, Cheng, X, Liu, C, Lv, L, Liu, C, Wang, Z, Du, B, Chen, R, Zhu, L, He, G, & Rice, b. glucanase Gene *Osg1* is Required for Callose Degradation in Pollen Development. Planta (2011). , 233, 309-323.

[32] Heslop-harrison, J. Cytoplasmic Connections between Angiosperm Meiocytes. Annals of Botany (1966a). , 30, 221-230.

[33] Heslop-harrison, J. Cytoplasmic Continuities during Spore Formation in Flowering Plants. Endeavour (1966b). , 25, 65-72.

[34] Godwin, H. The Origin of the Exine. New Phytologist (1968). , 67, 667-676.

[35] De Halac, N. I, & Harte, C. Female Gametophyte Competence in Relation to Polarization Phenomenon during the Megagametogenesis and Development of the Embryo Sac

in the Genus Oenothera. In: Mulcahy DL (Ed.). Gamete Competition in Plants and Animals. Amsterdam: North-Holland Publishers. (1975)., 43-56.

[36] Shivanna, K. R. Pollen Biology and Biotechnology. Plymouth: Science Publ. (2003).

[37] Barskaya, E. I, & Balina, N. V. The Role of Callose in Plant Anthers. Fiziologia Rastenil (1971)., 18, 716-721.

[38] Li, T, Gong, C, & Wang, T. RA68 is Required for Postmeiotic Pollen Development in Oryza sativa. Plant Molecular Biology (2010)., 72, 265-277.

[39] Izhar, S, & Frankel, R. Mechanism of Male-Sterility in *petunia*. I. The Relationship between pH, Callase Activity in the Anthers and Breakdown of Microsoprogenesis. Theoretical Applied Genetics (1971)., 41, 104-108.

[40] Warmke, H. E, & Overman, M. A. Cytoplasmic Male Sterility in Sorghum. 1. Callose Behavior in Fertile and Sterile Anthers. Journal of Heredity (1972)., 63, 103-108.

[41] Winiarczyk, K. Jaroszuk-S′ciseł J, Kupisz K. Characterization of Callase (b-1,3-D-glucanase) Activity during Microsporogenesis in the Sterile Anthers of *Allium sativum* L. and the Fertile Anthers of *A. atropurpureum*. Sexual Plant Reproduction (2012)., 25, 123-131.

[42] Shivaraj, B, & Pattabiraman, T. N. Natural Plant Enzyme Inhibitors. Characterization of an Unusual A-Amylase/Trypsin Inhibitor from Ragi (*Eleusine coracana* Geartn). Biochemical Journal (1981)., 193, 29-36.

[43] Elemo, G. N, Elemo, B. O, & Erukainure, O. L. Activities of Some Enzymes, Enzyme Inhibitors and Antinutritional Factors from the Seeds of Sponge Gourd (*Luffa aegyptiaca* M.). African Journal of Biochemical Research (2011)., 5, 86-89.

[44] Larson, D. A. Lewis jr CW. Cytoplasm in Mature, Nongerminated and Germinated Pollen. In: Breese Jr.S.S. (ed.). Electron microscopy. New York: Academic Press. (1962)., 2, 11.

[45] Waterkeyn, L, & Bienfait, A. On a Possible Function of the Callosic Special Wall in *Ipomoea purpurea* (L). Roth. Grana (1970)., 10, 13-20.

[46] Ford, J. H. Ultrastructural and Chemical Studies of Pollen Wall Development in the Epacridaceae. In : Brooks J, Grant PR, Muir M, Gijzel P, van Shaw G. (eds). Sporopollenin. London: Academic Press. (1971)., 686-707.

[47] Vijayaraghavan MR Shukla AKAbsence of Callose around the Microspore Tetrad and Poorly Developed Exine in *Pergularia daemia*. Annals of Botany (1977)., 41, 923-926.

[48] Ducker, S. C, Pettitt, J. M, & Knox, R. B. Biology of Australian Seagrasses: Pollen Development and Submarine Pollination in *Amphibolis antartica* and *Thalassodendron ciliatum* (Cymodoceaceae). Australian Journal of Botany (1978)., 26, 265-85.

[49] Pettitt, J. M. Reproduction in Seagrasses: Nature of the Pollen and Receptive Surface of the Stigma in the Hydrocharitaceae. Annals of Botany (1980)., 45, 257-271.

[50] Fitzgerald, M. A, Barnes, S. A, Blackmore, S, Calder, D. M, & Knox, R. B. Exine Formation in the Pollinium of Dendrobium. Protoplasma (1994)., 179, 121-130.

[51] Albert, B, Nadot, S, Dreyer, L, & Ressayre, A. The Influence of Tetrad Shape and Intersporal Callose Wall Formation on Pollen Aperture Pattern Ontogeny in Two Eudicot Species. Annals of Botany (2010)., 106, 557-564.

[52] Bhojwani, S. S, & Bhatnagar, S. P. The Embryology of Angiosperms. New Delhi: Vikas Publishing House; (1975).

[53] Gorska-brylass, A. The "Callose Stage" of the Generative Cells in Pollen Grains. Grana (1970)., 10, 21-30.

[54] Dunbar, A. Pollen Development in the *Eleoclzaris palrcrtris* Group (Cyperaceae). I. Ultrastructure and Ontogeny. Botaniska Notiser (1973)., 126, 197-254.

[55] Keijzer CJ Willemse MTMTissue Interactions in the Developing Locule of *Gasteria verrucosa* during Microgametogenesis. Acta Botanica Neerlandica (1988)., 37, 475-492.

[56] Zee, S. Y. Siu IHP. Studies on the Ontogeny of the Pollinium of a Massulate Orchid (*Peristylus spiranthes*). Review of Palaeobotany and Palynology (1990)., 64, 159-164.

[57] Schlag, M, & Hesse, M. The Formation of the Generative Cell in *Polystachia pubescens* (Orchidaceae). Sexual Plant Reproduction (1992)., 5, 131-137.

[58] Cresti, M, Blackmore, S, & Van Went, J. L. Atlas of Sexual Reproduction in Flowering Plants. Springer-Verlag: Berlin; (1992).

[59] Chebli, Y, & Geitmann, A. Mechanical Principles Governing Pollen Tube Growth. Functional Plant Science and Biotechnology, (2007)., 1, 232-245.

[60] Vervaeke, I, Londers, E, Piot, G, & Deroose, R. Proft MPD. The Division of the Generative Nucleus and the Formation of Callose Plugs in Pollen Tubes of *Aechmea fasciata* (Bromeliaceae) Cultured *in vitro*. Sexual Plant Reproduction (2005)., 18, 9-19.

[61] Malho, R. The Pollen Tube: A Cellular and Molecular Perspective. Berlin: Springer; (2006).

[62] Müller-stoll, W. E, Lerch, G, & Über, N. Entstehung und Eigenschaften der Kallosebildungen in Pollenschlauchen. Flora (1957)., 144, 297-472.

[63] Tsinger, N. V, & Petrovskaya-baranova, T. P. Formation and Physiological Role of Callose Pollen Tube Plugs. Soviet Plant Physiology (1967)., 14, 404-410.

[64] Kroh, M, & Knuiman, B. Ultrastructure of Cell Wall and Plugs of Tobacco Pollen Tubes after Chemical Extraction of Polysaccharides. Planta (1982)., 154, 241-250.

[65] Cresti, M, & Van Went, J. L. Callose Deposition and Plug Formation in *Petunia* Pollen Tubes *in situ*. Planta (1976)., 133, 35-40.

[66] Cresti, M, Ciampolini, F, & Sarfatti, G. Ultrastructural Investigations on *Lycopersicum peruvianum* Pollen Activation and Pollen Tube Organization after Self- and Cross Pollination. Planta (1980). , 150, 211-217.

[67] Jensen, W. A, & Fischer, D. B. Cotton Embriyogenesis: the Pollen Tube in the Stigma and the Style. Protoplasma (1970). , 69, 215-235.

[68] Rubinstein, A. L, Marquez, J, Suarez-cervera, M, & Bedinger, P. A. Extensin-like Glycoproteins in the Maize Pollen Tube Wall. Plant Cell (1995). , 7, 2211-2225.

[69] Giampiero, C, Faleri, C, & Casino, C. D. Emons AMC, Cresti M. Distribution of Callose Synthase, Cellulose Synthase, and Sucrose Synthase in Tobacco Pollen Tube is Controlled in Dissimilar Ways by Actin Filaments and Microtubules. Plant Physiology (2011). , 155, 1169-1190.

[70] Linskens, H. F, & Esser, K. Über eine Spezifische Anfarboung der Pollen Schlauche im Griffel und die Zahl der Kallosepfropfen nach Selbatung und Fremdung. Naturwisser (1957).

[71] Tupy, J. Callose Formation in Pollen Tubes and Incompatibility. Biologia Plantarum (1959). I: , 192-198.

[72] De Nettancourt, D, Devreux, M, Laneri, U, Cresti, M, Pacini, E, & Sarfatti, G. Genetical and Ultrastructural Aspects of Self- and Cross-Incompatibility in Interspecific Hybrids between Self-Compatible *Lycopersicum esculentum* and Self-Incompatible *L. peruvian m.* Theoretical Applied Genetics (1974). , 44, 278-288.

[73] De Nettancourt, D. Incompatibility in Angiosperms. Berlin: Springer-Verlag; (1977).

[74] Heslop-harrison, J, Knox, R. B, & Heslop-harrison, Y. (1974). Pollen-wall proteins: exine-held fractions associated with the incompatibility response in Cruciferae. Theoretical Applied Genetics, , 44, 133-137.

[75] Sastri, D. C, & Shivanna, K. R. Role of Pollen- Wall Proteins in Intraspecific Incompatibility in *Saccharum benegalens*. Phytomorphology (1979). , 29, 324-330.

[76] Vithanage HIMVGleeson PA, Clarke AE. The Nature of Callose Produced during Self-Pollination in *Secale cereale*. Planta (1980). , 148, 498-509.

[77] Franklin-tong, V. E. Franklin FCH. Gametophytic Self-Incompatibility in *Papaver rhoeas* L. Sexual Plant Reproduction (1992). , 5, 1-7.

[78] Ünal, M. Callose Formation and Incompatibility in the Pollen Tubes of *Petunia hybrida*. Marmara University, Journal of Pure and Applied Sciences (1988). In Turkish).

[79] Shivanna, K. R, Heslop-harrison, Y, & Heslop-harrison, J. The Pollen-Stigma Interaction: Bud Pollination in the Cruciferae. Acta Botanica Neerlandica (1978). , 27, 107-119.

[80] Sood, R, Parabha, K, & Gupta, S. C. Is the 'Rejection Reaction' Inducing Ability in Sporophytic Self-Incompatibility Systems Restricted Only to Pollen and Tapetum? Theoretical Applied Genetics (1982). , 63, 27-32.

[81] Shivanna, K. R, & Johri, B. M. The Angiosperm Pollen: Structure and Function. New Delhi: Wiley Eastern Ltd; (1985).

[82] Dickinson, H. G, & Lewis, D. Cytochemical and Ultrastructural Differences between Intraspecific Compatible and Incompatible Pollinations in *Raphamts*. Proceedings of the Royal Society Biological Sciences (1973). , 183, 21-38.

[83] Singh, A, & Paolillo, D. J. Role of Calcium in the Callose Response of Self-Pollinated Brassica Stigmas. American Journal of Botany (1990). , 77, 128-133.

[84] Elleman, C. J, & Dickinson, H. G. Identification of Pollen Components Regulating Pollination-Specific Responses in the Stigmatic Papillae of *Brassica oleracea*. New Phytologist (1996). , 133, 196-205.

[85] Bouman, F. Ovule In: Johri BM. (ed.). Embryology of Angiosperms. Berlin: Springer-Verlag; (1984).

[86] Bell, P. R. Megaspore Abortion: A Consequence of Selective Apoptosis? International Journal of Plant Sciences (1996). , 157, 1-7.

[87] Rodkiewicz, B, & Gorska-brylas, A. Occurence of Callose in the Walls of Meiotically Dividing Cells in the Ovule of Orchis. Naturwissen (1967).

[88] Rodkiewicz, B. Callose in the Cell Wall during Megasporogenesis in Angiosperms. Planta (1970). , 93, 39-47.

[89] Kuran, H. Callose Localization in the Wall of Megasporocytes and Megaspores in the Course of Development of Monosporic Embryo Sac. Acta Societatis Botanicorum Poloniae (1972). , 41, 519-534.

[90] Rodkiewicz, B, & Bednara, J. Cell Wall Ingrowth and Callose Distribution in Megasporogenesis in some Orchidaceae. Phytomorphology (1976). , 26, 2276-2281.

[91] Kapil, R. N, & Tiwari, S. C. Plant Embriyological Investigations and Fluoresecence Microscopy: An Assessment of Integration. International Review of Cytology (1978). , 53, 291-331.

[92] Russell, S. D. Fine Structure of Megagametophyte Development in *Zea mays*. Canadian Journal of Botany (1979). , 57, 1093-1110.

[93] De Halac, I. N. Fine Structure of the Nucellar Cells during Development of the Embryo Sac in *Oenothera biennis* L. Annals of Botany (1980). , 45, 515-521.

[94] Schulz, P, & Jensen, W. A. Prefertilization Ovule Development in *Capsella*: The Dyad, Tetrad, Developing Megaspore, and Two-Nucleate Gametophyte. Canadian Journal of Botany (1986). , 64, 875-884.

[95] Folsom, M. W, & Cass, D. D. Embryo Sac Development in Soybean: Ultrastructure of Megasporogenesis and Early Megagametogenesis. Canadian Journal of Botany (1989). , 67, 2841-2849.

[96] Webb, M. C. Gunning BES. Embryo Sac Development in *Arabidopsis thaliana*. I. Megasporogenesis, Including the Microtubular Cytoskeleton. Sexual Plant Reproduction (1990)., 3, 244-256.

[97] Raghavan, V. Molecular Embryology of Flowering Plants. Cambridge: Cambridge University Press; (1997).

[98] Yu, H. S, Hu, S. Y, & Russell, S. D. Sperm Cells in Pollen Tubes of *Nicotiana tabacum* L.: Three-Dimensional Reconstruction, Cytoplasmic Diminution, and Quantitative Cytology. Protoplasma (1992)., 168, 172-183.

[99] Jensen, W. A, & Fisher, D. B. Cotton Embryogenesis; the Entrance and Discharge of the Pollen Tube in the Embryo Sac. Planta (1968)., 78, 158-183.

[100] Vijayaraghavan, M. R, & Bhat, U. Synergids Before and After Fertilization. Phytomorphology (1983)., 33, 74-84.

[101] Willemse MTMvan Went JL. The Female Gametophyte. In: Johri BM (ed). Embryology of Angiosperms. Berlin: Springer. (1984)., 159-196.

[102] Gupta, P. K, Balyan, H. S, Sharma, P. C, & Ramesh, B. Microsatellites in Plants: A New Class of Molecular Markers. Current Science (1996)., 70, 45-54.

[103] Ryals, J, Neuenschwander, U, Willits, M, Molina, A, Steiner, H. Y, & Hunt, M. Systemic Acquired Resistance. Plant Cell (1996)., 8, 1809-1819.

[104] Donofrio, N. M, & Delaney, T. P. Abnormal Callose Response Phenotype and Hypersusceptibility to *Peronospora parasitica* in Defense-Compromised *Arabidopsis nim1-1* and Salicylate Hydroxylase Plants. Molecular Plant-Microbe Interactions (2001)., 14, 439-50.

[105] Benhamou, N. Ultrastructural Detection of β-1,3-glucans in Tobacco Root Tissues Infected by *Phytophthora parasitica* var. nicotianae using A Gold-Complexed Tobacco β-1,3-glucanase. Physiological and Molecular Plant Pathology (1992)., 41, 315-370.

[106] Delmer, D. P, Volokita, M, Solomon, M, Fritz, U, Delphendahl, W, & Herth, W. A Monoclonal Antibody Recognizes a 65 kDa Higher Plant Membrane Polypeptide which Undergoes Cation Dependent Association with Callose Synthase *in vitro* and Colocalizes with Site of High Callose Deposition *in vivo*. Protoplasma (1993)., 176, 33-42.

[107] Lucas, W. J, Ding, B, & Van Der Schoot, C. Plasmodesmata and the Supracellular Nature of Plants. New Phytologist (1993)., 125, 435-476.

[108] Vatén, A, Dettmer, J, Wu, S, Stierhof, Y. D, Miyashima, S, Yadav, S. R, Roberts, C. J, Campilho, A, Bulone, V, Lichtenberger, R, Lehesranta, S, Mähönen, A. P, Kim, J. Y, Jokitalo, E, Sauer, N, Scheres, B, Nakajima, K, Carlsbecker, A, Gallagher, K. L, & Helariutta, Y. Callose Biosynthesis Regulates Symplastic Trafficking during Root Development. Developmental Cell (2011)., 21, 1144-1155.

[109] Samuels, A. L, Giddings, T. H, & Staehelin, A. L. Cytokinesis in Tobacco BY-2 and Root Tip Cells: A New Model of Cell Plate Formation in Higher Plants. Boulder: University of Colorado; (1995).

[110] Apostolakos, P, Livanos, P, & Galatis, B. Microtubule Involvement in the Deposition of Radial Fibrillar Callose Arrays in the Stomato of the Fern *Asplenium nidus* L. Cell Motility and The Cytoskeleton (2009). , 66, 342-349.

[111] Barratt, D. H, Koelling, K, Graf, A, Pike, M, Calder, G, Findlay, K, Zeeman, S. C, & Smith, A. M. Callose Synthase *GSL7* is Necessary for Normal Phloem Transport and Inflorescence Growth in *Arabidopsis*. Plant Physiology (2011). , 155, 328-341.

[112] Bacic, A, Fincher, G. B, & Stone, B. A. Chemistry, Biochemistry and Biology of (1-3)-β-Glucans and Related Polysaccharides. USA: Academic Press; (2009).

[113] Kauss, H. Callose Biosynthesis as a Calcium-Regulated Process and Possible Relations to the Induction of Other Metabolic Changes. Journal of Cell Science (1985). Supp., 2, 89-103.

[114] Kauss, H. Ca^{2+} Dependence of Callose Sythesis and the Role of Polyamines in the Activation of 1,3-β-glucan Synthase by Ca^{2+}. In: Trewavas AJ (Ed.). Molecular and Cellular Aspects of Calcium in Plant Development. Plenum Press. (1987). , 131-136.

[115] Bhuja, P, Mclachlan, K, Stephens, J, & Taylor, G. Accumulation of 1,3-β-D-glucans, in Response to Aluminum and Cytosolic Calcium in *Triticum aestivum*. Plant and Cell Physiology (2004). , 45, 543-549.

[116] Østergaard, O, Melchior, S, Roepstorff, P, & Svensson, B. Initial Proteome Analysis of Mature Barley Seeds and Malt. Proteomics (2002). , 2, 733-739.

[117] Köhle, H, Jeblick, W, Poten, F, Blashek, W, & Kauss, H. Chitosan-Elicited Callose Synthesis in Soybean Cells as a Ca^{2+}-Dependent Process. Plant Phsiology (1985). , 77, 544-551.

[118] Andrawis, A, Solomon, M, & Delmer, D. P. Cotton Fiber Annexins: A Potential Role in the Regulation of Callose Synthase. Plant Journal (1993). , 3, 763-772.

[119] Schlüpmann, H, Bacic, A, & Read, S. M. A Novel Callose Synthase from Pollen Tubes of *Nicotiana*. Planta (1993). , 191, 470-481.

[120] Iglesias, A, Rosenzweig, C, & Pereira, D. Prediction Spatial Impacts of Climate in Agriculture in Spain. Global Environmental Change (2000). , 10, 69-80.

[121] Messiaen, J, Nérinckx, F, & Van Cutsem, P. Callose Synthesis in Spirostanol Treated Carrot Cells is not Triggered by Cytosolic Calcium, Cytosolic pH or Membrane Potential Changes. Plant Cell Physiology (1995). , 36, 1213-1220.

[122] Tang, X, Xie, M, Kim, Y. J, Zhou, J, Klessig, D. F, & Martin, G. B. Overexpression of *Pto* Activates Defense Responses and Confers Broad Resistance. Plant Cell (1999). , 11, 15-29.

[123] Kohler, B, & Blatt, M. R. Protein Phosphorylation Activates the Guard Cell Ca^{2+} Channel and is A Prerequisite for Gating by Abscisic Acid. Plant Journal (2002)., 32, 185-194.

[124] Hughes, J. E. Gunning BES. Glutaraldehyde-Induced Deposition of Callose. Canadian Journal of Botany (1980)., 58, 250-257.

[125] Vaughn, K. C, Hoffman, J. C, Hahn, M. G, & Staehelin, L. A. The Herbicide Dichlobenil Disrupts Cell Plate Formation: Immunogold Characterization. Protoplasma (1996)., 194, 117-132.

[126] Luna, E, Pastor, V, Robert, J, Flors, V, Mauch-mani, B, & Ton, J. Callose Deposition: A Multifaceted Plant Defense Response. Molecular Plant Microne Interactions (2011)., 24, 183-193.

[127] Vardar, F, Ismailoglu, I, Inan, D, & Ünal, M. Determination of Stress Responses Induced by Aluminum in Maize (*Zea mays*). Acta Biologica Hungarica (2011)., 62, 156-170.

[128] Wissemeier, A. H, & Horst, W. J. Effect of Light Intensity on Manganese Toxicity Symptoms and Callose Formation in Cowpea (*Vigna unguiculata* (L.) Walp. Plant and Soil (1992)., 143, 299-309.

[129] Vardar, F. Studies on the development and programmed cell death in the anthers of *Lathyrus undulatus* Boiss. PhD Thesis. Marmara University, Turkey; (2008).

Chapter 15

Antibiotic Susceptibilities and SDS-PAGE Protein Profiles of Methicillin-Resistant Staphylococcus Aureus (MRSA) Strains Obtained from Denizli Hospital

Göksel Doğan, Gülümser Acar Doğanlı,
Yasemin Gürsoy and Nazime Mercan Doğan

Additional information is available at the end of the chapter

http://dx.doi.org/10.5772/55457

1. Introduction

Soon after two years of introducing methicillin, *S. aureus* strains developed resistance to methicillin by through the gain of the mecA gene (MRSA). At first *S. aureus* strains were exclusively related to hospital acquired (HA) MRSA, but as from 1990s, community acquired (CA) MRSA came into view [1].

In both HA-MRSAs and CA- MRSAs are refered to as a significant factor of serious infections in high morbidity and mortality including bacteremia, pneumonia, endocarditis, osteomyelitis and toxic shock syndrome [2,3,4,5,6]. The factors that increase the prevalence of nosocomial bacteremia are the increase in older age groups in society, life period prolongation of people with chronic diseases, widespread use of immunosuppressive drugs, increase in interventional procedures for the purposes of diagnostic and therapeutic. Generally, some of staphylococ infections are nasocomial, other infections have occured by depending on MRSAs. The colonization rate with MRSA has increased in parallel duration of hospitalization. These strains have been found resistant against penicillins, combinations of betalactam/betalactamase inhibitory, sephalosporins, combinations of monobactames and carpenemes. To identify the resistance of staphylococcus's against methycillin antibiotic, those methods as of disc diffusion, tube dilution or microdilution, agar scanning, agar dilution, automatise susceptibility tests, DNA hybridisation technics and polimeraze chain reaction have been used [7,8,9]. The aim of this study is to identify antibiotic susceptibility and specificity of MRSAs isolated from various clinic samples with various methods including disc diffusion, SDS-PAGE and DNase test.

2. Methicillin resistant *Staphylococcus aureus*

2.1. General properties

S. aureus (including MRSA strains) are clusterforming, facultative aerobic, Gram-positive cocci (at 0.5-1.7 μ of diameters) with intrinsic ability to ferment carbohydrates, producing white to deep yellow pigmentation on solid culture media [2].

50% of cell wall of Staphylococci has composed from peptidoglycan. Peptidoglycan chains consist of alternative polysaccharide subunits included N-acetyl glucosamines and N-acetyl muramik acid. These chains are cross linkage by pentaglycine bridges that are specific for *S.aureus* and tetra peptide chains binded with N- acetyl muramik acid. Peptidoglycan can show endotoxin properties and structural differences among strains can lead to extensive intravenous coagulation [10,11].

Most researchers demonstrated that MRSAs caused various diseases ranging from soft, superficial dermatological diseases to acute and potentially fatal systemic enervations [2,12,13]. Some MRSAs live as a normal flora member in human mucose membrans and skins, others lead to ichor, abscess formation, various piogen infections and fatal septicemia. MRSA strains have also been detected in domestic animals and birds such as horses, cattle, chickens and dogs as well as associated individuals [2].

Staphylococcus aureus is coagulase positive and major patogen for humans. In general pathologic Staphylocci hemolysis the blood, coagulates the plasma, and also produces various extracellular enzymes and toxins. They have developed quickly against antimicrobial drugs [14].

2.2. Culture properties

Staphylococci grows easily aerobic or microaerofilic conditions. Optimal temperature is 37°C for these bacteria. Colonies of them are orbicular, sleek, bouffant and brilliant in solid media. In general, *S.aureus* has colonie colours that change from white to golden yellow. However, in many colonies, pigment occurs by those bacteria after long incubation time. It does not occur under anaerobic conditions or in broth [14].

2.3. Growing properties

Staphylococci have produced catalase variously then Streptococci. Staphylococci fermentate carbohydrates slowly by constituting acid, but they do not produce gases. On the other hand, pathogenic Staphylococci have generated so many extracellular substances. Even though, Staphylococci are durable against conditions of dry air, temperature (50°C, 30 m) and 9% of NaCI, but they can be inactivated easly with powerful chemicals such as 3% of hexaclorofen. Other one theme, these bacteria are sensetive against many of antimicrobial drugs. Resistant separates several of categories;

Mechanism of methicillin resistant: The resistant agaist beta-lactame antibiotics (methicillin, oxacillin, nafcillin, kloxacillin and dikloxacillin) not having been hyrolysed with beta-lactamase enzyme has denominated as methicillin resistant. Thus, it is clear that the resitant is chromosomal and is not with beta-lactamase enzyme inactivated the antibiotic [15,16].

PBP 2a (PBP 2′): Alhough methicillin sensitive *S. Aureus* (MSSA) has five types of penicillin binding proteins (PBP), in addition these proteins, methicillin resistant *S. Aureus* (MRSA) has also a different penicillin binding protein named as PBP 2′ or PBP 2a. This protein has 78 kDa of molecular weight [17]. PBP 2a shows lower affinity against beta-lactame antibiotics then other PBPs. Hence, the enzyme is single trancepeptidase that has the ability to continue of peptidoglycan synthesis by showing high affinity in presence of beta-lactame antibiotics [13,18]. The gene encoded PBP 2a is 2.1 kb and named *mecA*. Though, all of MRSAs have this gene, but there is no this gene at MSSA strains. The emergence of methicillin resistant phenotypeclly has been able to show variability among bacteria. The phenotypically expiration of methicillin resistant is possible in two ways; homogen and heterogen [17]. In homogen resistant, all of cells show high levels of resistance in presence of high methicillin consentrations by growing [19,11]. In hetrogen resistance, even though all cells have *mecA* gene had information that needs for methicillin resitance, only some cells show resistance.

a. ***mecR1-mecI sistemi:*** The *mecA* have been controled with two regulator genes. Those genes are *mecR1* and *mecI*. Also these genes are similar to *blaR1* and *blaI,* which are regulatory genes of beta-lactamase, in terms of structure, fonction and mechanism of regulation. *MecI* and *mecR1* have the same regulator role for *mecA*. *MecR1* encodes a signal stimulant protein, while *mecI* encodes a protin suppressed the *mecA* [15,16]

b. Other factors affected resistant phenotype:

   - Beta-lactamase plasmid: Production of beta-lactamase enzyme is encoded by *blaZ* gene and is controled by genes of *blaR1* and *blaI* which are antireceptor and receptor, recpectively. *BlaR1* which is a transmembrane protein binds to beta-lactame in presence of it and leads to start the synthesyse of beta-lactamase enzyme by providing signal transmission from out of cell to inside of cell [20]. At the same time, it has been thought that genes of *blaR1* and *blaI* have had a role for occuring of methicillin resistant phenotypically [17].

   - Fem Factors: The obtaining sensitive strains from methicillin resistance strains by tranposones via inactivation had led to identification of genes beyond of *mec*. These genes placed out of *mec* gene region had defined as "auxiliary" or "factors essential for the expression of methicillin resistance" or shortly "fem" genes [21]. Both MRSA and MSSA strains have fem factors variously from *mec*A gene. Also, it indicated that some conditions increased the occuring of methicillin resistant were correlated with modifications at cell autolysis.

2.4. Enzymes and toxins

Staphylococci can lead to diseases by large diffusion at tissue and producing many extracellular substances. Some of these extracellular substances are enzymes, others are toxins. Most toxins are under genetic control of plasmids. Some of them can be under both kromosomal and ekstrakromosomal control [22,23,24,25].

2.5. Coagulase and clumping factor

S.aureus produces coagulase being an enzyme providing coagulation of the plasma. Coagulase that can be droped out freely binds the prothrombin and initiates polymerization of fibrin. It can also accumulate the fibrin at suface of Staphylocci. It thinks that products of coagulase are similar to invasive patogenic power.

Clumping Factor which is responsible for binding of organism to fibrin and fibrinogen-is a surface component of *S.aureus*. When clumbing factor comes up with plasma, *S.aureus* forms clumps. Clumping Factor is discret from coagulase [22,25].

2.6. Enzymes

Other enzymes produced by Staphylococcus's are sthapylokinase, proteinase, DNase and enzymes having different properties such as ß-lactamase.

2.7. Exotoxins

Alfa toxin is a heterogen protein acting by depending on large spectrum of eucariotic cell membrans. α toxin is a power hemolysin (a substance that causes the fragmentation of erytrosit). ß toxin have reduced the sphingomyelin, therefore it is toxic for many cells included human red blood cells. Additionally, an other toxin, δ is heterogen. It fractionates the biologic membrans and can have a role at diarrheal patients because of *S.aureus*.

2.8. Leukocidin

This toxin of *S.aureus* has two components. It affects white blood cells in humans and rabbits. These two components have moved synergistic like γ toxin at the membrane of white blood cells. The toxin is an important virulance factor in community acquired MRSA (CA-MRSA) strains.

2.9. Toxic shock syndrom toxin

Many *S.aureus* strains isolated from patients with toxic shock syndrome produce the toxic shock syndrome toxin-1 (TSST–1) also namely enterotoxin F. TSST–1 is the super antigen and binds the MHC-II molecules that leads to T cell stimulation TSST–1. This toxin is related to febrile, shock and multisystem involvement which are scope skin disease.

2.10. Diagnostic laboratory tests

2.10.1. Gram staining

S. Aureus bacteria appears violet colour and looks like bunch of grapes by gram staining. It is imposible to separate pathogenic organism (*S.aureus*) from saprophytic organisms (*S.epidermitis*) by gram staining.

2.10.2. Catalase test

MRSAs produce catalase, which converts hydrogen peroxide into water and oxygen. The catalase test differentiates the staphylococci from the streptococci [14].

2.10.3. Susceptibility tests

At choosing of advisable antibiotic drug associated with therapy of infection, a number of factors such as potential infectious agents, antibiotic susceptibility, host factors that may affect the activity of the drug in vivo, the location of the infection, pharmacokinetic and pharmacodynamic properties of the drug should be evaluate [26]. Generally, *in vitro* procedures applied for determination of antimicrobic activity of an antibiotic is named as susceptibility tests. Susceptibility tests apply in the cases of not foreseeable susceptibility against antibacterial agent which will be applied at treatment of aerob and facultative anaerob bacteria which are clinically important. Susceptibility against antimicrobic drugs can be detected with a lot of methods. In most, inhibitor activity of drugs (bacteriostatic) evaulates in applied method. The applied methods with this purpose can consider of; 1. dilution methods in liquid and solid media; 2. disc diffusion method; 3. gradient diffusion (E-test) method; 4. the detection of enzymes which inactivate antimicrobic agents [26].

At disc diffusion method, paper discs is absorbed a specific amount of antibiotic place onto plate inoculed with the test microorganism. Thus, antibiotic absorbed by disc diffuses into agar and inhibits the growing of bacteria at effect levels of antibiotic. At the end of this situation, a circular inhibition zone where does not grow bacteria occurs at ambient of the disc. The categories of susceptibility as of sensitive, medium and resistance identify by measuring diameter of this zone. The limit values related to these categories detect for every antimicrobic agent by regarding accescible serum levels [26,27]. For example, Staphilococci are *mec*A positive and are resistant against methicillin at Müller-Hinton agar contented 6 of μg/mL of oxasilin and 4% of NaCl.

2.11. Community and hospital acquired MRSA infections

Molecular epedemiology of community aquired MRSA (CA-MRSA) is tolerably different from hospital acquired MRSA (HA-MRSA). CA-infections commonly cause of skin and soft tisue infections, bacteremia and endocardit [2].

Panton-Valentine leukocidin (PVL) gene encoded a toxin which is responsible from virulance of bacteria and type 4 SCC*mec* genetic component frequently are presence at CA-MRSA isolates [22,16]. HA-MRSA isolates generally have type I, II or III of staphylococcal casette chromosome (SCC*mec*) genetic component. This gene domain is responsible from showing resistant of bacteria against antibiotics made from beta-lactam and even other drugs such as clindamycin, gentamicin and florocinolon. Characterisation of the staphylococcal cassette chromosome (SCC) mec type has led to better discrimination of hospital acquired MRSA (HA-MRSA) and community acquired MRSA (CA-MRSA) [28]. SCCs are mobile elements characterized by association of a *mec complex* and *ccr genes* coding for integration into or excision from the chromosome. Three types of SCC (types I, II and III) were originally described in hospital-acquired MRSA strains (HA-MRSA), most of them isolated before 1990. A fourth type (type IV) was recently described, first in community-acquired MRSA isolates (CA-MRSA) and then in several MRSA backgrounds, including hospital isolates [29].

To compare HA-MRSA strains with CA-MRSA, It needs to examine several aspects. Innitially, chromosomal elements for meticillin resistance in community-associated strains are chromosome cassette mec (SCCmec) types IV or V, being smaller and more active than SCCmec types I–III found in hospital-acquired MRSA. In HA-MRSA, the larger gene elements are correlated with reduced bacterial ability as well as decreased toxin generation. Also, the PVL toxin is more common in CA-MRSA than in MSSA. Another thing, increased expression of certain virulence determinants which can cause more acute disease (e.g. phenol-soluble modulins-PSMs-) is available in CA MRSA. The last one,, while all S. aureus strains have an aptness to generate biofilms, it suggest that variations in biofilm matrix in CA-MRSA compared to other strains. But, there is no sufficient evidence in the literature that any of MRSA strain sample has a larger capability to cause invasive infection than MSSA strains [7].

2.12. Clinic Infections

2.12.1. Skin and soft tisue infections

CA-MRSA strains can be infected skin and soft tissue infections, which characteristically occur in healthy people without preconditions. For instance, the US had one of the biggest CA-MRSA epidemic, with one strain named USA300, being liable for most of infections. In 2005, 13.7% of all invasive MRSA infections in the US were community associated. [30]. Skin, soft tisue and bone infections seems at most. These infections can be confined from a localized infektion to more general infections such as cellulite, impedigo, folliculit, boll, carboncul and surgical wound infection. Staphylococcal bone marrow dermatitis (osteomyelitis) occurs typically at young children because of bacteremia. More severe manifestations can include necrotizing pneumonia, pyomyositis, sepsis, osteomyelitis and necrotizing fasciitis [7]. Even though, some of *S.aureus* infections corellate with development of TSS, nowadays most of patients have skin and soft tissue infections with this disease. For instance, Staphylococcal scalded skin syndrome seems at most in young children.It is less common in adults and older children. The reason is that some of toxins (exfoliative toxins; ETA and ETB) bind with GM4-like glycolipids in newborns sensitive epidermis. GM4-like glycolipids are not available in adult and children [31,32] Figure 1 shows a sample of skin and soft tisue infection of MRSA strains.

2.13. Systemic infections

2.13.1. Pneumonia

At 1918 in registries, obtained from influence pandemia of young individuals, most of deaths related with bacterial super infections that *S.aureus* strains lead to those infections. Recently, *S.aureus* isolates produced PVL toxin has relevanted to infections of skin and soft tisue such as pnömonia at healthy young people. PVL is a bi-component exotoxin transmitted by bacteriophages that is encoded by two genes, *luk* FPV and *luk* S-PV. PVL genes are carried by

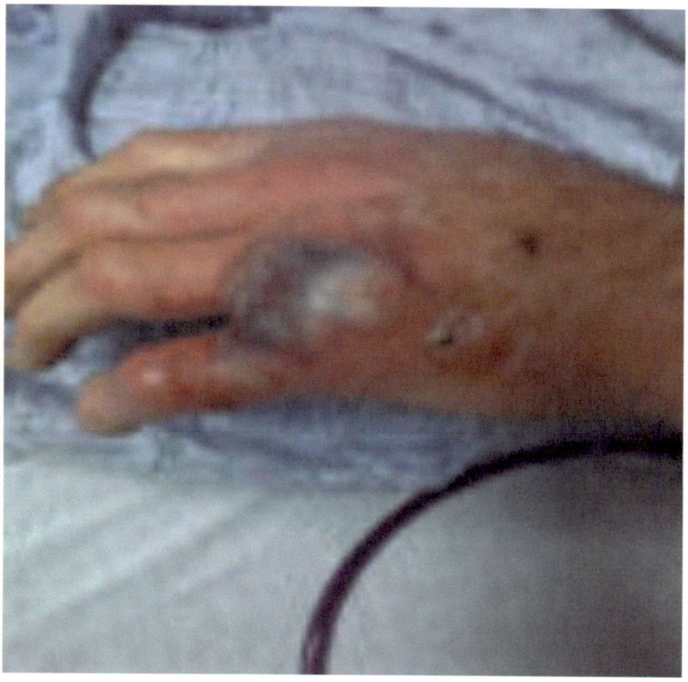

Figure 1. Skin and Soft tisue Infection of MRSA [33]

nearly every CA-MRSA strain as well as a small proportion of clinical MSSA strains. This suggests that PVL has an important role in fitness, transmissibility and virulence, but the role of PVL in the pathogenesis of CA-MRSA infections is controversial [7]. PVL is a toxin fragmented speedy the white blood cells. Also, these strains can be contained other virulance factors and toxins. Consequently, this kinf of infections have high rates of death.

2.13.2. Treatment

It is necessary the using of a penicillin which is resistant against β-lactamase in bacteremia, endocartidis, pneumonia and other infections which occur by *S.aureus* strains for long times. Vancomycin has been prefered at methicillin resistant strains. If the infections are because of *S.aureus* wich not produce β-lactamase, penicillin G has to choose for those infections. *S.aureus* strains izolated from clinic infections which are resistant against penicillin G always *produce* penicillinases. Those strains are generally sensitive against penicillins wich are resistant β-lactamases, cephalosporins or vancomycin. Resistant of methicillin is independent from producting of β-lactamase.

Resistant of drugs such as penicillin, tetracyclin, aminoglycosid and, erytromycin which has detected by plasmids can be transfered to other staphylococci by transduction and conjugation. Antibiotics such as linezolid, daptomycin and dalfopristin can be used at serious staphylococcal or enterococcal infections of patients which have common drug resistance.

3. Material and method

3.1. MRSA isolates

Thwenty-six isolates, which were isolated from intencive care unit (ICU) between September 2009-February 2010, were clinical isolates from ICU patients in Denizli Hospital. The isolates were identified as MRSA in hospital before obtaining. These isolates were obtained from tracheal aspirates, catheter tip, wounds, urine, blood, and effluxion, in a total of 26 strains were taken into account. Colonies were also checked by Gram-staining. Isolates were also identified by growth on Dnase test agar with methyl gren agar by DNase test. Table 1 shows the isolates and their origins.

Code of Strains	Source	Code of Strains	Source
MRSA 1	tracheal aspirates	MRSA 14	tracheal aspirates
MRSA 2	effluxion	MRSA 15	tracheal aspirates
MRSA 3	tracheal aspirates	MRSA 16	tracheal aspirates
MRSA 4	blood	MRSA 17	tracheal aspirates
MRSA 5	blood	MRSA 18	urine
MRSA 6	catheter tip	MRSA 19	tracheal aspirates
MRSA 7	blood	MRSA 20	blood
MRSA 8	blood	MRSA 21	tracheal aspirates
MRSA 9	tracheal aspirates	MRSA 22	catheter tip
MRSA 10	blood	MRSA 23	blood
MRSA 11	urine	MRSA 24	wound
MRSA 12	tracheal aspirates	MRSA 25	blood
MRSA 13	tracheal aspirates	MRSA 26	wound

Table shows MRSA samples obtained from 26 of patients, Denizli hospital

Table 1. MRSA strains and isolation resources

3.2. Media

Tryptic soy broth (TSB) medium (g/l:pepton from casein 17, pepton from soy meal 3, D(+)glucose 2.5, NACL Dipotassium hydrogen phosphate) was used for cultering MRSA strains at the study of antibiotic susceptibility. Tryptic soy agar (TSA) solid medium (g/l: pepton from casein 15.0; pepton from soymeal 5.0; Sodium chloride 5.0; agar-agar 15.0) was used for antibiogram tests. DNAase test agar with methyl green medium was used to determinate the DNAase activity. All of media were autoclaved at 121 ^{0}C'de for 15 min. and stored at 4 ^{0}C until using.

3.3. Antimicrobial susceptibilities

To determinate multiple antibiotic resistan of MRSA trains, antibiotic susceptibilities were investigated by disc diffusion method. Susceptibility to methicillin by disc diffusion had allready determined by cefoxitin (30 μg) discs before samples taking from hospital. The zone of inhibition was interpreted after 24 h of incubation at 35 ^{0}C. Plates were read at 24 and 48 h of incubation at 37 ^{0}C. In addition to cefoxitin (FOX, 30 μg), the following antibiotics were tested: vancomycin (VA, 30 μg), tetracycline (TE, 30 μg), erythromycin (E, 15 μg), clindamycin (DA, 2 μg), rifampicin (RA, 5 mcg), linezolid (LZD, 30 μg),, sulfamethoxazole / trimethoprim (SXT, 25 mcg), penicillin-G (P, 10 unit), amikacin (AK, 30 mcg), seforoksimsodyum (CXM, 30 mcg), Novobiosin (NV, 5 μg), ampicillin (AM, 10 mcg) and gentamicin (CN, 10 mcg) antibiotics.

3.4. Extraction of Whole Cell Proteins (WCPs)

The method of Laemmli [34] was used by a little modification for electrophoresis. After overnight incubation at 37 ^{0}C for 24 h. in 5 ml of TSB (Merc) media, samples were centrifuged for 20 min at 6000 rpm. The pellets were washed three times with sterile distilled water and stirred after adding 25 μl SDS sample buffer (0.06 M Tris, 2.5 % glycerol, 0.5 % SDS, 1.25 % β-mercaptoethanol and 0.001 % bromophenol blue). The proteins were denatured in boiling water for 10 min. Samples stayed in eppendorf tubes were uploaded to electrophoresis apparatus.

4. SDS-PAGE

Denatured whole cell proteins were analyzed by SDS-PAGE according to Laemmli. This method used 4 % acrylamide stacking gel and 10 % acrylamide separating gel. MBI Fermentas SM0661 kit was used as molecular weight standard in SDS-PAGE. Electrophoresis was performed with buffer system in a Biolab gel apparatus model V20-CDC. The gel was run at 150 V for 2 h at stacking gel, 200 V for 4 h at sperating gel until the bromophenol blue had reached the bottom. Gels were then stained with Coomassie Brilliant Blue R 250 (Sigma).

4.1. Determination of DNase activity

Following overnight incubation at 37 ^{0}C for 24 h. in TSB (Merc) media, 26 of MRSA strains were inoculated a full loop of cells to petridishes where place DNase test agar with methyl green media and were applied the spot test. Inoculeted cells were incubated for overnight at 37 ^{0}C for 24 h. After incubation, 1 N of HCl was dumped onto plates which grow MRSA colonies. It was checked whether achromatic color zone occur or not. The colonies occurring achromatic color zone were accepted as DNase positive strains, others were accepted DNase negative strains.

5. Results

5.1. Antimicrobial susceptibilities

Antimicrobial susceptibility testing was performed as recommended by the National Committee on Clinical Laboratory Standards [35,36]. MRSA samples that we used in our study were activated by culturing freshly at 37 ^{0}C for 24 h. two times. 100 μl from these activared fresh culture samples were done smear cultivation to petridishes of TSA medium. Antibiotic discs were fixed up to surface of the media by using Disc diffusion method under steril conditions. The samples were incubated at 37 ^{0}C for 24 h. and the diameters of zone were measured.

In general, It was determinated that all of strains showed resistance against all of antibiotics. No zone of inhibition has been seen only against cefoxitin (FOX, 30 μg) antibiotic. It was observed that the zone did not occur except a few strains and strains were resistant against penicilin, amikacin (AK, 30 mcg), sulfamethoxazole / trimethoprim (SXT, 25 mcg), ampicillin (AM, 10 mcg), (CN, 10 mcg), erythromycin (E, 15 μg) and rifampicin (RA, 5 mcg) antibiotics. Beyond linezolid (LZD, 30 μg) which have started clinic using also in our country recently and used alternatively as an antimicrobial agent against glikopeptits in M-R strains, it was determinated that MRSA strains used in this study were resistant against this antibiotic. Even though it was detected that there was no resistance against vancomycin (VA, 30 μg) for MRSA infection in many studies, the sensitivity of vancomycin (VA, 30 μg) decreased significantly against MRSA strains in our study. Table 2 shows the results of antibiotic susceptibility.

5.2. Determination of DNase activity

Acording to the DNase tests, three of strains are DNase negative, the rest of 26 strains are DNase positive. Strains were 11.54% DNase negative and 88.46% DNase positive. Table 2 shows the results of DNase activity (Also, see figure 3).

5.3. SDS-PAGE

With regard to SDS PAGE analyzes whole cell proteins (WCPs) of MRSA strains showed the similar protein profile bands. Figure 4 and 5 show the band profiles obtained from WCPs (Also, see figure 4).

Code of	Antibiotics														Dnaz
Strains	VA 30	TE 30	E 15	DA 2	RA 5	LZD 30	FOX 30	SXT 25	P 10	AK 30	CXM 30	NV 5	AM 10	CN 10	Activity
MRSA1	R	R	R	R	R	R	R	R	R	R	R	R	R	R	Positive
MRSA2	R	R	R	R	R	R	R	R	R	R	R	R	R	R	Positive
MRSA3	R	R	R	R	R	R	R	R	R	R	R	R	R	R	Positive
MRSA4	R	R	R	R	R	R	R	R	R	R	R	R	R	R	Positive
MRSA5	R	R	R	R	R	R	R	R	R	R	R	R	R	R	Positive
MRSA6	R	R	R	R	R	R	R	R	R	R	R	R	R	R	Positive
MRSA7	R	R	R	R	R	R	R	R	R	R	R	R	R	R	Positive
MRSA8	R	R	R	R	R	R	R	R	R	R	R	R	R	R	Positive
MRSA9	R	R	R	R	R	R	R	R	R	R	R	R	R	R	Positive
MRSA10	R	R	R	R	R	R	R	R	R	R	R	R	R	R	Positive
MRSA11	R	R	R	R	R	R	R	R	R	R	R	R	R	R	Negative
MRSA12	R	R	R	R	R	R	R	R	R	R	R	R	R	R	Positive
MRSA13	R	R	R	R	R	R	R	R	R	R	R	R	R	R	Positive
MRSA14	R	R	R	R	R	R	R	R	R	R	R	R	R	R	Positive
MRSA15	R	R	R	R	R	R	R	R	R	R	R	R	R	R	Negative
MRSA16	R	R	R	R	R	R	R	R	R	R	R	R	R	R	Positive
MRSA17	R	R	R	R	R	R	R	R	R	R	R	R	R	R	Positive
MRSA18	R	R	R	R		R	R	MS	R	R	R	R	R	R	Negative
MRSA19	R	R	R	R	R	R	R	R	R	R	R	R	R	R	Positive
MRSA20	R	R	R	R	R	R	R	R	R	R	R	R	R	R	Positive
MRSA21	R	R	R	R	R	R	R	R	R	R	R	R	R	R	Positive
MRSA22	R	R	R	R	R	R	R	R	R	R	R	R	R	R	Positive
MRSA23	R	R	R	R	R	R	R	R	R	R	R	R	R	R	Positive
MRSA24	R	R	R	R	R	R	R	R	R	R	R	R	R	R	Positive
MRSA25	R	R	R	R	R	R	R	R	R	R	R	R	R	R	Positive
MRSA26	R	R	R	R	R	R	R	R	R	R	R	R	R	R	Positive

R; Resistant, MS; Medium Sensetive, S; Sensetive (No sensetive strains in our study)

Table 2. Antibiotics susceptibility and DNase activity of MRSA strains

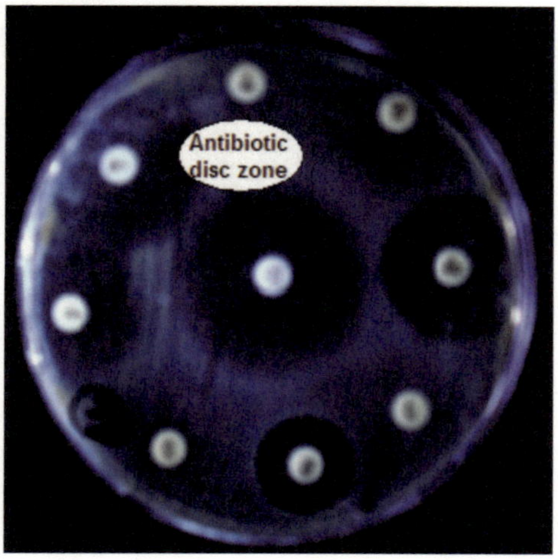

Figure 2. MRSA-24 antibiotic inhibition zones

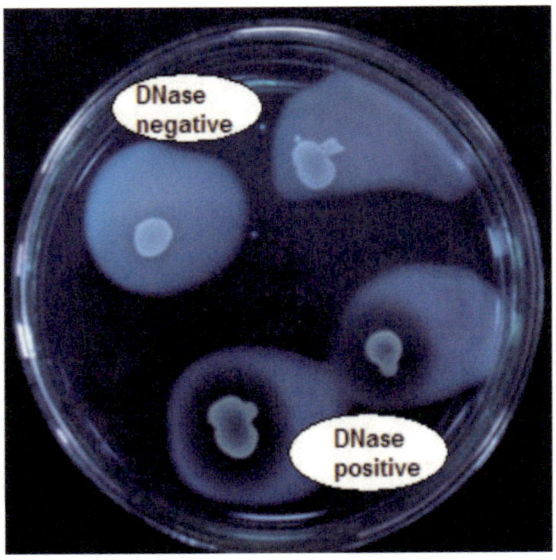

Figure 3. DNase activity test

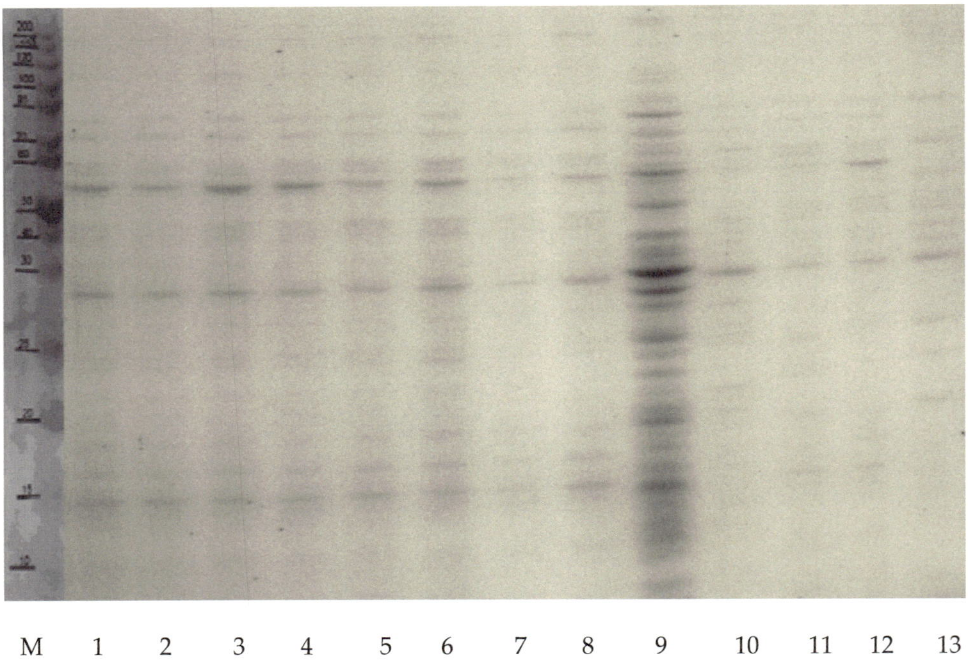

Figure 4. Whole cell protein profiles of MRSA strains by SDS-PAGE. Line 1-13: MRSA strains from ICU; Line M: Molecular weight standard in kD.

http://dx.doi.org/10.5772/55457

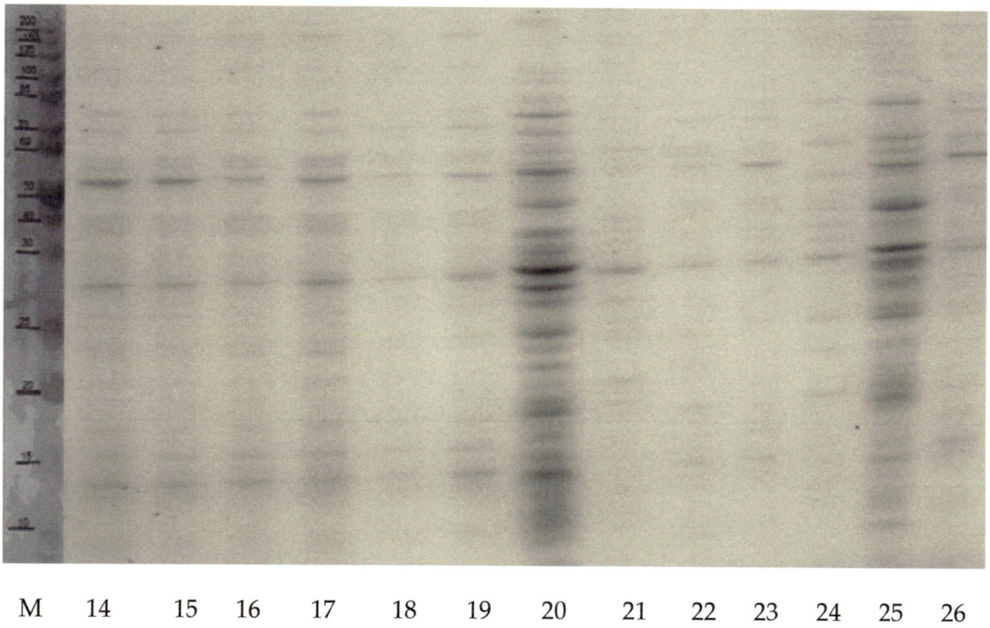

Figure 5. Whole cell protein profiles of MRSA strains by SDS-PAGE. Line 14-26: MRSA strains from ICU; Line M: Molecular weight standard in kD.

6. Discussion

Most of methods have been applied to determinate the MRSA strains. In the present study, SDS- PAGE was used for typing MRSA strains obtained from the various wards of patients in ICU. By SDS-PAGE (WCPs), all of the 26 MRSA strains, of which 11 from tracheal aspirat, 8 from blood, 2 from urine, 2 from wounds, 2 from catheter tip and the other one from effluxion were compared proteins profiles each other. Results of this study in MRSA strains by SDS-PAGE and previous studies obviusly indicate that valuable epidemiological informations can be demonstrated with electrophoretic methods. It is reported that WCPs can not be used because of the high similarities between their band patterns examined in the differentiation of MRSA strains [37]. In order to overcome this problem, it is necessary to make SDS-PAGE with the use of FPs and by N-PAGE using WCPs. Also this problem can dissolve when 5-7.5 % gel concentration uses in SDS-PAGE as opposed to 10% gel concentration [37]. İn this study we applied only SDS-PAGE with use WCPs because of inadequate time of study term.

By using various antibiotic discs, in study of antibiotic susceptibility, generally all of the MRSA strains showed multiple drug resistance. The high level morbidity and mortality of MRSA infections has caused to trace the prevalence of multiple antibiotic resistant staphylococci mainly on the brink of MRSA. In Turkey between 1996-1999, the average of resistant against methicillin was detected 47,5 %. Vancomicin being glycopeptit antibiotic is very important because of methicillin resistant in staphylococcus's. Until now the resistance of glycopeptit was no informed in many studies which have done in our country [9,38]. In our study, we investigated that none of MRSA strains wree resistance against Vancomycin. Susceptibilities of antibiotic groups such as fucidic acid, sulfamethoxazole / trimethoprim, clindamycin, erithromycin, and quinolone have come into prominence because of alternativ treatment options of those antibiotics without glycopeptit antibiotics in patients having light and middle infections of MRSA and remediabled on erect pozition. SXT is an other antibiotic not to be β-lactam which uses in resistant staphilococcus's. Even though, susceptibility of SXT for MRSA strains was 81% in our study, it was 91% in study of Sengoz [19]. Also we found that rate of resistant strains for eritromycin antibiotic was 73%. In one study done in laboratory of clinic microbiology, Haydar Paşa Hospital, this rate for eritromycin was found 71%. In general it was considered that eritromycin antibiotic is not to be alternativ antibiotic option for treatment in MRSA's. Clindamycin is an alternativ antibiotic which can use in infections of staphylococcus. We found that resistant of clindamycin to MRSA strain was 23% in present study. A few studies which had been done in Turkey ; in study of Gonluugur resistant of clindamycin was 39%, in study of Dogan it was 54% [10,39].Linezolid is the first member of antibiotics which are from oksazolidinon group. Linezolids do not show the cross resistant with other antibiotics due to different effect mechanism of those antibiotics. Also, to resistant evolve is power against in vitro linezolid. Resistant evolving occurs typicaly with single nucleotid chancing in genes which encode the 23 S rRNA. In present study, susceptibility of linezolid was found 100%. It was found that linezolid antibiotic was effectiv and safe in 70% of facts with *S.aureus* infection which is not respondet or tolerant [40]. Unfortunately in our country, there is limeted number of study associated with Linezolid. This rate of resistant was 92% against gentamicin in our study.

In this study, we investigated antibiotic susceptibilities, DNase activity and protein profiles by SDS-PAGE of MRSA strains. It was determinate that MRSA strains were resistant against all of antibiotics. A significant decrease in Vancomicin susceptibility is particularly notable. Moreover, the strains were 11.54% DNase negative and 88.46% DNase positive. Also strains showed similarities of band pattern for protein profiles by SDS-PAGE. Studies of Sacilik et al. (1999) and Van Belkum et al. (1997) [41] supported that dissemination of MRSA strains in Turkish hospitals probably originated from the same clone. In order to demostrate such informations and to understand clearly, it is nessesary to make more molecular genetic analyzes and studies in many zones of Turkey.

Acknowledgements

We acknowledge Nilüfer AYDINLIK for her valuable assistance. We are also grateful personel of Denizli Hospital for MRSA samples.

Author details

Göksel Doğan*, Gülümser Acar Doğanlı, Yasemin Gürsoy and Nazime Mercan Doğan

*Address all correspondence to: gksldogan@hotmail.com

Pamukkale University, Faculty of Arts and Sciences , Department of Biology, Denizli, Turkey

References

[1] Goss, C.H., Muhlebach, M.S., 2011. *Staphylococcus aureus* and MRSA in cystic fibrosis. Journal of Cystic Fibrosis 10; 298–306

[2] Azaez Akande, O., 2010. Global trend of methicillin-resistant *Staphlococcus aureus* and emergingchallenges for control. Afr. J. Cln. Exper. Microbiol 11(3): 150-158.

[3] Rello, J., Diaz, E. 2003. Pneumonia in the intensive care unit. Crt. Care Med.; 31: 2544 - 2551.

[4] Graffunder. E.M., Venezia, R.A., 2002.Risk factors associated with nosocomial methicillin resistant *Staphylococcus aureus* (MRSA) infection including previous use of antimicrobials. J. Antimicrob. Chemother.; 49:999 - 1005.

[5] Gottileb, G.S., Fowler, V.G. Jr., Kong, L.K. et al. 2000. *Staphylococcus aureus* bacteremia in the surgical patients: a prospective analysis of 73 postoperrative patients who developed *Staphylococcus aureus* bacteremia at a tertiary care facility. J. Am. Coll. Surg.; 190:50 - 57.

[6] Mylotte, J.M., Tayara, A. 2000. *Staphylococcus aureus* bacteremia: predictors of 30 - day mortality in a large cohort. Clin. Infect. Dis.; 31: 1170 - 1174.

[7] Watkins, R.R., David, M.Z., Salata, R.A., 2012. Current concepts on the virulence mechanisms of meticillin-resistant *Staphylococcus aureus*. Journal of Medical Microbiology Papers in Press. Published June 28, 2012 as doi:10.1099/jmm.0.043513-0.

[8] Chang, S., Sievert, D.M., Hageman, J.C., 2003. Infection with vancomycin-resistant *Staphylococcus aureus* containing the vanA resistance gene. *N Engl J Med,*; 348:1342–1347

[9] Chang, F.Y., MacDonald, B.B., Peacock, J.E., Jr, 2003. A prospective multicenter study of *Staphylococcus aureus* bacteremia: incidence of endocarditis, risk factors for mortality, and clinical impact of methicillin resistance. *Medicine* ; 82:322–332.

[10] Cosgrove, S.E., Qi Y, Kaye K.S., 2005. The impact of methicillin resistance in *Staphylococcus aureus* bacteremia on patient outcomes: mortality, length of stay, and hospital charges. *Infect Control Hosp Epidemiol*; 26:166–174.

[11] Chambers, H.F., 1988. Methicillin-resistant staphylococci. Clin Microbiol Rev; 1:173-86.

[12] Moran, GJ., Amii, R.N., Abrahamian, F.M., Talan, D.A 2005. Methicillin resistant *Staphylococcus aureus* in community - acquired skin infections. Emerg. Infect. Dis; 11 (11): 928 - 930.

[13] Chambers, H.F., 1997. Methicillin resistance in staphylococci: molecular and biochemical basis and clinical implications. American society for clinical microbiology. 4; 781-91.

[14] http://sci.kufauniv.com/teaching/hazim/bacteria/strept.doc.

[15] Koneman, E.W., Allen, S.D., William, M.J., Schereckenberger, P.C., Winn, W.C., 2006. Gram-positive cocci, Part I: Staphylococci and related gram-positive cocci. Winn WC Jr et al (editors). Color atlas and textbook of diagnostic microbiology, 6th ed. Lippincott Williams and Wilkins; 623–71.

[16] Jorgensen, J.H., 1997. Laboratory issues in the detection and reporting of antibacterial resistance. Infect Dis Clin North Am; 11:785-802.

[17] Hartman, B.J., Tomasz, A., 1986. Expression of methicillin resistance in heterogeneous strains of *Staphylococcus aureus*. Antimicrob Agents and Chemother; 29:85-92.

[18] Kuwahara-Arai, K., Kondo, N., Hori, S., Tateda-suzuki, E., Hiramatsu, K,. 1996. Suppression of methicillin resistance in a *mec*A containing pre-methicilin-resistant *Staphylococcus aureus* strain is caused by the *mecI* mediated repression of PBP 2′ production. Antimicrob Agents Chemother; 40:2680-5.

[19] Gulay, Z., 1999. Gülay Z. Antimikrobiyal ilaçlara direnç. Mutlu G, İmir T, Cengiz T, Ustaçelebi Ş, Tümbay E, Mete Ö (eds). Temel ve Klinik Mikrobiyoloji. Ankara: Güneş Kitabevi, 1999:91-108.

[20] Maranan, M.C., Moreira, B., Boyle-Vavra, S., Daum, R.S., 1997. Antimicrobial resistance in staphylococci. Infect Dis Clin North Am; 11:813-49.

[21] Hackbarth, C.J., Chambers, H.F., 1993. *blaI* and *blaR1* regulate β-lactamase and PBP 2a production in methicillin resistant *Staphylococcus aureus*. Antimicrob Agents Chemother; 37:1144-9.

[22] Brooks, G.F., Carroll, K.C., Butel, J.S., Morse, S., 2007. The Staphylococci. In: Jawetz, Melnick and Adelberg's medical microbiology. 24th ed. New York; McGraw-Hill.

[23] Bronner, S., Monteil, H., Prévost. G,. 2004. Regulation of virulence determinants in *Staphylococcus aureus*: Complexity and applications. FEMS Microbiol Rev; 28:183.

[24] Mulligan, M.E., Murray-Leisure, K.A., Standiford, H.C., 1993. Methicillin- resistant *Staphylococcus aureus*: a consessus review of the microbiology, pathogenesis and epidemiology with implications for prevention and management. Am J Med; 94:313-28.

[25] Thorsherry, C., 1984. Methicillin-resistant (heteroresistant) Staphylococci Antimicrobic Newsletter 1; 6.

[26] Franklin, D.L., 1998. *Staphylococcus aureus* infections. *N EnglJ Med,*; 339:520-32.

[27] Novick RP, Schelievert P, Ruzin A. 2001. Pathogenicity and resistance islands of staphylococci. Microbes and Infect;3:585.

[28] Boye, K., Bartels, M.D., Andersen, I.S., Møller, J.A., Westh, H.,2007. A new multiplex PCR for easy screening of methicillin-resistant*Staphylococcus aureus* SCC*mec* types I–V. Clinical Microbiology and Infection Volume 13, Issue 7, pages 725–727.

[29] Donnio, P.Y., Preney, L., Gautier-Lerestif, A.L., Avril, J.L., Lafforgue, N., 2004. Changes in staphylococcal cassette chromosome type and antibiotic resistance profile in methicillin-resistant *Staphylococcus aureus* isolates from a French hospital over an 11 year period. Journal of Antimicrobial Chemotherapy (2004) 53, 808–813.

[30] Klevens, R.M. et al., 2007. Invasive methicillin-resistant *Staphylococcus aureus* infections in the United States, J. Am. Med. Assoc. 298, 1763–1771.

[31] Kirca, Catar, F., 2008. *Staphylococcus aureus* suslarinda metisilin direnci tanisinda kullanilan bazi fenotipik yöntemlerin karsilastirilmasi. Uzmanlık Tezi, Gazi Universitesi, Tip Fakultesi, Tibbi Mikrobiyoloji Anabilim Dali, Ankara, Turkiye.

[32] Murray, P.R., Rosenthal, K.S., Kobayashi, G.S., Pfaller M.A., 2002. *Staphylococcus* and related organisms. Mosby Inc. St. Louis: 202-216.

[33] www.havasteril.com/images/xx/uygulamalar.htm

[34] Laemmli, U.K., 1970. Cleavage of structural proteins during the assembly of head of bacteriophage T4. Nature (London), 227: 680-85.

[35] National Committee for Clinical Laboratory Standards, 2000a. Methods for dilution antimicrobial susceptibility test for bacteria that grow aerobically, 5th ed. Approved standard M7–A5. National Committee for Clinical Laboratory Standards, Wayne, Pa.

[36] National Committee for Clinical Laboratory Standards, 2000b. Performance standard for antimicrobial susceptibility testing. Document M100–S10. National Committee for Clinical Laboratory Standards, Wayne, Pa.

[37] Sacilik, S.C., Osmanoglu, O., Palbiyikoglu, U., Bengisun, J.S., Cokmus, C., 2000. Analysis of Methicillin Resistant *Staphylococcus aureus* Isolates by Polyacrylamide Gel Electrophoresis in an Intensive Care Unit of Ibni-Sina Hospital. Turk J Med Sci. 30 367-371.

[38] Pa, W., 1997. National Committee for Clinical Laboratory Standarts. Performance standarts for antimicrobial disc susceptibility tests. Approved standart M2-A5, National Committee for Clinical Laboratory Standarts, 1997.

[39] Ridenour GA, Wong ES, Call MA, 2006. Duration of colonization with methicillin resistant*Staphylococcus aureus* among patients in the intensive care unit: implications for intervention. *Infect Control Hosp Epidemiol,*; 27:271–278.

[40] Doganay M., 1998. Nozokomiyal sepsis: önemi ve tanımlar, Hastane İnfeksiyon Dergisi; 2(4):179-81.

[41] Van Belkum, A., Van Leeuwen, W., Werkooyen R., Sacilik, S.C., Cokmus, C., Verbrugh H., 1997. Dissemination of a single clone of methicillin-resistant *Staphylococcus aureus* among Turkish hospitals. J Clin Microbiol, 35: 978-81,

Chapter 16

Plant Responses at Different Ploidy Levels

Mustafa Yildiz

Additional information is available at the end of the chapter

http://dx.doi.org/10.5772/55785

1. Introduction

The term "ploidy" expresses the number of sets of chromosomes in a biological cell and marked by an "X". A diploid genotype carries two paired (homologous) sets of chromosomes in the nucleus of each cell, one from each parent (Figure 1a). "Polyploidy" is the multiplication of entire sets of chromosomes. In other words, polyploid genotype has more than two homologous sets of chromosomes in its cell. For example, tetraploid plants have four sets of chromosomes in their cells (Figure 1b). Polyploidy is common among flowering plants (angiosperms) and is a major force in plant speciation [1]. Almost 47%-70% of angiosperms are polyploid [1-3].

There are differences between diploid and polyploid plants from morphological, physiological, cellular and biochemical aspects. Polyploid plants have bigger cells and stomatas than diploid ones that result in thicker and big leaves, larger flowers and fruits. In general, autotetraploids have greater vegetative volume and larger seed weight but lower reproductive fertility than diploids, and flowering and fruit formation were often later in tetraploids than in diploids as reported by Stebbins [4]. Shoots of polyploid genotypes are thicker with short internodes and wider crotch angles. As the chromosome number increased, DNA content per cell, enzyme activity per cell and cell volume all increased [5, 6]. In addition, polyploids are used as sources of variability and new genotypes for plant improvement [7, 8].

Polyploid genotypes have shown resistance to biotic (pests and pathogens) and abiotic (drought and cold etc.) stress factors in some cases and this resistance enables them to have greater adaptability to wider ecological regions. This could be attributed to higher chromosome number and gene expression causing to increase in the concentration of particular secondary metabolites and chemicals that are responsible for defense mechanism. This increase in the concentration of particular secondary metabolites and chemicals enable polyploid genotypes to resist against biotic and abiotic stress factors, consequently to grow in the wide range of environments.

However, the effects of increased ploidy level cannot be anticipated all the time. In contrast to common knowledge that polyploid individuals are superior than the diploid ones from many aspects, in some cases polyploid plants can have slower growth rates [9] which could be attributed to difficulties in the cell cycle and slow cell division [10] causing to fewer cell number and smaller organs. For example, it was reported that the overall chlorophyll content in polyploid plants are higher than diploid ones with lower chromosome numbers [5, 6, 11], while chlorophyll a, chlorophyll b and total chlorophyll contents of tetraploid sugar beet genotypes ('AD 440' and 'CBM 315') in our study were found to be lower than diploid ones ('Agnessa' and 'Felicita') [12].

Although there are studies reporting that seeds of tetraploid plants germinated faster with a higher percentage than those of diploids [13], in the study we conducted under greenhouse conditions, it was observed that germination and seedling growth of diploid sugar beet genotypes were much better than tetraploids. Our findings were parallel to the ones reporting that polyploid seeds might show lower germination and emergence percentage than diploids and this could be attributed to thicker seedcoat and weak seedling emergence [14] and weak embryo development [15].

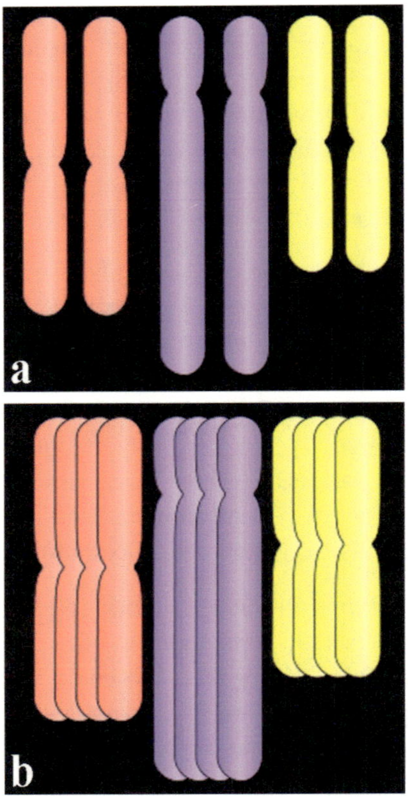

Figure 1. Diagram for cells at different ploidy levels. (a) Diploid (indicated by 2n = 2X) cell having two homologous copies of each chromosome, (b) Tetraploid (indicated by 2n = 4X) cell having four homologous copies of each chromosome

2. Growth pattern of genotypes at different ploidy levels

In a study conducted in sugar beet which is an important sucrose-producing crop worldwide in temperate regions and supplies about 20% of the world sugar consumption, two diploid ('Agnessa' and 'Felicita') and two tetraploid ('AD 440' and 'CBM 315') sugar beet genotypes were compared with respect to vegetative and generative characteristics such as seed germination, seedling growth, total chlorophyll and protein contents, root and sugar yields, and sugar content [12]. The size of epidermal cells in a field of view area on upper leaf surface of sterile seedlings were counted using clear fingernail polish, clear tape, a glass slide, and a microscope at 60X magnification. From these counts, the highest results regarding cell size were recorded in tetraploid genotypes (Table 1, Figure 2). Decreased cell number in polyploid genotypes was compensated for by increased cell size as reported by Doonan [16] and, Inze and De Veylder [17].

Genotypes	Cell Number	Cell Length (μm)	Cell Width (μm)	Approx. Cell Area (μm^2)
'Agnessa' (2X)	167.65 a	86.52 b	31.24 b	2702.88 b
'Felicita' (2X)	152.80 a	82.14 b	33.16 b	2723.76 b
'AD 440' (4X)	78.60 b	131.62 a	48.42 a	6373.04 a
'CBM 315' (4X)	72.40 b	128.24 a	52.16 a	6688.99 a

Values followed by the different letters in a column are significantly different at the 0.01 level

Table 1. Cell sizes in the upper leaf surface of 6-week-old sugar beet plants at different ploidy levels

Diploid genotypes gave higher results than tetraploids in seed germination percentage, root length and seedling height at 4th day and root length and seedling height at 14th day (Table 2). Polyploid seeds had lower germination and emergence percentages than diploid ones due to their thicker seedcoat and seedling emergence strength [14, 15].

In the first 6 weeks, diploid genotypes gave rise to the highest results with respect to plant height, root lenght, leaf length and width, approx. leaf area, plant fresh and dry weights, total chlorophyll content and protein percentage (Figure 3, Table 3). However, they were passed by tetraploid genotypes in the further stages of the development in the characters of plant height, root lenght, leaf length and width, approx. leaf area, plant fresh and dry weights (Figure 4, Table 4). These figures showed that tetraploid genotypes passed diploids vegetatively in the further developmental stages.

Plants developed from diploid seeds were more vital and well-grown. Plant height and root length scores in diploid genotypes were good indicators for vitality and growth. Leaf area which plays an important role on the photosynthetic acticity, was found higher in diploid genotypes in the first 6 weeks. High ploidy level does not result in increased shoot growth every time [18].

It was reported that the fresh weight increase was mainly due to cell enlargement by water absorption [19] and increase in dry weight was closely related to cell division and new material synthesis [20]. Dry weight increase in diploids was due to an increase in photosynthetic activity and carbohydrate metabolism resulting from increased water uptake by longer roots. Reduced fresh weight in tetraploids could be attributed to decreased water absorption as reported by Prado et al. [21]. Sullivan and Phafter [22] reported that seedling growth was affected by genotypic differences more than ploidy in diploid and autotetraploid *Secale cereale*. Lower results in morphological characters in the first developmental stages of tetraploid genotypes could be attributed to slow cell division as reported by Comai [10].

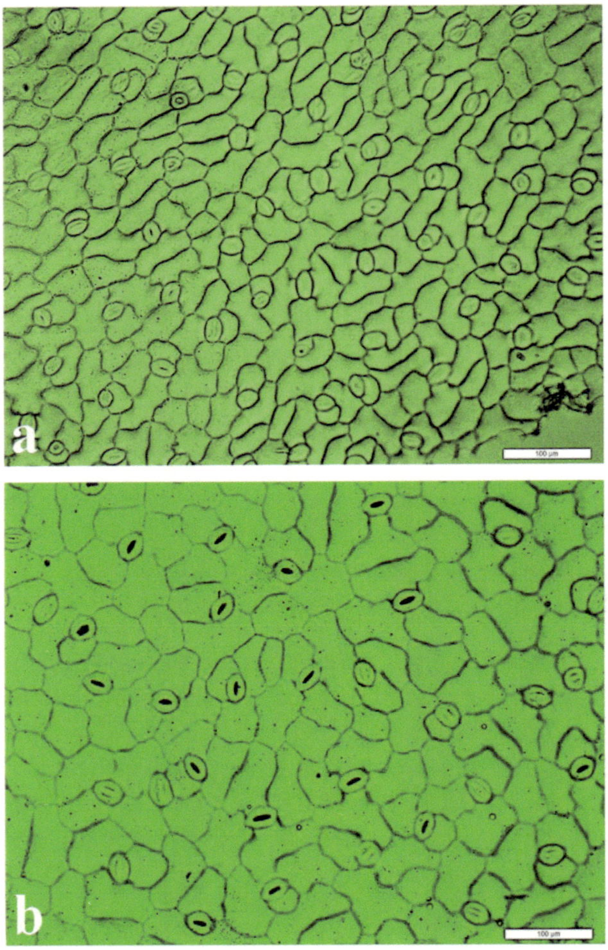

Figure 2. Cells and stomatas from the upper leaf surface of 6-week-old sugar beet seedlings. (a) Diploid genotype 'Felicita' and (b) Tetraploid genotype 'AD 440'

Genotypes	DAY 4			DAY 14	
	Germination (%)	Root Length (cm)	Seedling Height (cm)	Root Length (cm)	Seedling Height (cm)
'Agnessa' (2X)	75.10 a	7.40 a	6.34 a	12.67 a	9.05 a
'Felicita' (2X)	89.10 a	8.45 a	7.00 a	13.96 a	9.52 a
'AD 440' (4X)	60.10 b	5.05 b	5.74 a	7.50 b	6.21 b
'CBM 315' (4X)	60.10 b	5.86 b	5.49 a	7.52 b	7.38 b

Values followed by the different letters in a column are significantly different at the 0.01 level

Table 2. Germination and seedling growth in diploid and tetraploid sugar beet genotypes

Chlorophyll content which is accepted as an indicator of photosynthetic capacity of tissues [23-25], was again found higher in diploid plants. It was thought that this could be due to the fact that photosynthetic capacity of the tissue in diploids was higher because of higher chlorophyll content, water and nutrient uptake from the soil with their roots. Higher photosynthetic capacity resulted in higher protein content in diploids. The number of phosynthetic cells per unit leaf area decreases with increasing ploidy level [26]. Although chloroplasts [27, 28] and chlorophyll content [5] are higher in polyploid genotypes, increase tendency of chlorophyll content by increasing ploidy level is not always apparent. For instance, chlorophyll content remained constant in different ploidy levels of *Atriplex confertifolia* [26].

Polyploid plants may show high-ploidy syndrome that could be explained by costly cell cycle and slow cell division at higher ploidy levels. That means in some cases, diploid genotypes can show superior characteristics than tetraploid ones.

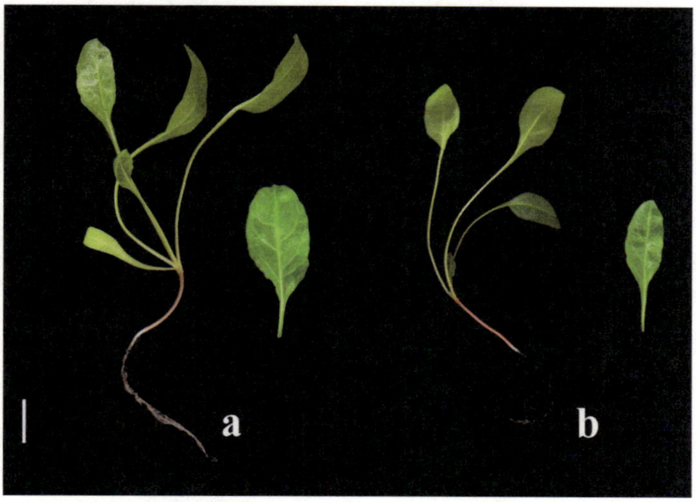

Figure 3. Development of seedlings from seeds of (a) diploid ('Felicita') and (b) tetraploid ('AD 440') genotypes 6 weeks after study initiation (Bar = 3 cm)

Genotypes	Vegetative Characters							Generative Characters	
	Plant Height (cm)	Root Length (cm)	Leaf Length (cm)	Leaf Width (cm)	Approx. Leaf Area (cm²)	Plant Fresh Weight (g)	Plant Dry Weight (g)	Total Chlorophyll Content (μg/g fresh tissue)	Protein (%)
'Agnessa' (2X)	18.53 a	21.40 a	5.13 a	3.04 a	16.51 a	11.81 a	2.50 a	894.07 b	18.45 a
'Felicita' (2X)	19.47 a	19.34 a	5.75 a	3.14 a	18.06 a	9.10 a	2.78 a	1035.47 a	21.07 a
Mean	19.00	20.37	5.44	3.09	17.28	10.45	2.64	964.77	19.76
'AD 440' (4X)	15.01 b	13.46 b	5.00 a	2.34 b	11.70 b	6.19 b	1.18 b	815.99 b	6.33 b
'CBM 315' (4X)	15.14 b	14.95 b	4.96 a	2.49 b	12.35 b	4.69 b	0.94 b	679.82 c	2.90 b
Mean	15.07	14.20	4.98	2.41	12.02	5.44	1.06	747.90	4.61

Values followed by the different letters in a column are significantly different at the 0.01 level

Table 3. Development of seedlings from seeds of diploid and tetraploid genotypes 6 weeks after study initiation

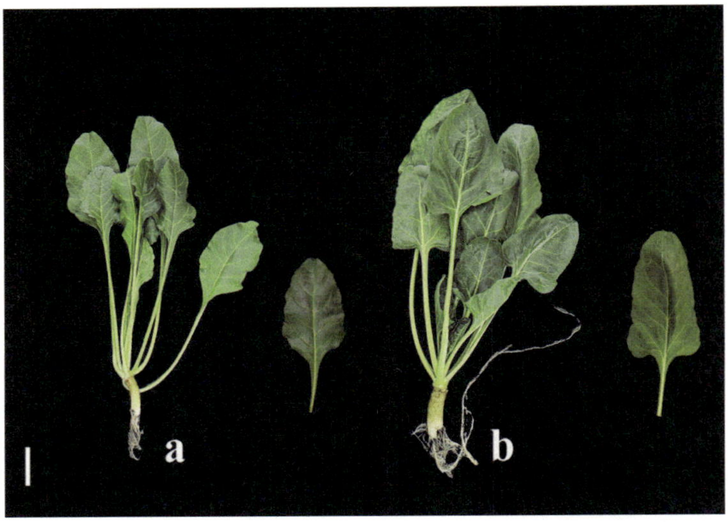

Figure 4. Development of seedlings from seeds of (a) diploid ('Felicita') and (b) tetraploid ('AD 440') genotypes 10 weeks after study initiation (Bar = 5 cm)

In general, tetraploids have higher vegetative growth but lower reproductive fertility than diploids. Thus, in our study, tetraploid genotypes passed diploid ones 10 weeks after study initiation regarding vegetative characters such as plant height, root length, leaf length and width, approximate leaf area, plant fresh and dry weights [12]. Data related to generative characters such as total chlorophyll content and protein percentage were the highest in diploid

http://dx.doi.org/10.5772/55785

genotyes (Table 4). Root and sugar yields, and sugar content obtained from field trials 6 months after study initiation were again found the highest in diploids (Table 5). Polyploids flower and fruit later than diploids as reported by Stebbins [4].

Genotypes	Vegetative Characters							Generative Characters	
	Plant Height (cm)	Root Length (cm)	Leaf Length (cm)	Leaf Width (cm)	Approx. Leaf Area (cm²)	Plant Fresh Weight (g)	Plant Dry Weight (g)	Total Chlorophyll Content (µg/g fresh tissue)	Protein (%)
'Agnessa' (2X)	20.5 b	29.0 b	13.4 b	7.3 b	97.8 b	286.6 b	42.9 b	1571.5 a	20.46 a
'Felicita' (2X)	27.3 b	33.8 b	14.9 b	6.9 b	102.8 b	306.1 b	51.6 b	1533.8 a	21.77 a
Mean	23.90	31.40	14.15	7.10	100.30	296.35	47.25	1552.65	21.11
'AD 440' (4X)	37.0 a	42.9 a	18.7 a	9.7 a	181.4 a	357.1 a	77.3 a	1210.6 b	16.10 b
'CBM 315' (4X)	33.0 a	44.8 a	18.1 a	8.8 a	159.3 a	381.1 a	77.6 a	1276.5 b	17.39 b
Mean	35.00	43.85	18.40	9.25	170.35	369.10	77.45	1243.55	16.74

Values followed by the different letters in a column are significantly different at the 0.01 level

Table 4. Development of seedlings from seeds of diploid and tetraploid genotypes 10 weeks after study initiation

Genotypes	Root Yield (tones/ha)	Sugar Content (%)	Sugar Yield (tones/ha)
'Agnessa' (2X)	74.46 a	14.88 a	11.08 a
'Felicita' (2X)	68.48 a	16.21 a	11.10 a
'AD 440' (4X)	54.40 b	12.85 b	6.99 b
'CBM 315' (4X)	58.66 b	12.07 b	7.08 b

Values followed by the different letters in a column are significantly different at the 0.01 level

Table 5. Sugar content, root and sugar yields in diploid and tetraploid genotypes

3. Regeneration capacity of genotypes at different ploidy levels under *In vitro* conditions

Genetic variation is a prerequisite for successful plant breeding. *In vitro* culture techniques seem to offer certain advantages in this respect through somatic hybridization, induction of mutants and selection of disease free and disease resistant plants [29].

In a study conducted in sugar beet, it was aimed to examine the effect of the ploidy level on *in vitro* explant growth, adventitious shoot regeneration, rooting and plantlet establishment from petiole segments of two inbred lines ('ELK 345' - diploid and 'CBM 315' - tetraploid) [30]. Petioles were used as explant and 1 mg l^{-1} BAP and 0.2 mg l^{-1} NAA as the combination of growth regulators for shoot regeneration in accordance with studies reporting that the most responsive explant for *in vitro* culture of sugar beet was petiole [31-37] and the combination of the plant growth regulators was 1 mg l^{-1} BAP and 0.2 mg l^{-1} NAA [37]. The results clearly showed that there were sharp and statistically significant differences in all parameters examined between lines at different ploidy levels. The study was set in three parallels to confirm the accuracy of the study.

The tetraploid line 'CBM 315' had a higher fresh weight than the diploid line 'ELK 345' in all three experiments (Table 6). In all experiments, the differences in fresh weight between the diploid and the tetraploid lines were statistically significant ($p < 0.05$). Dry weight scores were again found to be higher in the tetraploid line, and the differences between these lines were statistically significant at 0.01 level in all experiments (Table 6). The highest mean of fresh and dry weights of petiole explants was recorded from the tetraploid line as 0.254 g and 0.023 g. In the diploid line, the mean fresh and dry weights of petioles were noted as 0.172 g and 0.012 g (Table 6). The difference between fresh and dry weights signifies the tissue water content. From these results, the tissue water content was calculated as 0.231 g (0.254-0.023) in the tetraploid line 'CBM 315', and 0.160 g (0.172-0.012) in the diploid line 'ELK 345'.

The cells with high ploidy levels have bigger vacuoles [38] that play an important role in regulating the osmotic pressure of the cell [39]. Higher osmotic pressure of the cell in polyploid plants, as reported by Tal and Gardi [40], could cause higher tissue metabolic activity by increasing water and hormone uptake from the medium. Cell enlargement by water absorption, cell vacuolation, and turgor-deriven wall expansion is the main reason of fresh weight increase, as reported by Dale [19]. The increase in dry weight was closely related to cell division and new material synthesis [20]. Thus, increase in the fresh and dry weights of petiole explants of the tetraploid line in our study at the end of culture were chiefly due to an increase in the absorption of water and other components from the basal medium via the high cell osmotic pressure. On the contrary, lower osmotic pressure of the diploid line caused a decline in fresh and dry weights of petioles by decreasing the absorption of water and other components from the medium. Results about tissue water content clearly showed that the tetraploid line had higher osmotic pressure, which caused higher absorption of water and other components from the medium. Higher results of all parameters in the study could be attributed to higher cell osmotic pressure of the tetraploid line 'CBM 315'. Yildiz and Ozgen [41] have reported that increasing tissue water content, which caused higher tissue metabolic activity, resulted in higher results of all parameters examined.

The increase in ploidy level leads to a larger cell that has a higher growth rate [38]. Tetraploid genotypes had a higher water content [40] and more organic solutes than diploid genotypes [42]. Warner and Edwards [26] have reported that the chromosome number determines the size of leaves, the size of cells, the number of chloroplasts per cell, and amounts of photosynthetic enzymes and pigments in cell. As the chromosome number increased, DNA content per

		Fresh Weight (g)		Dry Weight (g)		Water Content (%)		Dry Matter Content (%)	
		'ELK 345' 2X	'CBM 315' 4X	'ELK 345' 2X	'CBM 315' 4X	'ELK 345' 2X	'CBM 315' 4X	'ELK 345' 2X	'CBM 315' 4X
1st experiment		0.168±0.009	0.226±0.011	0.012±0.001	0.023±0.002	92.83±0.410	89.76±0.410	7.17±1.147	10.24±1.147
	t value	4.226*		4.621**		2.561*		2.561*	
2nd experiment		0.161±0.091	0.251±0.028	0.012±0.001	0.022±0.002	92.34±0.361	91.34±0.275	7.66±0.361	8.66±0.275
	t value	3.120*		4.542**		2.165ns		2.165ns	
3rd experiment		0.187±0.017	0.284±0.019	0.013±0.0003	0.023±0.001	92.76±0.654	91.77±0.258	7.24±0.654	8.23±0.258
	t value	3.794*		6.708**		1.401ns		1.401ns	
Mean[1]		0.172	0.254	0.012	0.023	92.64	90.96	7.36	9.04

Significantly different from zero at * $p < 0.05$ and ** $p < 0.01$

[1] Mean of three experiments

Table 6. Fresh and dry weights, water and dry matter contents of petiole explants of 'ELK 345' (diploid) and 'CBM 315' (tetraploid) lines 5 weeks after culture initiation on MS medium containing 1 mg l^{-1} BAP and 0.2 mg l^{-1} NAA

cell, enzyme activity per cell, cell volume, and photosynthesis per cell all increased. It was also reported that the photosynthetic capacity of larger cells in polyploid plants are higher than smaller cells with lower chromosome numbers [5, 6, 43].

In all experiments, the highest results were obtained from petiole explants of the tetraploid line in the parameters of shoot regeneration percentage, shoot number per petiole, shoot length, total shoot number per Petri dish, number of shoots rooted, and the percentage of shoots rooted. During culture, petiole explants of the tetraploid line were observed to grow faster than the ones of the diploid line. By the end of the culture, petiole explants of the tetraploid line were bigger and well developed, and the number of shoots regenerated was also higher (Figure 5a-b) than the diploid line (Figure 5c). The differences between petiole explants of the diploid and tetraploid lines for all parameters examined were statistically significant at $p < 0.01$, with the exception of shoot regeneration percentage in all experiments which was different at $p < 0.05$ (Table 7, Table 8) [30].

Shoot primordias on petiole explants appeared in the first week of the culture in the tetraploid line while they developed 16 days after culture initiation in the diploid line. The highest mean shoot regeneration percentage and mean shoot number per petiole was recorded as 69.99% and 20.23 in the tetraploid line while it was 45.57% and 12.61 in the diploid line (Table 7). Regenerated shoot length was again found to be higher in the tetraploid line 5 weeks after culture initiation. The mean shoot length was found as 2.8 cm in the tetraploid line, while it was 2.0 cm in the diploid line. The mean total shoot number per Petri dish, which can be determined by shoot regeneration percentage and shoot number per petiole, was recorded as 141.77 in the tetraploid line and 57.50 in the diploid line (Table 7).

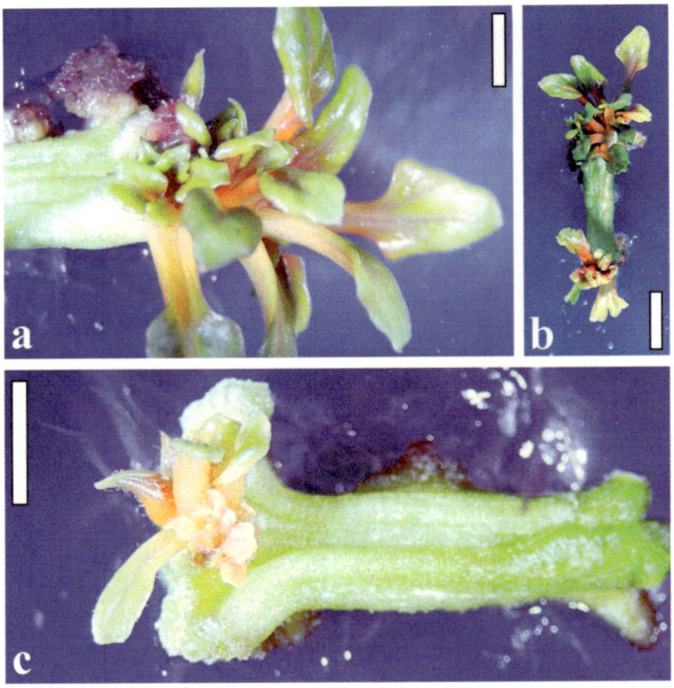

Figure 5. *In vitro* shoot regeneration from petiole explants of (a-b) 'CBM 315' (4X) and (c) 'ELK 345' (2X) line 5 weeks after culture initiation (Bars = 0.5 cm in a and c, 1 cm in b).

Shoots regenerated from petiole explants of the diploid and tetraploid lines were rooted on MS medium containing 3 mg l^{-1} IBA for 2 weeks. The best results were observed in shoots regenerated from petiole explants of the tetraploid line in all three experiments (Table 8). From the results, it is evident that shoots regenerated from petioles of the tetraploid line were more capable of establishing new plantlets than the ones grown from petioles of the diploid line (Figure 6a). Of the 70 shoots transferred to rooting medium, 61.3 shoots (87.62%) from tetraploid line 'CBM 315' and 51.7 shoots (73.81%) from the diploid line 'ELK 345' were rooted successfully (Table 8). Transferred plants reached harvest maturity in the field and no morphological abnormalities were observed.

4. *In vitro* susceptibility of genotypes to *Agrobacterium tumefaciens* infection at different ploidy levels

Agrobacterium-mediated transformation has been widely used for the introduction of foreign genes into plants and consequent regeneration of transgenic plants [44]. *A.tumefaciens* naturally infects the wound sites in dicotyledonous plants. Virulent strains of *A.tumefaciens*, when interacting with susceptible dicotyledonous plant cells, induce diseases known as crown gall

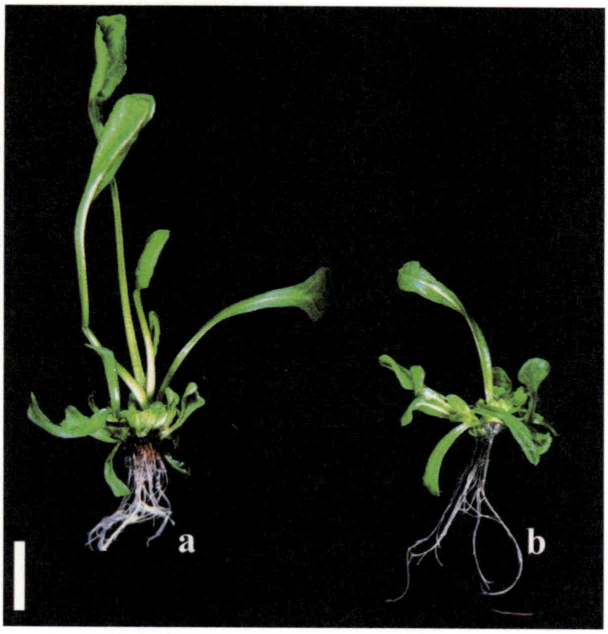

Figure 6. *In vitro* rooting and plantlet development from petiole explants of (a) 'CBM 315' (tetraploid) and (b) 'ELK 345' (diploid) line (Bar = 1.5 cm).

		Shoot Regeneration (%)		Shoot Number per Petiole		Shoot Length (cm)		Total Shoot Number per Petri Dish	
		'ELK 345' 2X	'CBM 315' 4X	'ELK 345' 2X	'CBM 315' 4X	'ELK 345' 2X	'CBM 315' 4X	'ELK 345' 2X	'CBM 315' 4X
1st experiment		40.0±5.773	66.7±3.333	12.53±0.617	22.80±1.106	2.2±0.577	3.2±0.153	50.12±9.181	152.73±14.589
	t value	3.957*		8.105**		6.124**		5.917**	
2nd experiment		46.7±3.333	70.0±5.774	13.70±0.656	19.70±0.929	1.9±0.153	2.7±0.058	63.67±3.844	138.97±12.305
	t value	3.368*		5.276**		3.703**		4.104**	
3rd experiment		50.0±5.774	73.3±3.333	11.60±0.625	18.20±0.557	1.8±0.100	2.5±0.115	58.70±9.650	133.60±8.426
	t value	3.501*		7.889**		4.583**		5.847**	
Mean[1]		45.57	69.99	12.61	20.23	2.0	2.8	57.50	141.77

Significantly different from zero at * $p < 0.05$ and ** $p < 0.01$

[1] Mean of three experiments

Table 7. Adventitious shoot regeneration from petiole explants of 'ELK 345' (diploid) and 'CBM 315' (tetraploid) 5 weeks after culture initiation on MS medium containing 1 mg l^{-1} BAP and 0.2 mg l^{-1} NAA

[45]. This strain contains a large megaplasmid (more than 200 kb), which plays a key role in tumor induction and for this reason it was named Ti (Tumor inducing) plasmid. The expression

		Number of Shoots Rooted		% of Shoots Rooted	
		'ELK 345' 2X	'CBM 315' 4X	'ELK 345' 2X	'CBM 315' 4X
1st experiment		53±1.155	64±1.000	75.71±1.648	91.43±1.430
	t value	7.201**		6.662**	
2nd experiment		52±1.528	59±1.155	74.28±2.181	84.29±1.648
	t value	3.656*		3.709*	
3rd experiment		50±1.528	61±1.399	71.43±2.181	87.14±1.648
	t value	5.745**		5.692**	
Mean[1]		51.7	61.3	73.81	87.62

Significantly different from zero at $^{*}p < 0.05$ and $^{**}p < 0.01$

[1] Mean of three experiments

Table 8. *In vitro* root development of shoots regenerated from petiole explants of 'ELK 345' (2X) and 'CBM 315' (4X) lines on rooting medium enriched with 3 mg l^{-1} IBA 2 weeks after culture initiation.

of T-DNA genes of Ti-plasmid in plant cells causes the formation of tumors at the infection site. Two genetic components of bacteria, virulence genes (*vir*) and chromosomal genes (*chv*), are directly involved in the transfer of T-DNA from *Agrobacterium* to plant cells [44]. The molecular basis of *Agrobacterium*-mediated transformation is the transfer and stable integration of a DNA sequence (T-DNA) from the *Agrobacterium tumefaciens* Ti (tumor-inducing) plasmid into the plant genome leading to plant cell transformation [46, 47].

In a study conducted by Yildiz et al. [48], it was aimed to determine the susceptibility level of two sugar beet lines to wild-type *Agrobacterium tumefaciens* infection and ploidy effect on gene transfer efficiency under *in vitro* conditions. To evaluate the susceptibility of sugar beet lines at different ploidy levels against *Agrobacterium* infection, tumor formation was scored using the virulent strains 'A281' and 'A136NC'.

Among two lines used in the study, 'CBM 315' gave the highest results in three parameters studied in 'A281' wild strain. In 'CBM 315', tumor induction percentage, tumor diameter and number of tumors per explant were scored as 94%, 3.88 mm and 7.78, respectively (Figure 7). 'CBM 315' was followed by 'ELK 345' as 62% in tumor induction percentage, 1.80 mm in tumor diameter and 4.03 in number of tumors per explant (Table 9). In 'A136NC' wild strain, the highest values in tumor induction percentage, tumor diameter and number of tumors per explant were obtained from 'CBM 315' as 96%, 4.24 mm and 8.13 whereas lowest results were recorded from line 'ELK 345' as 73%, 2.14 mm and 4.36, respectively (Table 9).

The virulence of the bacterium depends on the strain and its interaction with the host plant. Various plant species differ greatly in their susceptibility to infection by *Agrobacterium tumefaciens* or *Agrobacterium rhizogenes* [49-53].

Even within a species, different cultivars or ecotypes may show vastly different degrees of susceptibility to tumorigenesis by particular *Agrobacterium* strains [54-56]. These differences have been noted in rice [57], maize [58], various legumes [55], aspen [56], cucurbits [59], *Pinus* species [60], tomato [61], *Arabidopsis* [62], grape [63], and other species. Although some differences in transformation frequency may be attributed to environmental or physiological factors, a genetic basis for susceptibility has clearly been established in a few plant species [62, 64- 66].

Several researchers have reported that susceptibility to *Agrobacterium* transformation of various tissues, organs and cell types within a plant may differ. De Kathen and Jacobsen [67] reported that only dedifferentiating cells near the vascular system of cotyledon and epicotyl sections of *Pisum sativum* were susceptible to *Agrobacterium* transformation. Sangwan et al. [68] showed that only dedifferentiating mesophyll cells were competent for transformation in *Arabidopsis* cotyledon and leaf tissues.

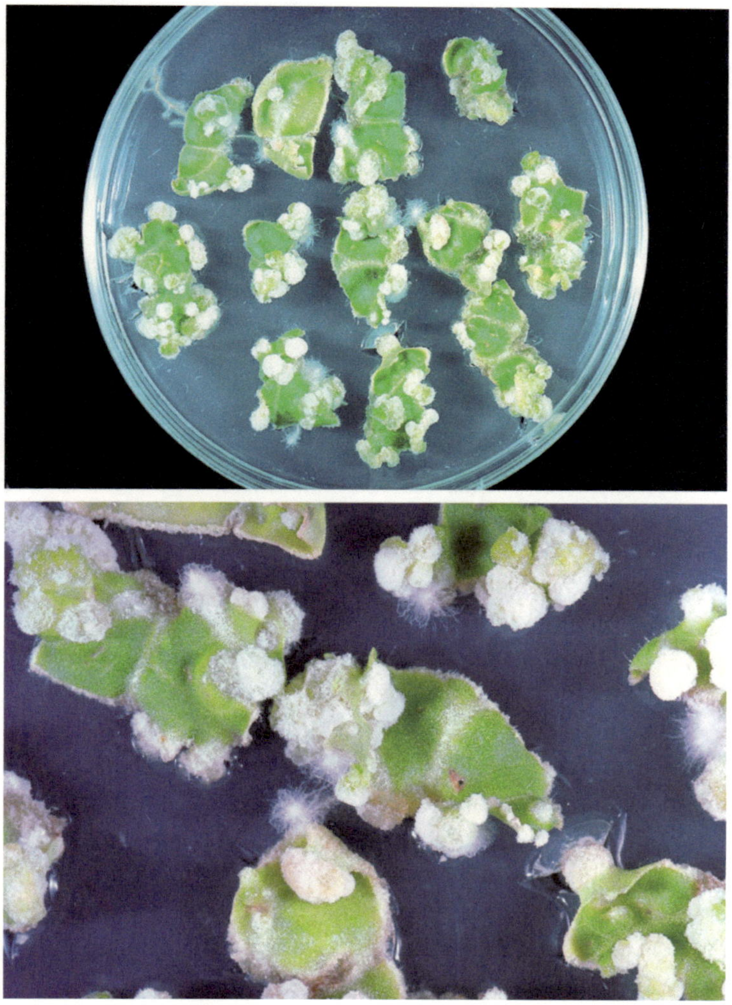

Figure 7. *In vitro* tumor formation caused by 'A281' virulent strain of *Agrobacterium tumefaciens* on leaf-disc explant of tetraploid sugar beet line 'CBM 315'

Genotype	A281			A136NC		
	Tumor Induction (%)	Tumor Diameter (mm)	No of Tumors / Explant	Tumor Induction (%)	Tumor Diameter (mm)	No of Tumors / Explant
'ELK 345' (2X)	62	1.80	4.03	73	2.14	4.36
'CBM 315' (4X)	94	3.88	7.78	96	4.24	8.13
t values	7.849**	5.881**	6.208**	3.994**	8.502**	7.808**

Each value is the mean of 3 replications with 12 explants

** Significantly different at the 0.01 level

Table 9. Response of two sugar beet lines at different ploidy levels to *Agrobacterium tumefaciens* virulent strains 'A281' and 'A136NC' 4 weeks after leaf-disc inoculation

The host-range limitation is perhaps the greatest disadvantage of *Agrobacterium*-mediated transformation although it is the most common used vector for the introduction of foreign genes to many crop plants, especially to dicotyledonous. The results were in accordance with the previous studies indicating strain and genotype differences [69-71].

From the results, it could be concluded that sugar beet lines have susceptibility to *Agrobacterium* infection with different levels. Moreover, if Table 9 was examined carefully, an interesting point came to attention that the difference in tumor induction might be related to ploidy level. Actually, in both strains of *Agrobacterium,* the highest results were obtained from 'CBM 315' which was tetraploid. Analysis showed that 'CBM 315' to be more beneficial for tumor induction and more susceptible to *Agrobacterium tumefaciens.*

It was reported that increased ploidy levels resulted in bigger cell size [72]. As it is known *Agrobacterium* infects cells at wound sites and size of the cells in this sites may influence transformation efficiency. The difference between diploid and tetrapoloid sugar beet lines with respect to wild-type *Agrobacterium tumefaciens* susceptibility might be related to ploidy levels. To our knowledge, this was the first report indicating that gene transfer efficiency might be affected from cell size at wound sites. However, this finding must be verified repeatedly by detealed studies.

5. Plant cellular response to salt stress at different ploidy level

The number of chlorophyll-containing chloroplasts increases from diploids to polyploids. Chlorophyll content and other proteins were shown to almost double from diploid to polyploid plants [40]. The cells with high ploidy level have bigger vacuoles and vacuole plays an important role in regulating osmotic pressure of the cell [38]. Higher cell osmotic pressure in polyploid plants cause to high tissue metabolic activity by increasing water and hormone uptake from the medium. Additionally, the increase in ploidy level leads to larger cell that has high growth rate. Polyploid genotypes have a higher water content and organic solutes than diploid genotypes [42]. Chromosome number determines the size of leaves, the size of cells, the number of chloroplasts per cell and amounts of photosynthetic enzymes and pigments in cell [26]. As chromosome number increased, DNA content per cell, enzyme activity per cell, cell volume and photosynthesis per cell are all increased. In general, photosynthetic capacity of larger cells in polyploid plants is higher than smaller cells with lower chromosome numbers [5, 6, 43].

In a study conducted by Yildiz et al. [73], the responses of sugar beet genotypes at different ploidy levels to salt stress were evaluated. Diploid ('Felicita') and tetraploid ('AD 440') sugar beet genotypes were grown in pots, 1-month-old seedlings were treated with NaCl at different concentrations (0, 50 and 150 mM). Four days after NaCl application, cytological observations (the number of cell and stomata in the field of view area, lengths and widths of cells and stomatas) and 8 days after, seedling and root lengths were recorded.

Root lengths of both genotypes increased by increasing NaCl concentrations. Root length was recorded as 7.25 cm in diploid genotype 'Felicita' at 150 mM NaCl while it was 7.90 cm in tetraploid genotype 'AD 440'. Seedling lengths also increased by increasing NaCl concentration. Seedling length was the highest in diploid genotype as 11.25 cm while it was only 7.90 in tetraploid genotype (Table 10). Damages of increasing NaCl concentration were seen clearly in the leaves of seedlings. At higher NaCl concentrations, tissue necrosis was observed (Figure 8).

It was observed that cell number decreased by increasing NaCl concentration in both genotypes. However, decrease rate in cell number was higher in diploid genotype than tetraploid. This was most probably due to bigger cell size in tetraploid genotype and consequently there was few cells in the unit area. Lower cell number could be attributed to slow cell division as reported by Comai [10]. Cell length and width increased by increasing NaCl concentration. However, the highest values related to cell length and width were recorded in 150 mM NaCl concentration in diploid genotype as 40.28 μm and 29.14 μm while they were realized in 50 mM NaCl in tetraploid genotype 'AD 440' as 70.56 μm and 49.13 μm. In diploid genotype 'Felicita', approx. cell area was recorded as 652.59 μm^2 in control (0 mM NaCl) while it was 1173.75 μm^2 in 150 mM NaCl treatment. Approx. cell area was found almost two times more in diploid genotype when NaCl concentration was 150 mM. On the other hand, in tetraploid genotype 'AD 440', approx. cell area was found as 1372.14 μm^2 in 0 mM NaCl (control) treatment whereas it was 3466.61 μm^2 in 50 mM NaCl. The highest results in the parameters of cell length, cell width and approx. cell area were noted from 50 mM NaCl treatment in tetraploid genotype (Table 11).

Genotype	Root Length (cm)			Seedlings Length (cm)		
	0 mM NaCl	50 mM NaCl	150 mM NaCl	0 mM NaCl	50 mM NaCl	150 mM NaCl
'Felicita' (2X)	5.25 b	5.50 b	7.25 a	8.75 b	10.75 a	11.25 a
'AD 440' (4X)	6.05 b	6.83 ab	7.90 a	5.80 b	7.33 ab	7.90 b

Values followed by the different letters in a row are significantly different at the 0.01 level

Table 10. The effect of different concentrations of NaCl on sugar beet seedling development 8 days after salt treatment

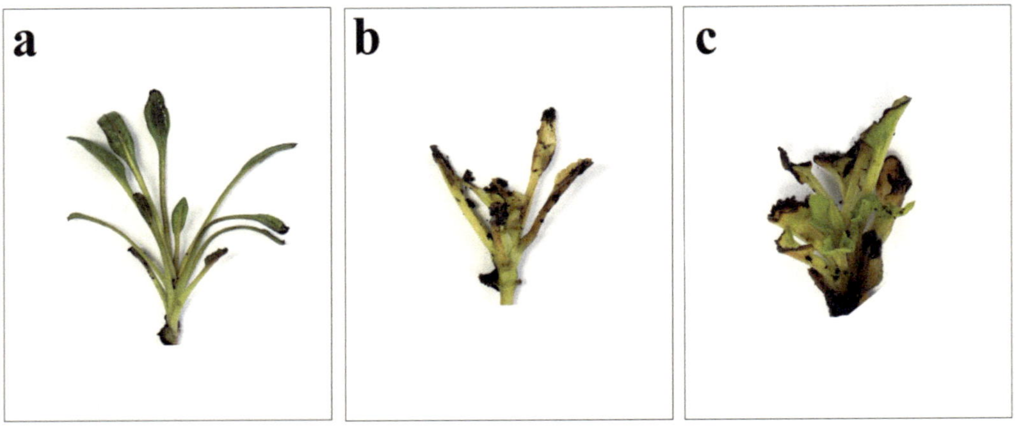

Figure 8. Sugar beet leaf development of cv. 'Felicita' 8 days after salt treatment (a) 0 mM NaCl (control), (b) 50 mM NaCl and (c) 150 mM NaCl

Number of stomata decreased by increasing NaCl concentration and this decrease was compensated by increased stomata size as reported by Inze and De Veylder [16]. Higher NaCl concentration increased stomata length and decreased stomata width in tetraploid genotype 'AD 440'. The highest stomata area was recorded from 150 mM NaCl treatment in diploid genotype while it was noted from 50 mM in tetraploid (Table 11).

The highest cell and stomata numbers were recorded from 0 mM NaCl treatment in both genotypes. And also cell and stomata numbers decreased by increasing NaCl concentration. However, this decrease in cell and stomata numbers were observed sharper in diploid genotype than in tetraploid one. The difference in cell and stomata numbers between 0 and 150 mM NaCl treatments was higher in diploid than in tetraploid. This could be due to the fact that tetraploid genotype 'AD 440' was more resistant to salt stress than diploid genotype 'Felicita' (Table 11). In other characters (cell and stomata lengths, cell and stomata widths, approx. cell and stomata areas), the highest values were recorded from 150 mM NaCl treatment in diploid genotype while they were noted from 50 mM NaCl treatment in tetraploid genotype. Since many characters in 150 mM NaCl concentration were almost the same as in 0 mM NaCl, it could be concluded that tetraploid genotype 'AD 440' was more resistant to salt stress than diploid one.

	Cell Number			Cell Length (μm)			Cell Width (μm)			Approx. Cell Area (μm²)		
Genotype	0 mM NaCl	50 mM NaCl	150 mM NaCl	0 mM NaCl	50 mM NaCl	150 mM NaCl	0 mM NaCl	50 mM NaCl	150 mM NaCl	0 mM NaCl	50 mM NaCl	150 mM NaCl
'Felicita' (2X)	162.70 a	124.50 b	70.70 c	31.71 b	27.14 b	40.28 a	20.58 b	19.28 b	29.14 a	652.59 b	523.25 b	1173.75 a
'AD 440' (4X)	84.60 a	52.40 c	69.30 b	54.58 b	70.56 a	44.85 b	25.14 b	49.13 a	30.85 b	1372.14 b	3466.61 a	1383.62 b
	Stomata Number			Stomata Length (μm)			Stomata Width (μm)			Approx. Stomata Area (μm²)		
Genotype	0 mM NaCl	50 mM NaCl	150 mM NaCl	0 mM NaCl	50 mM NaCl	150 mM NaCl	0 mM NaCl	50 mM NaCl	150 mM NaCl	0 mM NaCl	50 mM NaCl	150 mM NaCl
'Felicita' (2X)	18.80 a	18.20 b	7.30 c	26.28 b	21.42 b	28.57 a	18.85 b	18.85 b	20.56 a	495.37 b	440.39 c	538.54 a
'AD 440' (4X)	13.50 a	11.30 b	9.50 b	36.56 b	38.84 a	37.63 b	22.42 b	23.99 a	21.70 c	877.07 b	881.29 a	842.82 c

Values followed by the different letters in a row are significantly different at the 0.01 level

Table 11. Cellular responses to salt stress of sugar beet genotypes at different ploidy levels

6. Conclusion

Polyploidy is a common phenomenon in nature. There are differences between diploid and polyploid plants from morphological, physiological, cellular and biochemical aspects. Although polyploid genotypes have several advantages over diploids, the effects of increased ploidy level cannot be anticipated all the time. This was seen clearly in the studies we conducted. From one hand, diploid genotypes found superior than tetraploids in the generative characteristics such as total chlorophyll and protein contents, root and sugar yields, and sugar content under field conditions, on the other hand, regeneration capacity and susceptibility to *Agrobacterium tumefaciens* infection of polyploids were found higher under *in vtiro* conditions. Moreover, when cellular responses were examined, tetraploid genotype seemed more resistant to salt stress than diploid counterpart. Thus, it should be considered that responses of polyploid genotypes may differ from mophological, physiological, cellular and biochemical aspects. That is why, in a research study, responses of both diploid and polyploid genotypes should be evaluated carefully for successful results.

Author details

Mustafa Yildiz

Address all correspondence to: myildiz@ankara.edu.tr

Department of Field Crops, Faculty of Agriculture, University of Ankara, Diskapi, Ankara, Turkey

References

[1] Grant V. Plant Speciation, 2nd ed. Columbia University Press, New York, New York, USA; 1981.

[2] Goldblatt P. Polyploidy in angiosperms: Monocotyledons. In: Lewis W.H. (Ed.), Polyploidy: Biological relevance, 219 – 239. Plenum Press, New York, New York, USA; 1980.

[3] Ramsey JR, Schemske DW. Pathways, mechanisms, and rates of polyploid formation in flowering plants. Annual Review of Ecology and Systematics 1998; 29: 467-501.

[4] Stebbins GL. Types of polyploids: their classification and significance. Advances in Genetics 1947; 1: 403–429.

[5] Molin WT, Meyers SP, Baer GR, Schrader LE Ploidy effects of isogenic populations of alfalfa II. Photosynthesis, chloroplast number, ribulose-1,5-bisphosphate carboxylase, chlorophyll, and DNA in protoplasts. Plant Physiology 1982; 70: 1710-1714.

[6] Warner DA, Ku MSB, Edwards GE. Photosynthesis, leaf anatomy, and cellular constituents in the polyploid C4 grass *Panicum virgatum*. Plant Physiology 1987; 84: 461-466.

[7] Jan CC Induced tetraploidy and trisomic production of *Heliantus annus* L. Genome 1988; 30: 647–651.

[8] Hussain SW, Williams WM, Woodfield DR, Hampton JG. Development of a ploidy series from a single interspecific *Trifolium repens* L&A macr: nigrescens Viv. F1 hybrid. Theoritical and Applied Genetics 1997; 94: 821–831.

[9] Ranney TG. Polyploidy: From evolution to new plant development. Proceedings of the International Plant Propagator's Society 2006; 56: 604-607.

[10] Comai L. The advantages and disadvantages of being polyploid. Nature Genetics 2005; 6: 836-846.

[11] Mathura S, Fossey A, Beck S. Comperative study of chlorophyll content in diploid and tetraploid black Wattle *(Acacia mearnsii*). Forestry 2006; 79(4): 381-388.

[12] Beyaz R, Alizadeh B, Gurel S, Ozcan SF, Yıldız M. Sugar beet (*Beta vulgaris* L.) growth at different ploidy levels. Caryologia 2013 (in press).

[13] Bretagnolle F, Thompson JD, Lumaret R. The influence of seed size variation on seed germination and seedling vigour in diploid and tetraploid *Dactylis glomerata* L. Annals of Botany 1995; 76: 607-615.

[14] Sung JM, Chiu KY. Hydration effect on seedling emergence strength of watermelon seeds differing in ploidy. Plant Science 1995; 110: 21-26.

[15] Kihara H. Triploid watermelons. Proceedings of the American Society for Horticultural Science 1951; 58: 217-230.

[16] Doonan J. Social control on cell proliferation in plants. Current Opinion in Plant Biology 2000; 3: 482-487.

[17] Inze D, De Veylder L. Cell cycle regulation in plant development. Annual Review of Genetics 2006; 40: 77-105.

[18] Pegtel DM. Effect of ploidy level on fruit morphology, seed germination and juvenile growth in scurvy grass (*Cochlearia officinalis* L. s.l., Brassicaceae). Plant Species Biology 1999; 14: 201-215.

[19] Dale JE. The control of leaf expansion. Annual Review of Plant Physiology 1988; 39: 267-295.

[20] Sunderland N. Cell division and expansion in the growth of the leaf. Journal of Experimental Botany 1960; 11: 68-80.

[21] Prado FE, Gonzalez JA, Gallardo M, Moris M, Boero C, Kortsarz A. Changes in soluble carbonhydrates and invertase activity in *Chenopodium quinoa* ("quinoa") developed for saline stress during germination. Current Topics in Phytochemistry 1995; 14: 1-5.

[22] Sullivan BP, Phafler PL. Diploid-tetraploid comparison in rye. III. Temperature effects on seedling development. Crop Science 1986; 26: 795-799.

[23] Pal RN, Laloraya MM. Effect of calcium levels on chlorophyll synthesis in peanut and linseed plants. Biochemie und Physiologie Pflanezen 1972; 163: 443-449.

[24] Wright GC, Nageswara RRC, Farquhar GD. Water use efficiency and carbon isotope discrimination in peanut under water deficit conditions. Crop Science 1994; 34: 92-97.

[25] Nageswara RRC, Talwar HS, Wright GC. Rapid assessment of specific leaf area and leaf nitrogen in peanut (*Arachis hypogaea* L.) using chlorophyll meter. Journal of Agronomy and Crop Science 2001; 189: 175-182.

[26] Warner DA, Edwards GE. Effects of polyploidy on photosynthetic rates, photosynthetic enzymes, contents of DNA, chlorophyll, and sizes and numbers of photosynthetic cells in the C_4 dicot *Atriplex confertifolia*. Plant Physiology 1989; 91: 1143-1151.

[27] Beck SL, Dunlop RW, Fossey A. Evaluation of induced polyploidy in *Acacia mearnsii* through stomatal counts and guard cell measurements. The South African Journal of Botany 2003a; 69: 563-567.

[28] Beck SL, Fossey A, Mathura S. Ploidy determination of black waffle (*Acacia mearnsii*) using stomatal chloroplast counts. Southern African Forestry Journal 2003b; 192: 79-92.

[29] Thirugnanakumar S, Manivannan K, Prakash M, Narasimman R, Anitha Vasline Y. In Vitro Plant Breeding. Agrobios, India; 2009.

[30] Yıldız M, Alizadeh B, Beyaz R. *In vitro* explant growth and shoot regeneration from petioles of sugar beet (*Beta vulgaris* L.) lines at different ploidy levels. Journal of Sugar Beet Research 2013 (in press).

[31] Tetu T, Sangwan RS, Sangwan-Norreel BS. Hormonal control of organogenesis and somatic embryogenesis in *Beta vulgaris* callus. Journal of Experimental Botany 1987; 38: 506-517.

[32] Detrez C, Tetu T, Sangwan RS, Sangwan-Norreel BS. Direct organogenesis from petiole and thin cell layer explants in sugar beet cultured *in vitro*. Journal of Experimental Botany 1988; 39: 917-926.

[33] Ritchie GA, Short KC, Davey MR. *In vitro* shoot regeneration from callus, leaf axils and petioles of sugarbeet (*Beta vulgaris* L.). Journal of Experimental Botany 1989; 40: 277-283.

[34] Toldi O, Gyulai G, Kiss J, Tarns I, Balazs E. Antiauxin enhanced microshoot initiation and plant regeneration from epicotyl-originated thin layer explants of sugar beet (*Beta vulgaris* L). Plant Cell Reports 1996; 15: 851–854.

[35] Grieve TM, Gartlan KMA, Elliott MC. Micropropagation of commercially important sugar beet cultivars. Plant Growth Regulation 1997; 21: 15-18.

[36] Zhang CL, Chen DF, Elliott MC, Slater A. Thidiazuron-induced organogenesis and somatic embryogenesis in sugar beet (*Beta vulgaris* L). In Vitro Cellular and Developmental Biology-Plant 2001; 37: 305–310.

[37] Yildiz M, Onde S, Ozgen M. Sucrose effects on phenolic concentration and plant regeneration from sugarbeet leaf and petiole explants. Journal of Sugar Beet Research 2007; 44: 1–15.

[38] Jibiki M, Kuno Y, Shinoyama H, Fujii T. Isolation and properties of large cell strains from a methanol-utilizing yeast, *Candida* sp. N-16 by colchicine treatment. The Journal of General and Applied Microbiology 1993; 39: 439-442.

[39] Guertin DA, Sabatini DM. Cell size control. Encyclopedia of Life Sciences. John Wiley & Sons Ltd.; 2005.

[40] Tal M, Gardi I. Physiology of polyploid plants: Water balance in autotetraploid and diploid tomato under low and high salinity. Physiologia Plantarum 1976; 38, 257-261.

[41] Yildiz M, Özgen M. The effect of a submersion pretreatment on in vitro explant growth and shoot regeneration from hypocotyls of flax (*Linum usitatissimum*). Plant Cell, Tissue and Organ Culture 2004; 77: 111-115.

[42] Reinink K, Biom-Zandstra M. The relation between cell size, ploidy level and nitrate concentration in lettuce. Physiologia Plantarum 1989; 76: 575-580.

[43] Wintermans JFGM, De Mots A. Spectrophotometric characteristics of chlorophylls *a* and *b* and their pheophytins in ethanol. Biochimica et Biophysica Acta 1965; 109: 448-453.

[44] Hooykaas PJJ, Schilperoort RA. *Agrobacterium* and plant genetic engineering. Plant Molecular Biology 1992; 19: 15-38.

[45] Nester EW, Gordon MP, Amasino RM, Yanofsky MF. Crown gall: a molecular and physiological analysis. Annual Review of Plant Physiology 1984; 35: 387-413.

[46] Bevan MW, Chilton MD. T-DNA of the *Agrobacterium* Ti and Ri plamids. Annual Review Genetics 1982; 16: 357-384.

[47] Binns AN, Thomashaw MF. Cell biology of *Agrobacterium* infection and transformation of plants. Annual Review of Microbiology 1988; 42: 575-606.

[48] Yildiz M, Koyuncu N, Ozgen M. *In vitro* susceptibility of two sugar beet (*Beta vulgaris* L.) lines in different ploidy levels to *Agrobacterium tumefaciens*. Proceedings of Sixth Field Crops Congress of Turkey, 5-9 September, Antalya, Turkey; 2005.

[49] DeCleene M, DeLey J. The host range of crown gall. Botanical Review 1976; 42: 389–466.

[50] Anderson A, Moore L. Host specificity in the genus *Agrobacterium*. Phytopathology 1979; 69: 320–323.

[51] Porter JR. Host range and implications of plant infection by *Agrobacterium rhizogenes*. Critical Reviews in Plant Sciences 1991; 10: 387–421.

[52] Schläppi M, Hohn B. Competence of immature maize embryos for *Agrobacterium*-mediated gene transfer. Plant Cell 1992; 4: 7–16.

[53] Van Wordragen MF, Dons HJM. *Agrobacterium tumefaciens*-mediated transfor-mation of recalcitrant crops. Plant Molecular Biology Reporter 1992; 10:12–36.

[54] Hood EE, Fraley RT, Chilton MD. Virulence of *Agrobacterium tumefaciens* strain A281 on legumes. Plant Physiology 1987; 83: 529–34.

[55] Schroeder HE, Schotz AH, Wardley-Richardson T, Spencer D, Higgins TJV. Transformation and regeneration of two cultivars of pea (*Pisum sativum* L.). Plant Physiology 1993; 101: 751–57.

[56] Beneddra T, Picard C, Nesme X. Correlation between susceptibility to crown gall and sensitivity to cytokinin in aspen cultivars. Phytopathology 1996; 86: 225–231.

[57] Liu CN, Li XQ, Gelvin SB. Multiple copies of *virG* enhance the transient transformation of celery, carrot, and rice tissues by *Agrobacterium tumefaciens.* Plant Molecular Biology 1992; 20: 1071–1087.

[58] Ritchie SW, Liu CN, Sellmer JC, Kononowicz H, Hodges TK, Gelvin SB. *Agrobacterium tumefaciens*-mediated expression of *gusA* in maize tissues. Transgenic Research 1993; 2: 252–265.

[59] Smarrelli J, Watters MT, Diba LH. Response of various cucurbits to infection by plasmid-harboring strains of *Agrobacterium*. Plant Physiology 1986; 82: 622–624.

[60] Bergmann B, Stomp AM. Effect of host plant genotype and growth rate on *Agrobacterium tumefaciens*-mediated gall formation in *Pinus radiata*. Phytopathology 1992; 82: 1456–1462.

[61] Van Roekel JSC, Damm B, Melchers LS, Hoekema A. Factors influencing transformation frequency of tomato (*Lycopersicon esculentum*). Plant Cell Reports 1993; 12: 644–647.

[62] Nam J, Matthysse AG, Gelvin SB. Differences in susceptibility of *Arabidopsis* ecotypes to crown gall disease may result from a deficiency in T-DNA integration. Plant Cell 1997; 9: 317–333.

[63] Lowe BA, Krul WR. Physical, chemical, developmental, and genetic factors that modulate the *Agrobacterium-Vitis* interaction. Plant Physiology 1991; 96: 121–129.

[64] Bailey M, Boerma HR, Parrott WA. Inheritance of *Agrobacterium tumefaciens* induced tumorigenesis of soybean. Crop Science 1994; 34: 514–519.

[65] Mauro AO, Pfeiffer TW, Collins GB. Inheritance of soybean susceptibility to *Agrobacterium tumefaciens* and its relationship to transformation. Crop Science 1995; 35: 1152–1156.

[66] Robbs S L, Hawes MC, Lin HJ, Pueppke SG, Smith LY. Inheritance of resistance to crown gall in *Pisum sativum*. Plant Physiology 1991; 95: 52–57.

[67] De Kathen A, Jacobsen HJ. Cell competence for Agrobacterium-mediated DNA transfer in *Pisum sativum* L. Transgenic Research 1995; 4: 184–191.

[68] Sangwan RS, Bourgeois Y, Brown S, Vasseur G, Sangwan-Norreel B. Characterization of competent cells and early events of *Agrobacterium*-mediated genetic transformation in *Arabidopsis thaliana*. Planta 1992; 188: 439–456.

[69] Owens LD, Cress DE.. Genotypic variability of soybean response to *Agrobacterium* strains harboring the Ti or Ri plasmids. Plant Physiology 1985; 77: 87-94.

[70] Warkentin TD, McHughen A. Crown gall transformation of lentil (*Lens culinaris* Medic.) with virulent strains of *Agrobacterium tumefaciens*. Plant Cell Reports 1991; 10: 489-493.

[71] Islam R, Malik T, Husnain T, Riazuddin S. Strain and cultivar specificity in the *Agrobacterium*-chickpea interaction. Plant Cell Reports 1994; 13: 561-563.

[72] Yıldız M. The effect of cell size and cell shape of sugar beet (*Beta vulgaris* var. *saccharifera*) on yield and sucrose concentration. M.Sc. Thesis, Ankara University, Graduate School of Natural and Applied Sciences, Department of Field Crops, Ankara, Turkey; 1994.

[73] Yildiz M, Erkilic EG, Kocak N, Telci C, Kurumlu S and Ozcan S. The response of sugar beet lines and cultivars (*Beta vulgaris* L.) with different ploidy levels to *in vitro* salinity stress. 1st National Congress on Agriculture and Exposition with International Participation, April 27-30, Eskisehir, Turkey; 2011.